Science

V6/ 15⁰⁰

110670371

Biological Effects of Radiations

SECOND EDITION

Biological Effects of Radiations

SECOND EDITION

Daniel S. Grosch

Department of Genetics
School of Agriculture and Life Sciences
North Carolina State University
Raleigh, North Carolina

Larry E. Hopwood

Department of Radiology
The Medical College of Wisconsin
Milwaukee, Wisconsin

ACADEMIC PRESS

New York   San Francisco   London   1979

A Subsidiary of Harcourt Brace Jovanovich, Publishers

COPYRIGHT © 1979, BY ACADEMIC PRESS, INC.
ALL RIGHTS RESERVED.
NO PART OF THIS PUBLICATION MAY BE REPRODUCED OR
TRANSMITTED IN ANY FORM OR BY ANY MEANS, ELECTRONIC
OR MECHANICAL, INCLUDING PHOTOCOPY, RECORDING, OR ANY
INFORMATION STORAGE AND RETRIEVAL SYSTEM, WITHOUT
PERMISSION IN WRITING FROM THE PUBLISHER.

ACADEMIC PRESS, INC.
111 Fifth Avenue, New York, New York 10003

United Kingdom Edition published by
ACADEMIC PRESS, INC. (LONDON) LTD.
24/28 Oval Road, London NW1   7DX

Library of Congress Cataloging in Publication Data

Grosch, Daniel S
    The biological effects of radiations.

    Includes bibliographies and index.
    1. Radiobiology. I. Hopwood, Larry E.,
joint author. II. Title.
QH652.G76   1979   574.1'915   79–51677
ISBN 0–12–304150–3

PRINTED IN THE UNITED STATES OF AMERICA

79 80 81 82   9 8 7 6 5 4 3 2 1

They were deliberating among themselves as to how they could give wings
to Death so that it could in a moment
penetrate everywhere both near and
far.

The Labyrinth of the World in Czech, 1623,
Jan Amos Komenský,
COMENIUS, LAST BISHOP OF
UNITAS FRATRUM BOHEMORUM

Contents

Preface

This book was conceived as a text–reference to serve both students and professionals in a variety of fields. Although developed for use in universities and technical institutions, this volume will be helpful to specialists and researchers in other fields who require a knowledge of the essentials involved in the biological response to radiation. In our own courses the enrollment includes botanists, ecologists, fish and game conservationists, geneticists, medical students, nuclear engineers, physicists, and veterinarians. Accordingly, the language of exposition is such that any educated individual can grasp the basic principles. Highly technical terms are used only to save space in certain summary paragraphs.

Our purpose is to present an organized survey of the diverse experiments in which living material has been exposed to ionizing and exciting types of radiations, a gamut which touches upon every facet of biology. Human and mammalian research is an important feature, but the considerable literature on lower organisms is given equal attention. Much of the latter information is not available in any other general presentation.

The story as it unfolds tells of the manner in which a minute amount of energy can damage vulnerable submicroscopic structure and be translated into alterations of the appearances and abilities of entire organisms. The consequence may even be seen in later generations and be reflected in changes in populations. The ultimate importance of the disruption of nucleic acid structures emerges not only for genetic disturbances but for uninherited somatic aberrations.

For the most part the second edition follows the outline of the first. The rationale was to start with simple systems and proceed through the order of increasing biological complexity. After two introductory chapters, the information is organized into sections on cellular topics, tissues and organs, organism responses, and finally the interrelations between organisms in contaminated areas. The titles of chapters given in the table of contents reflect their specific emphasis. As in the first edition an entire chapter is devoted to the consequences of mutations induced in populations. A new chapter has been added to present discoveries from experiments with cultured cells.

Advances in the last decade made in nearly every facet of radiation biology necessitated revision of and addition to all but a few topics in every chapter. Two sets of subject matter have been reorganized: (1) the DNA studies including its repair mechanisms are now collected in Chapter 4; (2) other restoration processes are combined with protective measures in Chapter 13 because of their common foundation in the cellular basis of organism survival. Unfortunately, not every topic fits cleanly into a discrete category, and in some cases a topic may appear in more than one chapter. Conversely, two topics in the same chapter may easily be categorized into separate pigeonholes, but their interrelationship may not yet be clarified. Both of these problems in presentation stem from the underlying unity of nature. The divisions necessary for organizing a book are man-made, and we recognize the provisional nature of their placement. For example, some of the first edition's systematic structure became untenable in the light of subsequent research.

Today's scientific paper tends to focus tightly upon a particular aspect selected from the partial disclosures of an earlier broad exploratory phase of investigation. In order to provide an adequate perspective for a reader's first encounter, we have referred to many of the early classic experiments before presenting current developments. The instructive value of the investigation has been a prime consideration in choosing examples from the enormous body of literature. Selection has been difficult. An inevitable result is that a book of reasonable length cannot do justice by direct reference to the work of all investigators whose contributions are significant. Accordingly, the cited references serve primarily as a guide to further readings. The monographs or symposia devoted to a single aspect merit special attention.

Some of the common abbreviations and symbols have undergone transition since the first edition was written. R is now commonly used instead of r for the roentgen unit of dosage. Another example is in the designation of radionuclides. In physical notation the atomic mass number now precedes the element's symbol, as in ^{32}P instead of the original P^{32} which is still the most convenient oral usage. Again, as this book is going to press new designations are being proposed. Instead of the curie (Ci), the International Commission on Radiation Units and Measurements suggests the becquerel (Bq) for an activity of one per second (s^{-1}). For the absorbed dose, the gray (Gy) represents a quantity of one joule per kilogram (J/kg), or the equivalent of 100 rads. Whether these and other new units will catch on with the practicing health physicist remains to be seen. They have not yet replaced the decades-old conventions in the open biological literature.

We would like to take this opportunity to acknowledge with thanks all the authors, editors, and publishers who have been exceedingly gracious and helpful in providing material upon which to base figures and tables.

Daniel S. Grosch
Larry E. Hopwood

PART I INTRODUCTION

Before we can fully appreciate experiments which demonstrate the biological effects of radiations, we need to understand something about the radiations and the units of measurement applied in quantitative work. The purpose of the first two chapters is to set the scene and to allow us to develop some definitions and concepts with a physical basis. A necessarily superficial treatment of physical aspects is given in Chapter 1, but specialized radiation biology appears in Chapter 2.

CHAPTER 1   The Radiations: Historical Considerations and Characteristics

The Era of Discovery: Radiations and Hazards

Our story begins in 1895 with Wilhelm Georg Roentgen's discovery of x rays which was followed closely by Henri Becquerel's demonstration of natural radioactivity. Each unwittingly performed biological experiments. Roentgen saw an image of the bones of his hand by interposing it between a vacuum tube and an improvised fluorescent screen. Since his various interests included photography, the substitution of a photographic plate for the barium platinocyanide coated cardboard was an obvious sequel. Tradition ascribes a domestic motive to the production of the classic picture of a skeletal hand with wedding ring. This prototypic radiograph may have convinced Mrs. Roentgen that long hours spent in the laboratory were not in vain.

Within a month after the January 1896 announcement of x rays, E. H. Grubbe, a Chicago tube manufacturer, experienced a serious radiation burn. The physician he consulted later referred to Grubbe a woman with recurrent breast cancer. Her treatment in early 1896 was probably the first therapeutic application of x rays. Grubbe's own experience fortunately caused him to use lead shielding to protect the rest of her body. While investigations into the applicability for selective destruction of cancers had begun, unfortunately not all scientists used adequate shielding. C. M. Dally, one of Edison's assistants, is believed to have been the first person in the United States to die from radiation-induced cancer (Brown, 1936). By 1922, as commemorated by the Hamburg, Germany, memorial, 169 radiological pioneers from many different countries had died as the result of their exposure to the subject of their investigations. Roentgen's habitual use of a zinc-lined box to

shield his equipment evidently protected him from serious consequences of his investigations.

Radiation injuries featured also in the early experiences with natural
radioactivity. Becquerel burned himself by carrying a sample of
uranium in his pocket. Both Marie and Pierre Curie received analogous
skin burns from radium; also both developed leukemia although a
traffic accident spared Pierre from the slower death experienced by
Marie. Daughter Irene and son-in-law Frederic Joliot-Curie were rav-
aged by radiation-induced tissue damage. In addition weakness and
debility were a constant complaint of the technicians and assistants in
the Curie laboratory (Wilson, 1972). Unequivocal evidence that radiation damage had occurred came in later years.

Early Basic Research

In addition to the electromagnetic rays, the discovery of alpha particles and neutrons occurred during the early 1900s. Biological experiments were begun using human skin, bacteria, plants, invertebrates,
and rodents. By 1906, the fundamental pattern of histological damage
was known. However, for many years basic research in radiation biology was reported in a scattering of specialty journals among the various
disciplines, including those medically oriented toward diagnostic
radiology. The majority of the biologists paid no attention. In 1927,
convincing evidence of gene mutation introduced a theme which predominated during the 1930s, but sustained general interest in
radiobiology was an aftermath of the atomic explosions of 1945. Full
appreciation of even the genetic investigations was delayed until after
these events. Although Muller reported his successful inductions of
mutations in 1927, it was not until 1946 that public recognition came
with the award of the Nobel Prize.

Due to the security restrictions associated with the development of
atomic energy, there was a publishing hiatus during and immediately
after World War II. In the early 1950s, declassification of extensive
information and a shift from military applications to fundamental questions stimulated a surge of publication. This included numerous symposia and edited compendia which tended to consolidate the research
reports of earlier years. New journals were founded. *Radiation Research*
appeared first in 1954, and the *International Journal of Radiation Biology*
followed in 1959. *Radiation Botany*, founded in 1961, was superseded
after 14 years by *Environmental and Experimental Botany*.

During the 1950s, discoveries were made in other areas, particularly molecular biology, which led to important progress in radiation biology during the 1960s. These included the translation of the genetic code, techniques to study the biochemistry and fine structure of cells, and methods for determining the survival of individual cells *in vitro* and *in vivo*. During the 1960s, a quantitative approach developed toward the understanding of factors which affect cell radiosensitivity.

Radiation Protection Standards

During World War I instructions for the safety of military personnel were issued, but many years elapsed before legislation opened the way for protection of civilians (Spear, 1953). In 1928, a Radiation Protection Committee was formed at the Second International Congress of Radiology. Subsequently the committee evolved into the International Commission on Radiation Protection (ICRP). A corresponding organization in the United States was the National Committee on Radiation Protection (NCRP), later to become the National Council on Radiation Protection. However, recommendations did not become law until the state enabling acts were passed in the 1950s and 1960s. This was not possible until the federal government released the preemptive power asserted in 1946 when Congress enacted legislation to remove the U.S. atomic energy program from military control to the civilian agency, the Atomic Energy Commission (AEC). Over the years the AEC relied on the advice and guidance of the NCRP. Finally, in 1972, authority was vested in the Environmental Protection Agency (EPA) to establish applicable environmental standards, with enforcement mainly in the hands of the state boards of health.

The Radiations

The term radiation indicates a physical phenomenon in which energy travels through space. Radiations are usually classified in two main groups: (1) the electromagnetic, and (2) the corpuscular or particulate rays. The former have energy alone. The latter have mass and energy. It is the energy that gives rise to the biological changes which will be discussed.

Figure 1.1 demonstrates how ultraviolet (uv) rays, x rays, and gamma (γ) rays form a continuous spectrum extending down from the familiar visible range of wavelengths. Our own sun is a source of a spectrum of radiations extending into x-ray wavelength. Ultraviolet rays can be

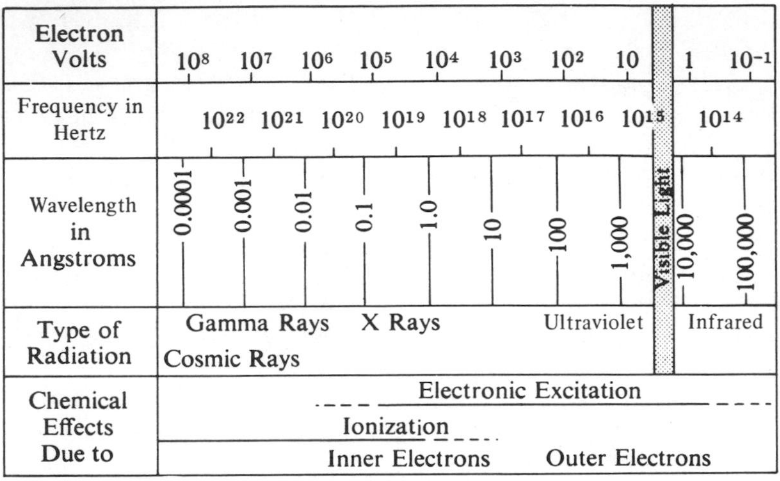

Electron Volts	10^8	10^7	10^6	10^5	10^4	10^3	10^2	10		1	10^{-1}
Frequency in Hertz	10^{22}	10^{21}	10^{20}	10^{19}	10^{18}	10^{17}	10^{16}	10^{15}		10^{14}	
Wavelength in Angstroms	0.0001	0.001	0.01	0.1	1.0	10	100	1,000	Visible Light	10,000	100,000
Type of Radiation	Gamma Rays　　X Rays						Ultraviolet			Infrared	
	Cosmic Rays										
Chemical Effects Due to				Electronic Excitation							
			Ionization								
				Inner Electrons			Outer Electrons				

Figure 1.1.　Chart of electromagnetic radiation.

produced artifically by special lamps, particularly of the tungsten–mercury arc type. X rays are produced in vacuum tubes when electrons accelerated in an electric field collide with a solid body, usually a tungsten target. Two types of radiation are produced: characteristic and continuous x rays. Characteristic radiation of "x-ray spectra" is produced when a target electron in a particular energy level is ejected and replaced by another. Its contribution to the total energy depends on the filtration and energy, and becomes less important at higher doses. Continuous radiation results from the loss of energy of the high speed electrons as they approach the target nucleus. This deceleration must be accompanied by loss of energy, in the form of photons with energy ranging from zero to the maximum potential of the x-ray tube. In recent years generators have been built which can produce x rays within the range of γ ray wavelengths. Therefore an early distinction between the two has broken down. Originally, x rays were simply those of high energy generated by man-made apparatus, and γ rays were the electromagnetic type given off by radioactive elements. A distinction that still holds is that x rays arise outside the atomic nucleus, while gamma rays come from within the nucleus.

A number of isotopes eject electrons. Streams of these negative particles are called beta (β) rays. Their velocity varies through a wide range, and the β rays from different isotopes differ in maximum energy. The E_{max} for ^{32}P is 1.71 MeV, for ^{14}C is 0.156, for ^3H is 0.018. In decay schemes, the notation $^A_Z H$ is used. A represents the atomic mass number and Z the atomic number.

$$^3_1\text{H} \xrightarrow{\beta^-} \, ^3_2\text{He} + \, _{-1}^{\;\;0}e$$

$$^{14}_{\;6}\text{C} \xrightarrow{\beta^-} \, ^{14}_{\;7}\text{N} + \, _{-1}^{\;\;0}e$$

$$^{32}_{15}\text{P} \xrightarrow{\beta^-} \, ^{32}_{16}\text{S} + \, _{-1}^{\;\;0}e$$

In a similar manner, positrons are emitted in the decay of a number of isotopes. Their properties are identical to those of electrons except for their positive charge. However, this charge assures a very short life of the order of 10^{-9} because the positron combines with an electron almost immediately. The annihilation energy is given off as a γ ray.
Alpha rays are given off by a few isotopes of high atomic weight, polonium and radon in particular.

$$^{210}_{\;84}\text{Po} \xrightarrow{\alpha} \, ^{206}_{\;82}\text{Pb} + \, ^4_2\text{He}$$

$$^{222}_{\;84}\text{Rn} \xrightarrow{\alpha} \, ^{218}_{\;84}\text{Po} + \, ^4_2\text{He}$$

Alpha rays are streams of positively charged particles, each of which contains 2 protons and 2 neutrons. Thus they resemble the nuclei of helium atoms. Figure 1.2 diagrams characteristic differences between alpha, beta, and gamma rays.
In isotopes where the ratio of neutrons to protons is low, the nucleus captures an orbital electron from the K level. The combination of this electron with a proton provides a neutron. Loss of the extranuclear electron leaves a vacancy which promptly is filled by an electron from a higher energy level. The excess energy is emitted as an x ray characteristic of the product atom.

$$^{55}_{26}\text{Fe} + \, _{-1}^{\;\;0}e \; \rightarrow \, ^{55}_{23}\text{Mn} + 5.3 \text{ keV} \times \text{ray}$$

Generators have been developed which can strip atoms of electrons to produce α rays as well as other types of charged particles. If hydrogen nuclei carrying one positive charge are stripped of their electrons, protons can be obtained—as a beam from the cyclotron, for example. Deuterons are nuclei from heavy hydrogen atoms. Indeed the ingenuity of physicists continues to provide various kinds of atomic fragments for study. However, we shall concern ourselves only with those rays with which significant biological investigation has been performed.

Neutrons, the particles which resemble protons in mass but carry no charge, are prepared by three methods: in nuclear reactors by fission, in particle accelerators when deuterons bombard tritium, and in neutron "howitzers" by dislodgment from target atoms (usually α rays striking beryllium). There are no significant naturally occurring neutron emitters on earth. Neutrons are a normal constituent of all kinds of matter except the common form of hydrogen, but ordinarily they remain locked into the nucleus. In the course of transformation induced by high-energy radiations, neutrons are released from nuclei. Depending on their rate of speed they are classed as either fast or slow. The energies involved are respectively above 100,000 eV and below 100 eV.

Through collisions with atomic nuclei, neutrons which started out fast are reduced in speed when passing through a substance, until their energy is equal to the mean energy of thermal agitation in the medium. They are then known as thermal or slow neutrons and can be captured by atomic nuclei, which may then become radioactive.

Terrestrial radioactivity from natural sources and extraterrestrial rays of cosmic origin are components of the radiation environment to which life on earth has always been exposed. Primary cosmic radiation consists of 79% protons (H nuclei), 20% α particles (He nuclei), and 1% assorted atomic nuclei (ranging from Li to Ni). These charged particles, which reflect the presumed relative abundance of elements in the universe, carry enormous energies and produce a variety of secondary particles or rays by atom-smashing interaction with the earth's atmosphere. The study of these interactions is a science in itself. For our purposes, it should suffice to state that the rays of cosmic origin have great penetrating power, contributing only a small fraction to the absorbed dose experienced by living organisms at ordinary altitudes. Furthermore, earth's magnetic field influences the charged cosmic particles so that they are deflected toward the poles and the intensity is greater toward the higher latitudes. The study of the high energy nuclei has become more important to biologists since man has ventured into space. On earth, the particles have been employed in radiation therapy.

Dissipation of Energy in Matter

A brief examination of atomic structure will help to explain how rays can penetrate matter. The various kinds of atoms serving as the building blocks of terrestrial things are each made up of a nucleus and orbital electrons. Most of the mass is concentrated in the nucleus, yet in relative terms the nucleus occupies a space only about that of a basketball in the center of a large gymnasium, or that of a printed period on a page near the middle of a large classroom. The rest is empty space through which the tiny, light electrons revolve at tremendous speeds. Their orbital configurations are many times the radius of the atomic nucleus. Thus the unoccupied territory is ample for a penetration by rays.

Radiations lose their energy in passing through materials. This energy may merely displace electrons from one orbital shell to another of higher energy to produce "excited" atoms. Ultraviolet light is classed as an exciting ray (Figure 1.1). It is chemically less efficient and biologically less effective than the ionizing rays which will be discussed. Also, since it is absorbed by the superficial tissues of macroorganisms, its genetic implications are limited.

Ionizing rays are so called because their principal means of dissipation of energy in passage through matter is the ejection of electrons from atoms in their path. When an electrically neutral atom has lost one or more of its orbital electrons, the atom is left positively charged, that is, *ionized*. An ionized atom is one eager for chemical reaction. The electron ejected at ionization eventually becomes attached to another atom, making the latter a negative ion. In its passage the electron produces secondary ionizations.

Since matter is made up of positively charged atomic nuclei and negatively charged electrons, we can easily appreciate the fact that electrically charged particles interact with the atoms in the molecules which surround their path. The charged particles of corpuscular rays may attract or repel electrons from their atomic orbits, depending upon their charge. It is more difficult to comprehend how electromagnetic radiations give up energy to the molecules through which they pass, although we may be aware of the packets of energy, called *quanta*. The shorter the wavelength, the richer in energy are the quanta, more than adequate to eject an electron from an atom. Here again we are dealing with a charged particle which upon its release from an orbit will travel through matter. On this basis, x rays and γ rays may be viewed as a means of releasing energetic electrons within irradiated material.

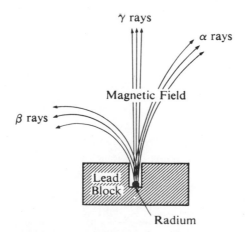

Figure 1.2.   Diagram of the deflection of α and β rays shown in the conventional manner, with the magnetic field pointing outward.

There are three distinct physical processes whereby a quantum of energy can release an electron from an atom: the photoelectric effect, the Compton effect, and the pair effect. Which of these three predominates depends on the energies of the rays and on the atomic number of the material traversed. The photoelectric and Compton effects are diagrammed in Figure 1.3.

At lower energies, all quanta are completely absorbed. Electrons are ejected from their atoms with energy equal to the difference between the initial energy of the photon and the binding energy of the ejected electron. Because the energy of a photon is transferred to an electron, this is called the *photoelectric effect*.

As energy levels increase, impinging quanta collide directly with orbital electrons to eject them, but only a fraction of the energy is used. The remainder is transformed into a new quantum of lower energy, in turn able to produce ions. The entire process is known as the *Compton effect*.

When the photon energy is at least 1.02 MeV, outright generation of particles can occur, especially when radiation traverses the atomic seat of strong forces (i.e., the electrostatic field of a nucleus of high Z). Simultaneously the photon disappears and a negatron and a positron appear—hence the term *pair production*. In other words, there has been a "materialization of energy." The energy required to create a particle is

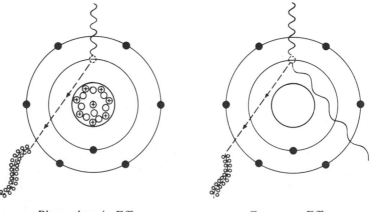

Photoelectric Effect   Compton Effect

Figure 1.3. Left: Photon strikes electron of an oxygen atom. Part of its energy is used for removal of electron to exterior of atom. Remainder of energy is imparted to electron. If it has enough energy, the electron produces ion pairs as it travels through the medium. Right: Photon loses only part of its energy to the electron and travels on in another direction with reduced energy. The electron produces ion pairs until attached.

calculated from the Einstein equation of the relationship between energy and mass, $E = mc^2$ in which m is the mass of an electron and c is the speed of light. The important influence of a high atomic number means that for a given photon energy, pair production occurs much more frequently in heavy metals than in the most common elements of living matter, H,C,N, or O.

Finally, at very high energies transmutation may occur when gamma rays are absorbed by atomic nuclei and cause subsequent neutron emission.

Neither charged nor electromagnetic, the neutron does not lose its energy to the electrons of atoms in the material traversed. Instead there are billiard-ball interactions with atomic nuclei. Primarily, collisions are with the nuclei of hydrogen atoms (i.e., protons) which are of similar mass. The recoil protons with acquired velocity are chiefly responsible for the ionizations produced in biological tissues. After loss of energy, slowed-down neutrons may enter atomic nuclei and, as mentioned above, render them unstable.

Linear Ion Density

Disturbance in the form of ionizations occurs along the pathways rays or particles have taken. This may actually be photographed in a cloud chamber (Figure 1.4). Ions produced in gas that is supersaturated with

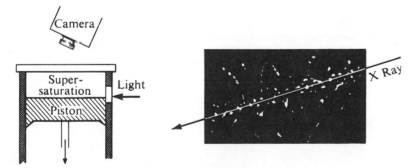

Figure 1.4. Left: Diagram of a Wilson cloud chamber. Gas saturated with water vapor is under pressure until the piston is suddenly withdrawn, to cause cooling and supersaturation. Right: An ionizing particle passing through the chamber immediately after the expansion produces a trail of ions to act as condensation nuclei for fine droplets of water. Long tracks diffusing from the ion trail are made by photoelectrons. The visible white streaks can be photographed if adequate illumination and a dark background are supplied.

water vapor act as condensation centers, thus rendering the ions visible.

Linear ion density is a distinguishing feature of an ionizing radiation from the biological standpoint. For one thing, particles of heavy mass and dense ion track are not very penetrating. Also, the effect of a small number of particles, each producing a large number of ions, is not necessarily the same as the converse, a large number of particles each producing few ions. Figure 1.5 shows linear ion density in relation to a virus particle, a matter to be considered in more detail in Chapter 2. Linear Energy Transfer (LET) serves as a formalized recognition of the average energy lost per unit length of track. It is usually expressed as keV/nm in biology, but as MeV/cm in health physics.

Dosage Representation

A typical biological experiment compares results in terms of damage to a particular structure or function obtained from a series of radiation doses. These may be expressed as (1) the exposure dose, or (2) the absorbed or delivered dose.

The *roentgen* (originally r, now R), a measure of ionization in air, is a unit of exposure dose for x rays or γ rays. It is defined as the quantity of x or γ rays which will produce 1 stat coulomb, that is, 1 electrostatic unit of electricity of either sign, in 1 cm³ of dry air at 0°C and standard atmospheric pressure. On the basis of the energy required to produce an ion pair in air, the roentgen may be translated into ergs per gram of air. This works out to about 90 ergs, really a minute amount of energy when one considers that 42 *million* ergs are required to raise 1 g of water 1°C. Is it not remarkable that a few hundred roentgens can kill a man?

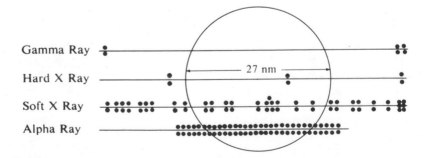

Figure 1.5.   Linear ion density in relation to a virus particle 27 nm in diameter. (From Gray, 1946.)

The roentgen was introduced by the International Commission on Radiological Units in 1928. In 1942, the atomic energy program was faced with the practical problem of calculating doses from mixtures of photon, alpha, beta, and neutron radiation. H. M. Parker of the Hanford project suggested a unit called the roentgen equivalent physical (*rep*) as a way to progress from the familiar R unit into the measurement of absorbed dose. Unfortunately, different authors used values ranging from 83 to 95 ergs/gram for absorption in air, water, or tissue. Finally the situation was resolved in 1953, when the rad was proposed at the Seventh International Congress of Radiology. As the unit of absorbed dose, the *rad* indicates the acquisition of a fixed amount of energy, 100 ergs per gram of the irradiated material.

The *rem* (roentgen equivalent man), a unit of dose equivalence, was added to the list, because a dose in rads from different types of radiation does not necessarily produce the same degree of biological effect. Thus:

$$\text{rem} = \text{dose in rads} \times \text{quality factor}$$

The quality factor (QF) relates the physical effects of another radiation or mixture of radiations to that of an electromagnetic radiation. In biology, the QF of the health physicist is known as the RBE, the relative biological effectiveness, usually calculated as the ratio of dose in rad to produce a given effect with x or γ rays to the dose in rad to produce the effect with another radiation under investigation.

For measuring *amounts* of a radioactive substance, the rate of its disintegration has been used rather than the radiation itself or its effects. The basic unit of rate of decay is the curie (Ci), that quantity of any radionuclide (nucleus exhibiting radioactivity) having a decay rate of 3.7×10^{10} disintegrations per second (dps). The unitary basis of this value is that 1 gram of pure radium is 1 curie of radium, and because of the 1620-year half-life, the decay rate does not decrease significantly during the time required for a biological experiment. For shorter-lived isotopes, the activity of samples must be specified for a certain date. Also, the number of disintegrations per unit time is not necessarily equal to the number of particles given off by the radionuclide unless the emanation is comprised entirely of only one type. Furthermore, disintegrations per unit time convey nothing about the energy or range of the radiation emitted. For example, 1 Ci of ^{210}Po next to the human skin would deliver all its energy via α rays to the first 1/1000 inch. In contrast, because of its β and γ rays, only about 0.02% of the energy from 1 Ci of ^{60}Co would be absorbed by the surface layer of the skin.

Biologically speaking, one curie is an enormous amount of

radioisotope. Two smaller units, the millicurie (mCi) and the microcurie (μCi), a thousandth and a millionth of a curie respectively, are used to measure significant amounts for living organisms. The maximum permissible amount of ^{32}P is 6 μCi for people occupationally exposed, while as little as 0.1 μCi is generally considered the limit to the body burden of ^{226}Ra. These are the amounts that within a lifetime will produce no noticeable deleterious effects. For permissible levels in air and water, measurements are in trillionths of a curie or picocuries (pCi).

Because of the complicated nature of neutron reactions, it is most convenient to measure and express the neutron flux. This is the number of neutrons impinging per unit area per unit of time.

Concluding Remarks

In this first chapter we have attempted a brief historical orientation as well as a presentation of the definitions and concepts which are considered basic and which shall be used throughout the book. The radiations, their linear ion densities, and their dosage representations can be given only brief introduction. Serious students will find recompense in consulting the selected references and the further sources of information which they suggest.

References

Brown, P. (1936). "American Martyrs to Science through the Roentgen Rays." Thomas, Springfield, Illinois.

Gray, L. H. (1946). Comparative studies of the biological effects of x rays, neutrons, and other ionizing radiations. *Br. Med. Bull.* **4**, 11–18.

Spear, F. G. (1953). "Radiations and Living Cells." Wiley, New York.

Wilson, M. (1972). The Curie tradition. *World*, December 5, pp. 33–36.

General References

Arena, V. (1971). "Ionizing Radiation and Life." Mosby, St. Louis, Missouri.

Attix, F. H., ed. (1972). "Radiation Dosimetry," 2nd ed., Suppl. I. Academic Press, New York.

Attix, F. H., and Roesch, W. C. (1968). "Radiation Dosimetry," 2nd ed., Vol. I. Academic Press, New York.

Bacq, Z. M., and Alexander, P. (1961). "Fundamentals of Radiobiology," 2nd ed., Chapter 1. Pergamon, Oxford.

Glasstone, S. (1967). "Sourcebook on Atomic Energy," 3rd ed., Van Nostrand: Reinhold, Princeton, New Jersey.

Hendee, W. (1973). "Medical Radiation Physics." Yearbook Publ., Chicago, Illinois.

Hollaender, A. (1954). "Radiation Biology," Vol. 1, Part 1, Chapters 1–6. McGraw-Hill, New York.

Johns, H., and Cunningham, J. (1973). "The Physics of Radiology," 3rd ed. Thomas, Springfield, Illinois.

Morgan, K. Z., and Turner, J. E. (1967). "Principles of Radiation Protection." Wiley, New York.

Shapiro, J. (1972). "Radiation Protection." Harvard Univ. Press, Cambridge, Massachusetts.

Shilling, C. W. (1964). "Atomic Energy Encyclopedia in the Life Sciences." Saunders, Philadelphia, Pennsylvania.

CHAPTER 2   Direct and Indirect Action on Living Matter

The purpose of this chapter is to explore the early steps between exposure to radiation and the first detectable indication of radiation injury in biological material. We shall first have to consider what substances are present to be ionized. This in turn introduces the problem of estimating direct action on molecules of biological importance which may be only sparsely represented, in contrast to action beginning in changes in unspecialized substances, especially water, which may be present in abundance. Finally, the characteristics of results in direct action phenomena are considered.

What Is Ionized?

Ionization is not a selective process. Any atom or molecule in the path of a radiation may be ionized. The predominant constituents of a complex system will stand the best chance of being ionized.

The chief constituent of living material in its functional state is water. In marine forms, water may comprise more than 96% of the organism. Many human tissues are made up of 70–80% water. Thus, we identify water as the most probable material in which the ionizations caused by radiation may occur. The resulting chemical products may react with biologically important organic molecules and thus be indirectly responsible for an observable effect.

Although simple at first thought, radiation research on water has proved to be difficult and there has been little agreement on exactly what happens to ionized water molecules. The chemical products of irradiated water include such things as H, OH, H_2O_2, and HO_2. Radiochemists, using ferrous sulfate as a test substance, have shown a total of four oxidizing equivalents produced for every molecule of water decomposed in the presence of air.

17

Strictly speaking, since the number of electrons is uneven, the ions formed through irradiation would be called free radicals to distinguish them from the more stable ions produced by the dissociation of salts. The presence of unpaired or odd electrons makes free radicals highly reactive. In water for example, the two ions formed by irradiation might be represented as

$$H_2O^+ = H_x^{\cdot\cdot} \cdot O \cdot {}_x^{\cdot\cdot}H$$

and

$$H_2O^- = H_x^{\cdot\cdot} \cdot O \cdot {}_x^{\cdot\cdot}H$$

by which we demonstrate that neither of these two ions has an oxygen with an octet of electrons for the outer orbit. The ionized water decomposes almost immediately:

$$H_2O^+ \rightarrow H^+ + OH^{\cdot}$$
$$H_2O^- \rightarrow OH^- + H^{\cdot}$$

The dot symbolizes the odd electron carried by a free radical. The reactions of these radicals (Figure 2.1) are responsible for the indirect action of radiation. As shown, free H can combine with oxygen in the living cell to produce additional H_2O_2 and HO_2. These and possibly other powerful oxidizing agents in proximity to delicate cell mechanisms are expected to interfere with balanced chemical activities. HO_2 may even abstract H ions from organic substances:

$$RH + HO_2^{\cdot} \rightarrow R^{\cdot} + H_2O_2$$

or an exchange reaction may occur

$$RH + HO_2^{\cdot} \rightarrow RO + H_2O$$

Also organic peroxides may be formed in biological systems.

In addition to the ionization of water with resulting free radical formation, the H bonds, double bonds, and SH groups of other molecules may be split to give rise to free radicals.

There is a smaller but very important probability that ionization may occur in a significant organic molecule such as an enzyme or a nucleic acid. This is termed *direct action* and is distinguished from the *indirect action*, mentioned above, by the receipt of energy directly from a ray rather than in chemical reaction with another molecule.

$$H + OH \rightarrow H_2O$$ Water reconstitution Deactivation reactions

$$\left.\begin{array}{l} H + H \rightarrow H_2 \\ OH + OH \rightarrow H_2O_2 \end{array}\right\}$$ Radical-radical reactions intratrack possibilities

$$\left.\begin{array}{l} OH + H_2 \rightarrow H_2O + H \\ H + H_2O_2 \rightarrow H_2O + OH \end{array}\right\}$$ Destruction of molecular products

$$\begin{array}{l} OH + H_2O_2 \rightarrow HO_2 + H_2O \\ HO_2 + HO_2 \rightarrow H_2O_2 + O_2 \end{array}$$ Free radical decomposition of H_2O_2 breaks the deactivation sequence and can lead to oxygen formation Radical reactions with molecules

$$HO_2 + OH \rightarrow H_2O + O_2$$ The competitive radical removal reaction also forms oxygen

$$\left.\begin{array}{l} H + O_2 \rightarrow HO_2 \\ HO_2 + e \rightarrow HO_2^- \\ HO_2^- + H^+ \rightarrow H_2O_2 \end{array}\right\}$$ With oxygen present as in biological experiments

Figure 2.1. When water is irradiated, a complicated chain of events ensues. Included are such reactions as shown. Whether intratrack combinations or others occur depends on the geometric distribution of the primary products.

Distinguishing between Direct and Indirect Action

When a biologically active material such as an enzyme is purified and irradiated dry, any action of radiation is necessarily of the direct type. On the other hand, when the material is irradiated in the functional hydrated state, the action can be either direct or indirect. Comparisons between dry and wet experiments can provide quantitative studies.

The radiation sensitivity of enzymes in wet and dry yeast cells has been compared by Hutchinson and associates (1957) (Table 2.1). These experiments were performed to study the mechanisms involved in the action of radiation, particularly the distance traveled by the chemically active intermediates responsible for indirect action. Free radicals were found to diffuse only 30 Å on the average, which means that the radicals do not spread widely throughout the cell (Hutchinson, 1957). Also it may explain the general reflection of dose with size of molecule— coenzyme A being a relatively small molecule. While considering dose, note the massive doses of radiation employed in this type of research— they are at least 10,000 times the doses lethal to mammals.

TABLE 2.1

Enzymes from Yeast Cells Irradiated under Wet and under Dry Conditions[a]

Enzyme	Radiation	Rate of energy loss (eV/100Å in protein)	37% Dose			
			Wet (particles/cm²)	Dry (particles/cm²)	Wet (megarads)	Dry (megarads)
Invertase	4-MeV deuterons	230	2.2×10^{12}	4.4×10^{12}	6.2 ± 0.5	12 ± 1
	8-MeV α particles	1000	0.44	0.91	5.4 ± 0.5	11 ± 1
	^{60}Co γ rays	~3			6 ± 0.5	11 ± 1
Alcohol dehydrogenase	4-MeV deuterons	230	0.40	10	1.1 ± 0.4	28 ± 5
	^{60}Co γ rays	~3			1.5 ± 0.4	20–40
Coenzyme A	4-MeV deuterons	230	1	70	3 ± 1	190 ± 30
	40-MeV α particles	250	<3	55	<9	160 ± 30

[a] From Hutchinson et al. (1957).

If oxidizing radicals are responsible for inactivation of enzymes, enzymes with SH groups might be especially vulnerable. The group led by Barrón (Barrón and Flood, 1950) provided early evidence along these lines. They not only formulated the oxidation of sulfhydryl groups, but also showed that the enzymes can be reactivated by supplying a compound, such as glutathione, which possesses sulfhydryl groups. On the other hand, if there was additional damage besides that to SH groups, reactivation was not demonstrable.

Viruses which can withstand desiccation lend themselves to the dry versus the wet type of experiment. In macroorganisms however, low concentrations of water are found only in plant seeds and animal cysts. Experiments have been performed with encysted *Artemia*, the brine shrimp. Figure 2.2 demonstrates the general principle that it takes much less radiation to damage well-hydrated (that is, wet) material. This may be verified in plant seeds. For example, barley seeds soaked for several hours are more radiosensitive than desiccated seeds. However, when Caldecott (1955) studied seeds stored at various vapor pressures he found that the phenomenon was not a simple one. There was a decreased sensitivity for seeds when water content was 4–8% above dry weight. This effect of moisture has proved to be most evident during

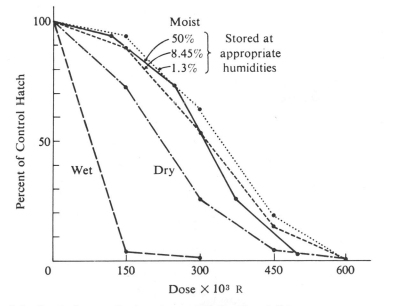

Figure 2.2. Survival curves for *Artemia* cysts irradiated with ^{60}Co γ rays at various water content values. (From Engel and Fluke, 1962; by permission of Academic Press, Inc.)

the postirradiation period and can be held to a minimum by immediate germination. Similar effects have been demonstrated recently for *Artemia* cysts (Snipes and Gordy, 1963). In both types of material a study of the signals of electron-spin resonance provide an explanation. Water vapor increases the rate of decay of the resonance pattern of free radicals. By neutralizing radiation-induced free radicals, water vapor can protect cysts or seeds from damage. However, much higher doses must be employed to obtain clear-cut results with *Artemia* cysts where "hatching" does not involve cell divisions than with plant seeds where much of the damage is correlated with chromosome aberrations induced in dividing cells. Radiations with dense ionization tracks are more effective than x or γ rays, and less energy is required to inactivate dry plant seeds and animal cysts. Iwasaki's (Iwasaki *et al.*, 1971) group demonstrated that fast neutrons were about twice as effective as ^{60}Co γ rays (RBE $\sim$ 2). Furthermore, cytological studies revealed that doses with no effect on hatching caused death during naupliar development when cells of the larva must divide. The neutrons in particular were responsible for severe chromosome abnormalities and depressed mitotic activity.

When drying is not feasible, the effects of dilution, protection, and freezing are useful tests for indirect action, if applicable. If the action is indirect, the number of molecules or organisms inactivated should be independent of the concentration (since a fixed number of free radicals is produced in water by a given amount of radiation).

A substance added to the system which could compete for the fixed number of radicals should reduce the number of test items inactivated. Dale (1942), among the first to postulate enzyme inhibition due to radiation products of water, was a pioneer in attempts to study the phenomenon by addition of protective agents. Results of a classic experiment are shown in Table 2.2. Note how the oxygen uptake decreases with decreasing concentrations of the protective agent.

The indirect effect should also be reduced by freezing since the diffusion of free radicals is hindered in ice. These methods, of course, cannot be extended to animals with homeostatic physiology. External changes are compensated and extensive internal tampering is not tolerated.

The Target Theory

In cases where direct action predominates, the results can be interpreted by the "Target Theory" or *Treffertheorie*. In this approach, a

TABLE 2.2
Inactivation of Alloxazinadenine Dinucleotide (D) by 8000 R of X Radiation in the Presence and Absence of Leucylglycine (L) as Protector[a]

Manometer	Contents		Volume of O_2 in first 10 min (μl)
	D	+ Protein + Substrate	28.6
2	(D + 10^{-4} mole L)[b]	+ Protein + Substrate	27.1
3	(D + 10^{-6} mole L)[b]	+ Protein + Substrate	19.3
4	(D + 10^{-7} mole L)[b]	+ Protein + Substrate	12.8
5	(D + 10^{-8} mole L)[b]	+ Protein + Substrate	10.0
6	(D)[a]	+ Protein + Substrate	10.7

[a] (Courtesy of W. M. Dale, with permission of the editors of the *Biochemical Journal*.)
[b] Denotes irradiation of contents in parentheses.

macromolecule no less important than the gene is viewed as the target in which an ionization is considered a "hit." However, the typical irradiation device cannot be aimed at specific molecules as a gun is sighted on a target. Rather it is more like directing arms fire into a target area which is out of sight.

From a physical basis the concept is attractive. We may view ionizing radiations as destructive agents whose action is localized in submicroscopic areas smaller than those obtainable by any other method. Within a minute volume, ionization releases an amount of energy so great as to almost certainly bring about significant chemical change.

Lea (1947), the outstanding exponent of the theory, recognized the single ionization type of action on the basis of three lines of evidence: (1) the curve plotted from experimental data should be exponential; (2) the effect of a given dose should be independent of time; and (3) the differences in yield should be in orderly relationship with the radiations differing in ion density. Lea emphasized that all criteria, not merely the shape of the dose–effect curve, must be met. Let us consider each of the criteria in detail.

Shape of the Curve. Points obtained by experiment should lie on a straight line within the error of the experiment. This would occur in a single-hit target effect since the number of hits is proportional to the number of ionizations, which in turn is proportional to the amount of radiation delivered. With low doses only a small proportion of targets are hit, and results plotted against dose fall on a straight line even on a simple arithmetic graph. If the dose is so large that the number of targets hit is a considerable proportion of those present, some targets

will be hit more than once. Thus, the number of targets influenced
would be less than the number of potentially effective hits, and yield
plotted against dose tends to fall off in a geometrical progression. The
curve obtained is exponential and may be converted into a straight line
if logarithms are used to represent the yield (Figure 2.3).

Survival curves and the use of Napierian logarithms have fostered the
adoption of the "37%" dose by advocates of the target theory. This dose
corresponds to an average of one hit per target and is based on the fact
that

$$e^{-D/D^0} = e^{-1} = 0.368$$

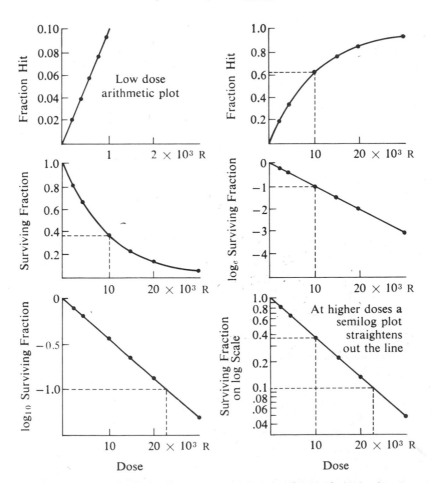

Figure 2.3 Methods of plotting experimental data for the single-ionization type of
action. (From Lea, 1947; by permission of Cambridge University Press.)

or approximately 37%. D represents dose, and D^0 the dose required to score one hit per organism. To state this more simply, a dose of radiation sufficient to inactivate all the available targets actually influences only 63% of them. This is based upon the exponential nature of the survival curve and is due to duplicating hits in many of the targets where one hit should suffice. This allows 37% of the targets to escape from damage.

By knowing the 37% dose and the number of ionizations produced per volume in tissue for a unit of radiation, it is possible to calculate the size of the target. For the refinement of this method and various necessary assumptions, refer to Lea's (1947) monograph.

Time-Intensity. The second criterion means that alterations in the dose rate should not influence the yield of the experiment. Thus, whether a certain amount of radiation is given in seconds, minutes, or hours, continuously or in fractions, a particular number of ionizations should result and the same number of targets should be hit.

Dependence on Type of Radiation. Because of differences in the number of ionizations per micron path, with heavily ionizing rays many ionizations may be produced in targets the size of biologically important molecules. Since one hit is considered to suffice in target action, the additional ionizations do not contribute to the biological effect although they do contribute to the dose delivered. This results in a reduction of yield per ionization, and more densely ionizing radiations are less effective. For equal effect, the dose increases from that of γ rays, through x rays, to α rays.

A catch phrase to help remember this order is; "The RBE decreases with increasing LET" for a single hit effect. As defined in Chapter 1, RBE is an abbreviation for Relative Biological Efficiency and LET is Linear Energy Transfer. If the RBE of α:x is 0.2:1 for inactivation of a virus particle, it means that five times as great a dose of alpha rays is required as that of x rays. Thus the alpha rays are relatively inefficient in this respect. However the reverse is found for many biological situations. For example, there is the 15:1 ratio of α:x effectiveness in chromosome breakage of *Tradescantia*. In general the ratio favors heavily ionized tracks for chromosome damage. Accordingly, if such damage explains many organ and organism phenomena, it follows that RBEs favor high LET in many important aspects of radiation biology. On the other hand, single-hit inactivation does not occur for any biological unit more complex than small viruses. In higher organisms, the cells show survival curves that necessitate the formulation of multitarget and multihit theories (see Chapter 6).

Inactivation of Viruses. The most striking success of the target approach came in radiation experiments with the smaller viruses. However, although viruses served as the first system on which to test the target theory, they also supplied examples of discrepancies in target size determinations.

Staphylococcus phage K inactivation is one example of this type of investigation. The survival curve was exponential (Figure 2.4). Although intensities differing in a ratio of 28:1 were employed, namely 1.34×10^4 R/min and 4.72×10^2 R/min, inactivation doses (the 37% approach) did not vary outside of the error of the experiments. When the inactivation doses for γ rays, x rays (1.5 Å), and α rays were compared, it was found that the dose increased in the order of ion density:

$$0.079 \times 10^6 \text{ R for } \gamma$$

$$0.109 \times 10^6 \text{ R for x}$$

$$0.45 \times 10^6 \text{ R for } \alpha$$

Target Size. The target diameter of *Staphylococcus* phage K was calculated in nm as 15.5 with γ rays, 15.9 with x rays, and 16.3 with α rays. Microscopic measurements place the diameter at 16 nm unhydrated, which corresponds nicely with target calculations.

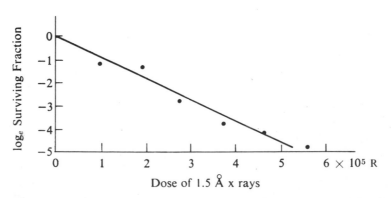

Figure 2.4. Survival curve for *Staphylococcus* bacteriophage K. (From Lea, 1947; by permission of Cambridge University Press.)

More significant discrepancies were noted with larger viruses. In particular, the large virus vaccinia is almost three times the largest size calculatable from radiation data. In the small viruses only a thin protein sheath encloses the nucleic acid, but in the vaccinia virus the biconcave inner core containing the nucleic acid is sandwiched between two lateral masses and enclosed in inner and outer membranes. Thus the original idea that the radiosensitive volume corresponded to the particle's physical volume is untenable. Better correspondence was found between the inactivation dose and the amount of nucleic acid (Kaplan and Moses, 1964). However, even on the basis of nucleic acid content, target size calculations are not in exact agreement with the dimensions obtained by electron microscopy.

Successes as well as discrepancies have been reported for macromolecules isolated from biological material. Target size calculated from irradiation data, and molecular weight determined by physical chemical methods check well for hemocyanin, ribonuclease, pepsin, and the pneumococcus transforming factor. Discrepancies were found for antigens and other types of molecules where specificity resides in only one part of the structure. For some molecules, different target sizes were found for different functional abilities, for example, milk clotting and casein digestion by chymotrypsin. Since the years of these early investigations, the interest of radiobiologists has waned and biophysicists have developed specialized areas of research. As indicated in Table 2.1, enzyme inactivations may require megarad doses.

Concluding Remarks

In this chapter we have introduced the concepts of direct and indirect action on biologically important macromolecules. The target theory which formalized analysis of direct action was presented, and inactivation of viruses was given as an example of a successful application of the approach. During the decade culminating in 1947, attention was devoted to the target idea with an intensity which almost prohibited other research activity. More recent investigations have revealed the complexities which must be considered in delineating the cellular target whose damage leads to death (see Chapters 4 and 5). In the following chapters we shall relate both direct and indirect action at the submicroscopic level to biological change recognized at both microscopic and macroscopic levels.

References

Barrón, E. S. G., and Flood, V. (1950). Studies on the mechanism of action of ionizing radiations. VI. The oxidation of thiols by ionizing radiation. *J. Gen. Physiol.* **33**, 229–241.

Caldecott, R. S. (1955). Effects of hydration on x ray sensitivity in *Hordeum. Radiat. Res.* **3**, 316–330.

Dale, W. M. (1942). The effect of x rays on the conjugated protein *d*-amino-acid oxidase. *Biochem. J.* **36**, 80–85.

Engel, D. W., and Fluke, D. J. (1962). The effect of water content and postirradiation storage on radiation sensitivity of brine shrimp cysts. *Radiat. Res.* **16**, 173–181.

Hutchinson, F. (1957). The distance that a radical formed by ionizing radiation can diffuse in a yeast cell. *Radiat. Res.* **7**, 473–483.

Hutchinson, F., Preston, A., and Vogel, B. (1957). Radiation sensitivity of enzymes in wet and dry yeast cells. *Radiat. Res.* **7**, 465–472.

Iwasaki, T., Maruyama, T., Kumamoto, Y., and Kato, Y. (1971). Effects of fast neutrons and ^{60}Co γ-rays on *Artemia. Radiat. Res.* **45**, 288–298.

Kaplan, H. S., and Moses, L. E. (1964). Biological complexity and radiosensitivity. *Science* **145**, 21–25.

Lea, D. E. (1947). "Actions of Radiations on Living Cells." Cambridge Univ. Press, London and New York.

Snipes, W. C., and Gordy, W. (1963). Radiation damage to *Artemia* cysts: Effects of water vapor. *Science* **142**, 503–504.

General References

Bacq, Z. M., and Alexander, P. (1955). "Fundamentals of Radiobiology," 1st ed., Chapter 2. Academic Press, New York.

Casarett, A. P. (1968). "Radiation Biology," Chapter 4. Prentice-Hall, Englewood Cliffs, New Jersey.

Pollard, E. C., Guild, W. R., Hutchinson, F., and Setlow, R. B. (1955). The direct action of ionizing radiation on enzymes and antigens. *Prog. Biophys. Biophys. Chem.* **5**, 72–108.

Ward, J. F. (1975). Molecular mechanisms of radiation induced damage to nucleic acids. *Adv. Radiat. Biol.* **5**, 181–239.

PART II   THE CELLULAR LEVEL

In the preceding two chapters, we encountered the idea that radiation produces rather indiscriminate effects on the atoms and small molecules that comprise the cell. We discovered that massive doses may have to be delivered to inactivate certain enzymes, whereas a single ionization may suffice to inactivate a virus particle. We will now consider radiation damage at the level of the subcellular components and the whole cell. Here, too, there will be both radioresistant and radiosensitive phenomena. To give organization to our approach, we shall work from the outside to the inside. After the survey of a broad range of possible radiation-induced events, the response of the single cell will be discussed. Since a universal environment for every cell does not exist, we will explore the various internal and external conditions that may alter the response of the cell to radiation.

CHAPTER 3 Cytosomal Effects and Cell Division

Microscopic examination of heavily irradiated cells gave early investigators some evidence of visible change. The vacuolization of cytoplasm and an intracellular accumulation of released fat are cytoplasmic changes which became well known to morphologists. Heilbrunn and Mazia (1936), Ellinger (1941, 1949), and Kimball (1955) provide a number of references. However, marked changes in physiology may not necessarily be reflected in the microscopic appearance of the cell. Permeability changes, viscosity changes, and effects upon the apparatus of cell division are phenomena best investigated by physiological methods. Historically there was a period during which permeability and viscosity studies were favored to such a degree that they occupied the attention of a majority of cell physiologists. Undoubtedly the hope of demonstrating a cytosomal basis of radiation sensitivity spurred many of the radiation experiments. However, it has been established that massive doses are necessary to produce significant changes, and along with advances in technology, the attention of physiologists has shifted toward explanations consistent with the disclosures of the electron microscope. Nevertheless, the results are valid and worthy of our consideration. On the other hand, we shall discuss a highly radiosensitive phenomenon, the time-course of cell division, in which the nucleus plays a part.

Permeability

The cell membrane and the cortex are involved in determining which materials pass in and out of the cell, as well as the rates of these processes. Despite the fact that at one time this aspect of cell physiology received more attention than any other, there has been a dearth of certain information on radiation effects. In 1936, Heilbrunn and Mazia summarized early work and presented a critique of experimental methods. Preferred evidence was given by plasmolysis of plant cells and chemical analysis of their vacuole contents, as well as by hemolysis, hematocrit, and chloride determination on vertebrate blood. The conclusion was that both ionizing and exciting types of radiation cause a definite increase in permeability.

Within a few years, techniques for measuring the rate of hemolysis had advanced, and it could be conclusively established that erythrocytes irradiated at substantial doses suffer osmotic disturbance. A series of papers published by Ting and Zirkle in 1940 is considered classic. However, these investigations were performed without the aid of radioactive tracers. Within a decade, the availability of radioisotopes and advances in instrumentation enabled investigators to perceive that passive diffusion is not the only process involved in cell permeability. Active transport and facilitated diffusion must also be considered. Induced changes in permeability to univalent cations soon became an established fact, but controversy developed over the relative importance of induced damage to the three components.

Irradiation was found to increase the migration of ^{42}K from both blood and yeast cells into the exterior (Hevesy and Zerahn, 1946). With careful attention to the physiological conditions, it was shown that the initial disturbance to erythrocytes after irradiation was not hemolysis but ionic leakage, especially of potassium (Sheppard and Stewart, 1952). Simultaneously and almost reciprocally, sodium penetrated. Exchange processes preceded osmotic catastrophe by as much as hours (Figure 3.1).

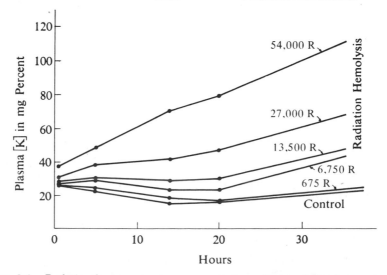

Figure 3.1. Prolytic plasma potassium concentration changes following exposure of human erythrocytes to various doses of x rays. (Courtesy of C. W. Sheppard.)

When plotted against dose, the rate of K loss proves to be roughly proportional to dose (Figure 3.2). Cold storage accentuates the phenomenon. No oxygen effect was found, and attempts to relate the radiation effect to such biochemical processes as glycolysis or cholinesterase activity were not successful. Therefore, disturbance of ion selectivity at the cell surface was postulated. If this can occur, local irradiation should produce local failure, as indeed has been accomplished (Figure 3.3).

Reciprocal sodium–potassium exchanges in erythrocytes, and permeability changes in plant cells may be produced by a number of disturbing influences other than irradiation. In recent years, permeability has become linked more closely to metabolic activity than to the physical characteristics of the cell membrane and cortex. However radiation-induced leakage of univalent ions is most pronounced at low temperatures where active transport does not function well. Also the rate of K^+ loss after complete inhibition of active transport by ouabain is trivial compared with that observed after irradiation. The mammalian

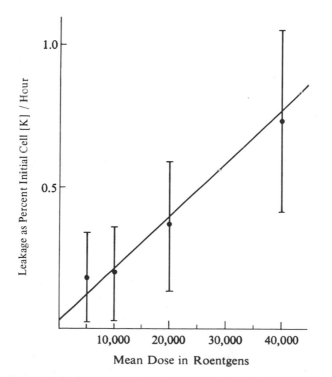

Figure 3.2. Potassium leakage rates plotted against x-ray dose for human erythrocytes. (Courtesy of C. W. Sheppard.)

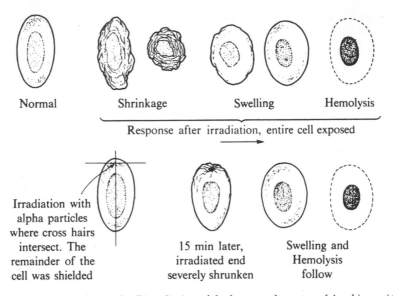

Figure 3.3. Total and partial cell irradiation of the large erythrocytes of *Amphiuma*. (After Buchsbaum and Zirkle, 1949.)

erythrocyte is considered the ideal cell in which to study the phenomenon, since the maintenance of gradients is uncomplicated by the presence of a nucleus. Other vertebrate tissue cells in which reciprocal K^+ and Na^+ flow has been studied include nerve, muscle, liver, ileum, and thymus lymphocytes. Results obtained with erythrocytes indicate that radiation disorganizes the lipoprotein structure of the cell membrane. Oxidation of membrane thiols and disruption of disulfide bonds occur, along with an increased susceptibility to proteolytic enzymes. Contributing to the hemolytic crisis is the formation of lipid peroxides concordant with the destruction of antioxidants in the membrane (Myers, 1970).

In a cultured mammalian cell system, Hopwood and Dewey (1976) found no effect of 1000 or 5000-rad doses on the V_{max} or K_m values for the facilitated diffusion of thymidine when the kinetic rates were determined 10 min after irradiation. The absence of effects on V_{max} and K_m values indicates that the number and binding affinity of the transport sites are not influenced by radiation. The synthesis or degradation of binding sites also did not appear to be changed by radiation, since the uptake kinetics were unaffected at 2.5 hours after 1000-rad doses.

The interpretation of prokaryotic cell responses is more difficult. In bacterial cells where DNA is attached to the cytoplasmic membrane, damage to the membrane may markedly influence reproductive survival.

Organelles

Altered permeability of the cell membrane and cortex is not the only important structural consideration. The semipermeability of intra-cellular membranes are important in separating enzymes from their substrates. In an early experiment, Bacq and Hervé (1952) used discol-oration of irradiated mushrooms to introduce this concept. Subse-quently, many radiobiologists have sought to demonstrate alterations in organelles following the irradiation of intact animals or isolated preparations. Decisive results were obtained only with high doses (Harris, 1970), especially in intact cells which contain mechanisms for protecting membranes against the oxidation of SH groups and the peroxidation of lipids. Isolated lysosomes are sensitive to doses not effective *in situ*. Kilo radiation absorbed doses to the microsomal frac-tion from the endoplasmic reticulum of liver cells produce lipid peroxides only after incubation in the absence of antioxidants.

Lysosomes are the most radiosensitive organelles. Since they are sacs which segregate enzymes capable of demolishing almost every type of cellular molecule, damage to their single membrane has serious conse-quences. The lysosomes of different tissues are not equally radiosensi-tive. Only 100 rads increased the permeability of lysosomal membranes of spleen cells, but no change in permeability or associated enzyme activity was evident after 850 rads to the whole body of ^{60}Co γ rays when other tissues of the rodents were considered (liver, heart, kidney, or adrenal glands) (Aikman and Wills, 1974).

Reports that the irradiation of cells changes the number, size, shape, and dry mass of their mitochondria are not uncommon, but alterations are usually transient. Often there are thousands per cell and only mas-sive doses provide clear evidence of induced change. For permeability, the most quoted report concerns the rate of swelling of flight muscle sarcosomes isolated from houseflies given doses from 25 to 100 krads (Carney, 1965). Swollen mitochondria are also evident in the moribund follicular epithelium of rat thyroids damaged by ^{131}I.

Target number experiments are not feasible for the thousands of mitochondria and ribosomes per animal cell, but the limited number of chloroplasts (10) in *Euglena* provided opportunity for inactivation studies of another organelle (Lyman *et al.*, 1961). The thirty hits per cytosome required for cell-bleaching indicated that three mutations per plastid must occur. This is consistent with other evidence that 30 DNA-containing extranuclear units control *Euglena* chloroplast development. Extended to higher plants with up to 40 plastids per cell, this implies that hundreds of sites must be inactivated to obtain a response which could be obtained by inactivation of a single nuclear gene controlling any of the steps in the chlorophyll pathway (although then expression is delayed until homozygosity is obtained). Indeed, over a million rads are required to decrease by 90% the chlorophyll content of an exposed tobacco leaf.

Protoplasmic Viscosity

The "submicroscopic" ground substance examined at electron microscope resolutions appears as a complex polyphasic mixture. The innumerable membranous and fibrous elements are suspended in a matrix which still is conveniently called protoplasm. Methods adapted from colloid chemistry characterized early attempts to demonstrate radiation induced changes in the cytoplasm (Sparrow, 1951). Changes were assessed by studying the movements of granules or inclusion particles under centrifugation. Heilbrunn and Mazia (1936) cite early investigations with many kinds of plant cells, marine eggs, and vertebrate tissues. Historically, the investigations formed part of an attack upon the reactivity of cells to all sorts of stimuli. A related concern was protoplasmic clotting, the response to cell membrane rupture which seals the opening.

The Heilbrunn group of investigators viewed the subject from the standpoint of a theory of stimulation involving calcium release from the cell cortex. Liquefaction followed by gelation fits this scheme, and was actually obtained, first for the plasma sol of *Amoeba dubia* after ultraviolet exposures, and later with x rays on *Spirogyra* filaments, although a certain amount of centrifugal force is required to break chloroplast moorings (Northen and MacVicar, 1940). Protoplasm was visualized as a network of protein molecules in which both dissociation and reassociation can be influenced.

Investigations extended to β rays and γ rays from radioisotopes yield patterns of initial liquefaction followed by reversion. Virgin and Ehrenberg (1953) centrifuged *Elodea* leaves after immersion for various times in solutions of ^{32}P, ^{35}S, or ^{22}Na. Only the highest doses of 23 rep/min obtained with ^{32}P at concentrations of 1150 μCi/ml caused nonreverting liquefaction. Interest in this type of research has flagged but new techniques like employing a spin label in magnetic resonance could revitalize viscosity studies (Keith and Snipes, 1974).

Perhaps the most striking demonstration of an effect on cytoplasmic structure is that found during the mitotic divisions subsequent to the fertilization of eggs from marine invertebrates (Figure 3.4). During the first cleavage division, the viscosity of irradiated eggs remains high for a period two to three times longer than the normal mitotic gelation (Wilson, 1950). Simultaneously, the progress of the spindle-mediated events is delayed to the same extent. In situations like the sea urchin *Arbacia*, where the sperm contributes the centrosome as well as a nucleus at fertilization, an effect on peripheral viscosity as well as that of division delay can be obtained in normal eggs fertilized with irradiated sperm.

Investigations with unfertilized eggs avoid this complication, but null effect as well as alteration in viscosity have been reported after irradiation. One explanation is that species differ in the degree of maturation attained in the ovary. For example, star fish (*Asterias*) eggs, in which viscosity change may be demonstrated, are in meiosis by the time they are obtained for irradiation work. However, those of the parchment worm *Chaetopterus* and *Arbacia* are not, and prove resistant to radiation-induced structural change. Apparently the physiological state during the division process is significant. In any event, appreci-

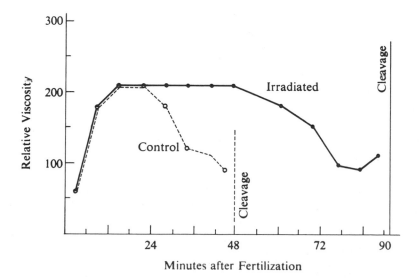

Figure 3.4. Viscosity of irradiated *Arbacia* eggs fertilized with normal sperm. Before fertilization, eggs received 10,000 R of x rays. (Courtesy of W. L. Wilson.)

able doses must be delivered to obtain a clear-cut phenomenon in
responsive material.

Effects on the Spindle

In a discussion of effects on the cytosome, the spindle must properly
be considered, since the main portion of the mitotic apparatus is believed to come from the cytoplasm. Analyses of isolated spindles indicate that the nucleus is simply not large enough to hold all the protein
required (Mazia, 1961). This does not deny that the nucleus may in
some way contribute in direction or as a source of material. It only states
that the protein is drawn from the cytoplasm at the time the mitotic
apparatus is forming. The protein molecules are aggregated by inter-
molecular bonding into a system of microtubules which electron microscopy has revealed in the peripheral cytoplasm of many kinds of
cells. Still unsettled is the way in which kinetochore microtubules
interact with continuous-spindle microtubules to generate poleward
movement of the chromosomes. At present, it is difficult to choose
between an assembly–dissembly hypothesis and the idea of microtubules sliding past each other.

Consistent with chemical analysis of the spindle are the observations
that the ultraviolet wavelengths capable of altering the spindle are those
typical of protein absorption. On the other hand, the achromatic figure
of animal cells seems relatively insensitive to ionizing radiations. When
8000 R of x rays were applied to the dividing grasshopper neuroblast
they had no effect on the structure or function of the spindle. Henshaw's (Figure 3.5) multipolar *Arbacia* cleavages, an indication of spindle disruption, occur after a threshold dose in the neighborhood of
60,000 R of x rays. In other animals, no visible changes occurred in

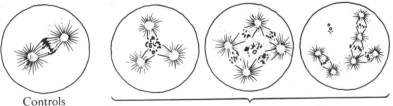

Controls
Normal bipolar
configuration

Examples of variations among irradiated
abnormal multipolar cleavage divisions

Figure 3.5. Mitotic configurations of *Arbacia* zygotes whose sperm had received 62,400 R
of x rays. (Courtesy of P. S. Henshaw.)

spindles given sizable doses. Carlson's (1954) review supplies a number of references on this point.

Significant localized disruption of the mitotic mechanism can result from microbeam applications of uv, protons, or α rays. When focused on the kinetochore, this type of probe can halt the positioning movements of the prometaphase chromosomes in relation to the spindle. The dose of uv used on the kinetochore is sufficient to destroy the end of the spindle. Here the particulate rays were less effective. Although 20 to 40 protons sufficed for kinetochore damage, many thousands were required to destroy the spindle's polar ends (Zirkle et al., 1955). Site radiation between the metaphase plate and a pole can cause a visibly distinguishable spot to appear (reduced birefringence) which moves to the pole at a velocity similar to that characteristic for chromosomes of the same cell (Forer, 1965).

In this section we considered formed spindles. Delayed division which involves many other more radiosensitive cell functions is discussed later in the chapter.

Relative Vulnerability of Nucleus and Cytosome

In making the transition from cytosomal considerations to effects in which the nucleus is involved we should stress a point demonstrable by direct experiment. Measured in terms of cell radiosensitivity, the most sensitive structure of the cell is the nucleus. This is expected because the nucleus is the coordinating and directing center of the cell. Furthermore, most cells capable of division possess a nucleus characterized by a limited number of chromosomes and structural genes, whereas the cytoplasm contains many multiples of its important structures. The redundancy in assemblies of structural devices for tranducing energy and manufacturing specialized molecules results not only in impressive cytoplasmic performances but also assures relative radiotolerance. Admittedly, repetitive sequences in nuclear DNAs have been demonstrated in the genomes of many types of animals. However, their interspersion with single-copy structural genes provides neither redundancy of the latter nor radiotolerance.

Convincing evidence comes from two types of experiments involving (a) cells with eccentric nuclei, and (b) nuclear transplantation. Fern spores were used in the earliest study wherein position of the nucleus made possible cytoplasmic exposure to α rays without penetration to the nucleus. More recently, the usefulness of the eccentric placement of wasp egg nuclei has been appreciated. Figure 3.6 contrasts the compara-

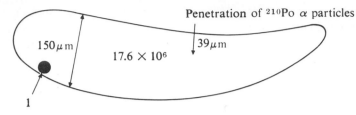

Figure 3.6. Comparative radiosensitivity of nucleus and cytoplasm of *Habrobracon* eggs. The average number of incident α particles required to lower hatchability to 37% is designated. The eccentric position of the nucleus in newly laid wasp eggs enables selective radiation of the cytosome, or nucleus, depending on orientation and shielding. (Based on investigations by von Borstel and Rogers, 1958).

tive radiosensitivity of the nucleus and cytoplasm of *Habrobracon* eggs. As shown, the nucleus is at the convex surface and is easily reached by short penetrating radiation if the egg is oriented toward the source of the rays. Over a million (10^6) more α particles must be delivered to the cytoplasm than to the nucleus in order to kill the same proportion of a sample of eggs. An impressive difference in radiosensitivity is also demonstrable between the anterior nucleated half of *Drosophila* eggs and the posterior nonnucleated half.

Delicate microsurgery has made possible the transplantation of nuclei from unirradiated into irradiated cells and vice versa. Experiments with protozoa and eggs of various lower animals point up the greater resistance of the cytoplasm to cell-inactivating injury. Transplantation of an irradiated nucleus to an unirradiated cell is typically lethal at doses from which an irradiated cell provided with a nucleus from an unirradiated cell survives. The presence of a nucleus protects cell fragments from cytolytic effects evident on enucleate fragments. Conversely, a cell with all its cytoplasm is less vulnerable to nuclear damage than one from which half the cytoplasm has been removed. Since this can be shown even for amebas which spread as a thin layer on any surface, the effect is not one of shielding. An uninterrupted flow of information from the nucleus is important for the direction of cytoplasmic repair activities. Also, reverse flow plays a part in the repair of nuclear damage. Heavily irradiated amebas were rescued from death and enabled to divide by injections of cytoplasm from nonirradiated cells (Daniels and Breyer, 1970).

Much simpler experiments in nuclear transfer may be set up by using members of the order Hymenoptera in which normal males can be parthenogenetically produced from unfertilized eggs. By heavily irradiating females and then mating them to normal males, it is possible to produce "motherless" sons. These individuals develop from the sperm nucleus operating in irradiated cytoplasm (Whiting, 1946). Visible evidence of the degeneration of the egg nucleus can be obtained with a microscope, and genetic evidence of the paternity of the sons is acquired by means of marker genes. Obviously the cytoplasm has not been irrevocably damaged if a sexually mature adult can develop from it. Only massive radiation doses cause cytoplasmic destruction so severe that the functioning of an untreated nucleus is not compensatory (Whiting, 1949).

Cleavage Delay

Both nuclear and cytoplasmic materials are involved in cell division, and its time course can be easily influenced by radiations.

Henshaw (1940) and associates pioneered in an extensive series of studies on the mitotic rate after irradiation. While exploiting the fact that large samples of eggs from marine animals go through cleavage synchronously, they found that the time required for 50% of the eggs to cleave was a feasible endpoint. The most radiosensitive period of the cleaving *Arbacia* zygote corresponded to the period of greatest viscosity and permeability. In cytological terms, this occurs when pronuclei have come together, but before there is visible evidence of prophase. A second peak in radiosensitivity is noted in early prophase.

Irradiation of either sperm, eggs, or both, delayed postfertilization division. Experiments with halved eggs suggested that the nucleus is involved. Irradiation of a nucleated half-egg imparts the same cleavage delay as irradiation of the whole egg. Furthermore, no delay occurs for a nonnucleated cytoplasmic mass which has been irradiated and later fertilized (Henshaw, 1938).

The duration of delay increases with increasing doses. Thus, it is a graded rather than an all-or-none action. Also, impermanence of the delay implies that the effect is one from which recovery occurs. In its various aspects this contrasts with the target type effect as Lea (1947) himself appreciated. Rather than a single ionizing event in a localized area, many ionizations in an appreciable volume seem necessary to produce the effect. Lea found it necessary to allow both for radiation received and for the recovery occurred by a given moment when he attempted to express the phenomenon mathematically.

The general principles have been verified independently on the regulative eggs of other species of sea urchins (Miwa *et al.*, 1939) and on the mosaic eggs of molluscs (Cather, 1959). A prolongation of prophase is typical in a variety of experimental materials in addition to invertebrate eggs. On the other hand, when investigations were extended to other types of cells the entire cell cycle came under scrutiny, not merely cytokinesis. Events in mitotically active tissues are discussed in subsequent sections. Here we restrict the discussion to fertilized eggs.

At lower doses adequate to induce significant cleavage delay, the DNA synthesis in both control and irradiated *Arbacia* eggs occurs at the same rate and begins simultaneously for the first cleavage (Rao and Hinegardner, 1965). Therefore neither rate nor initiation of DNA synthesis has been changed. In contrast, protein synthesis plays an important role as demonstrated in puromycin inhibition studies, but whatever messenger-RNA is required for the radiosensitive protein's synthesis is already present in the unfertilized egg and cannot be influenced by actinomycin D (Rustad and Burchill, 1966).

Mitotic Activity in Tissues

Delayed division has been studied in many other experimental materials such as bacteria, plant root tips, and rapidly dividing animal tissues. However, the experimental procedures and methods of scoring are different from those used on marine eggs. Bacteriologists employ turbidimetry to determine the number of cells attained by a culture in a given period of time. In plant and animal tissues, counts may be made to determine the number of cells in midmitosis after specific amounts of time have elapsed following irradiation. Results are compared with suitable controls. Interpretation is complicated by the fact that not all of the individual cells are in the same stage of development at the time of irradiation.

The most direct approach in tissues has been made by Carlson (1954) and associates (1949) who used hanging drop preparations of grasshopper neuroblasts. An incubation chamber encloses the lower part of a microscope, so that observations of living cells can be made at a constant temperature for an extended period of time. It is possible to see all internal structures and identify all the stages of mitosis. Again prophase was found to be the most sensitive stage in division; however, the sensitivity was manifested somewhat later than in *Arbacia* ova. As in the ova, an inhibition of protein synthesis by puromycin blocks the mitotic progress of neuroblasts both into and out of midmitosis.

In grasshopper neuroblasts, the critical period occurs shortly before the breakdown of the nuclear membrane, when the cell shape is beginning to change and the cytoplasmic viscosity is falling rapidly. When all cells past this stage have completed mitosis, a period exists during which no division stages are visible in the tissue. The length of this period depends on the dose of radiation. If mitotic ratio is plotted against time since irradiation, a characteristic curve is obtained (Figure 3.7). This curve features a compensatory surge due to two classes of cells entering division when mitotic activity reappears. One class consists of cells which were in a relatively insensitive stage at the time of irradiation. These divide about when they normally would. A second class consists of cells whose development was delayed. As these two classes enter mitosis together the mitotic activity is higher than that in unirradiated material. Canti and Spear (1927, 1929) provided an early demonstration of this in cultured chick tissue. A family of curves was obtained in which the decline phase was enhanced and the recovery phase depressed with increases in dose up to a level where irreversible cell damage of other types became appreciable.

Qualitatively speaking, we may expect these kinds of curves when any proliferative tissue of animal or plant origin is irradiated. Quantitative differences appear when radiation doses are compared. For example, the mitotic activity of grasshopper neuroblasts is reduced to a much

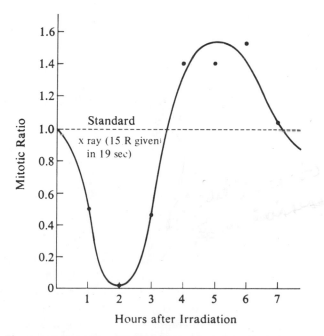

Figure 3.7. The proportion of grasshopper neuroblasts in mitosis in comparison with control values. (Courtesy of J. Gordon Carlson.)

greater degree than that of chick fibroblasts given the same amount of radiation. Measured when the effect is maximum, the efficiency of a radiation is different for different kinds of cells. Dose-effect predictions for a tissue cannot be made from experiments with unrelated tissues. Equally fallacious is a conclusion that relative radiosensitivities measured by one effect are necessarily correlated with radiosensitivities determined by another.

In the mitotic cycles of acridian neuroblasts, avian fibroblasts, and mammalian carcinoma cells, there exists a critical period before which acute doses of radiation can cause simulated reversion from defined to undefined chromatin threads (Carlson, 1969). At least 250 R delivered 5 min before the nuclear membrane disappears in dividing neuroblasts produces a reference standard of reversion associated with division delay. In all other materials investigated to date, the relative duration of visible prophase is less accommodating, and the exact timing difficult to determine.

Dose Rates

The relative effectiveness of different rates of delivery is a matter of both theoretical and practical interest. Grasshopper neuroblasts have provided an excellent demonstration of the kind of results which can be expected (Figure 3.8). Various doses were given at two different dose rates. At lower doses results were not significantly different. As the dose increased the more intense radiation was significantly more effective in lowering the mitotic counts.

Subsequently, another set of experiments was run using 0.25 R/min, an especially low dose rate for this type of experiment. At exposures totaling 32 R and more, recovery processes appeared to keep pace with the radiation effects (Carlson, 1950).

The mitotic activity of animal cells reaches a minimum sooner than 6 hours after irradiation. In contrast, the rate of decrease of mitotic activity is generally slower in plants, where the minimum may not be reached until a day after treatment. This is probably correlated with the length of the mitotic cycle which tends to be shorter in animals.

The interval between treatment and disappearance of midmitotic stages tends to be greater than the time required to complete mitosis normally. In grasshopper (*Chortophaga*) neuroblasts when normal mitosis takes 26 min, mitotic stages disappear from irradiated ganglia after 50 min. In bean (*Vicia*) root tips mitosis takes 2½ hours and stages disappear in 9 to 12 hours.

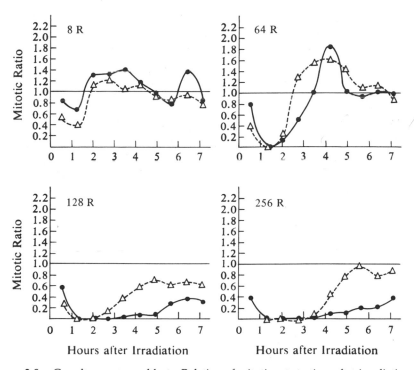

Figure 3.8. Grasshopper neuroblasts. Relation of mitotic rate to time after irradiation at two different dosage rates: △ = 2 R/min and ● = 32 R/min. The normal number of cells in mitosis is shown by the horizontal line. The proportion of dividing cells at successive times after irradiation is compared with the control level. (Courtesy of J. Gordon Carlson.)

Analysis of Mitotic Delay in Cultured Cells

Cells cultured from vertebrate tissues have provided evidence that progress through mitosis can be modified by radiation delivered at any period during the entire cell cycle. Unfortunately, some investigators have used the term *mitotic delay* loosely in referring to failures in division and colony formation, rather than restricting it to a retardation directly observed. Strictly speaking we are concerned with an induced block in the G_2 phase. Other phenomena such as the prolongation of the DNA S phase will be discussed elsewhere.

When mitotic delay "of the classical sense" was considered for mouse leukemic cells, an assessment by five different methods demonstrated that the block induced by 200 rads of x rays occurred in the middle of the G_2 stage (Doida and Okada, 1969). This is similar to the time of the puromycin block but quite different from the times when DNA or RNA synthesis is switched off.

Various destructive or perturbative techniques have been used to synchronize cultured cell lines, but these introduce additional complications to the interpretation of the radiation effects. The mitotic selection procedure for cell cycle analysis provides a less complicated situation. It is based on the tendency of mammalian cells growing in monolayers to round up and become loosely attached as they enter mitosis (Terasima and Tolmach, 1963). Therefore, shaking the medium removes mitotic cells from the culturing surface, and they can be poured out for cytological examination. After replacement of the medium and further incubation, the procedure can be repeated. Periodic sampling of the culture after inhibitory treatment provides data which reflects the time limits during which the sensitive biochemical events are vulnerable.

The transition period for the x-ray-induced G_2 block is identified as the point beyond which cells are not delayed by irradiation. This point, late in G_2, moved closer to mitosis as the radiation dose was increased. Hypothetically this corresponds to the time of completion of the final assembly of the protein structure essential for division. Disrupting either synthesis or assembly of the specific precursor would interfere with the time course of division. Dewey and Highfield (1976) explain the maximum mitotic delay induced in early G_2 in terms of the abundance of precursor substance offering the greatest probability for maximum damage, but admit an alternate possibility that G_2 is more sensitive to delay than G_1 because there is less time for repair before the scheduled time for the start of division. Although protein synthesis has been considered relatively insensitive to radiation, the synthesis of a specific protein necessary for mitosis may not be. Evidence has been provided by diverse materials: urchin eggs, insect neuroblasts, mammalian cells, and cultured pea roots (Van't Hof and Kovacs, 1970).

Concluding Remarks

The main point in this chapter is the relative radiotolerance of cytoplasmic constituents. This concept has been developed in several ways. First we surveyed the experiments in which membranes, organelles, and ground substances were exposed. Then we considered the contrast in results when either the nucleus or the cytosome was preferentially exposed. Finally we emphasized the complex events of mitosis which involve both nuclear and cytoplasmic components. Interference with the process expresses itself as delayed division, perhaps the most sensitive of the easily demonstrated effects of radiation. Still obscure is the specific trigger mechanism or the molecular conditions which serve as a tripping device. However, subsequent chapters on DNA damage and chromosomal aberrations introduce matters which can contribute to delayed progress through the cell cycle.

Although significant in its own right for posing problems in tissue development and maintenance, the lengthening of the intermitotic period introduces opposing factors which can influence the yield of mutations from a particular dose of radiation. More time between divisions allows greater opportunity for repair mechanisms to complete their work. On the other hand, more time means that more energy can be absorbed from a chronic exposure to cause the accumulation of more defects before fixation or elimination. These matters are not yet resolved. In plant experiments where lower temperatures were used to lengthen the cell cycle, the decrease in temperature could have interfered with the efficiency of the repair processes.

References

Aikman, A. A., and Wills, E. D. (1974). Studies on lysosomes after irradiation. *Radiat. Res.* **57,** 403–415 and 416–430.

Bacq, Z. M., and Alexander, P. (1955). "Fundamentals of Radiobiology." Academic Press, New York.

Bacq, Z. M., and Hervé, A. (1952). Protection chimique contre le rayonnement. *Bull. Acad. R. Med. Belg.* [6] **18,** 13–58.

Buchsbaum, R , and Zirkle, R. E. (1949). Shrinking and swelling after alpha irradiation of various parts of large erythrocytes. *Proc. Soc. Exp. Biol. Med.* **72,** 27–29.

Canti, R. G., and Spear, F. G. (1927). The effect of gamma irradiation on cell division in tissue culture in vitro. *Proc. R. Soc. London, Ser. B* **102,** 92–101.

Canti, R. G., and Spear, F. G. (1929). The effect of γ radiation in cell division in tissue culture *in vitro. Proc. R. Soc. London, Ser. B* **105,** 93–98.

Carlson, J. G. (1950). Effects of radiation on mitosis. *J. Cell. Comp. Physiol.* **35,** Suppl. 1, 89–101.

Carlson, J. G. (1954). Immediate effects on division, morphology, and viability of the cell. *In* "Radiation Biology" (A. Hollaender, ed.), Chapter 11. McGraw-Hill, New York.

Carlson, J. G. (1969). X-ray-induced prophase delay and reversion of selected cells in certain avian and mammalian tissues in culture. *Radiat. Res.* **37,** 15–30.

Carlson, J. G., Snyder, M. L., and Hollaender, A. (1949). Relation of gamma dosage rate to mitotic effect in the grasshopper neuroblast. *J. Cell. Comp. Physiol.,* **33,** 365–372.

Carney, G. C. (1965). Swelling and shrinkage properties of housefly sarcosomes after *in vivo* exposure to x-rays. *Radiat. Res.* **25,** 637–645.

Cather, J. N. (1959). The effects of x radiation on the early cleavage stages of the snail, *Ilyanassa obsoleta*. *Radiat. Res.* **11**, 720–731.

Daniels, E. W., and Breyer, E. P. (1970). Rescue of supralethally x-irradiated amoebae with nonirradiated cytoplasm. *Radiat. Res.* **41**, 326–341.

Dewey, W. C., and Highfield, D. P. (1976). G_2 block in Chinese hamster cells induced by x-irradiation, hyperthermia, cycloheximide or actinomycin D. *Radiat. Res.* **65**, 511–528.

Doida, Y., and Okada, S. (1969). Radiation induced mitotic delay in cultured mammalian cells (L5178Y). *Radiat. Res.* **38**, 513–529.

Ellinger, F. (1941). "The Biologic Fundamentals of Radiation Therapy." Am. Elsevier, New York.

Ellinger, F. (1949). Fundamental biology of ionizing radiation. *In* "Atomic Medicine" (C. F. Behrens, ed.), Chapter 6. Thomas Nelson, New York.

Forer, A. (1965). Local reduction of spindle fiber birefringence in living *Nephrotoma suturalis* (Loew). *J. Cell Biol.* **25**, 95–117.

Harris, J. W. (1970). Effects of ionizing radiation on lysomes and other intracellular membranes. *Adv. Biol. Med. Phys.* **13**, 273–287.

Heilbrunn, L. V., and Mazia, D. (1936). The actions of radiations on living protoplasm. *In* "Biological Effects of Radiation" (B. M. Duggar, ed.), pp. 625–676. McGraw-Hill, New York.

Henshaw, P. S. (1938). The action of x-rays on nucleated and nonnucleated egg fragments. *Am. J. Cancer* **33**, 258–264.

Henshaw, P. S. (1940). Further studies on the action of roentgen rays on the gametes of *Arbacia punctulata*. A series of 6 papers. *Am. J. Roentgenol., Radium Ther. Nucl. Med.* **43**, 899–933.

Hevesy, G., and Zerahn, K. (1946). The effect of Roentgen rays and ultraviolet radiation on the permeability of yeast. *Acta Radiol.* **27**, 316–327.

Hopwood, L. E., and Dewey, W. C. (1976). Effect of x-irradiation on the transport of thymidine into asynchronous and S-phase CHO cells. *Int. J. Radiat. Biol.* **29**, 279–286.

Keith, A. D., and Snipes, W. (1974). Viscosity of cellular protoplasm. *Science* **183**, 666–668.

Kimball, R. F. (1955). The effects of radiation on protozoa and the eggs of invertebrates other than insects. *In* "Radiation Biology" (A. Hollaender, ed.), Vol. 2, Chapter 8. McGraw-Hill, New York.

Lea, D. E. (1947). "Actions of Radiations on Living Cells." Cambridge Univ. Press, London and New York.

Lyman, H., Epstein, H. T., and Schiff, J. A. (1961). Studies of chloroplast development in *Euglena. Biochim. Biophy. Acta.* **50**, 301–309.

Mazia, D. (1961). Mitosis and the physiology of cell division. *In* "The Cell: Biochemistry, Physiology, Morphology" (J. Brocher and A. E. Mirsky, eds.), Vol. 3, pp. 80–412. Academic Press, New York.

Miwa, M., Yamashita, H., and Mori, K. (1939). The action of ionizing rays on sea urchin. *Gann* **33**, 1–12 and 323–330.

Myers, D. K. (1970). Some aspects of radiation effects on cell membranes. *Adv. Biol. Med. Phys.* **13**, 219–234.

Northen, H. T., and MacVicar, R. (1940). Effects of x rays on the structural viscosity of protoplasm. *Biodynamica* **3**, 28–32.

Rao, B., and Hinegardner, R. T. (1965). Analysis of DNA synthesis and x-ray-induced mitotic delay in sea urchin eggs. *Radiat. Res.* **26**, 534–537.

Rustad, R. C., and Burchill, B. R. (1966). Radiation-induced mitotic delay in sea urchin eggs treated with puromycin and actinomycin D. *Radiat. Res.* **29,** 203–210.

Sheppard, C. W., and Stewart, M. (1952). The direct effects of radiation on erythrocytes. *J. Cell. Comp. Physiol.* **39,** Suppl. 2, 189–215.

Sparrow, A. H. (1951). Radiation sensitivity of cells during mitotic and meiotic cycles with emphasis on possible cytochemical changes. *Ann. N.Y. Acad. Sci.* **51,** 1508–1540.

Terasima, T., and Tolmach, L. J. (1963). Growth and nucleic acid synthesis in synchronously dividing populations of HeLa cells. *Exp. Cell Res.* **30,** 344–362.

Ting, T. P., and Zirkle, R. E. (1940). Permeability of x-rayed erythrocytes. *J. Cell. Comp. Physiol.* **16,** 197–206, 269–276, and 277–283.

Van't Hof, J., and Kovacs, C. J. (1970). Mitotic delay in two biochemically different G_1 cell populations in cultured roots of pea (*Pisum sativum*). *Radiat. Res.* **44,** 700–712.

Virgin, H. I., and Ehrenberg, L. (1953). Effects of β and γ-rays on the protoplasmic viscosity of *Helodea densa* cells. *Physiol. Plant.* **6,** 159–165.

Von Borstel, R. C., and Rogers, R. W. (1958). Alpha particle bombardment of the *Habrobracon* egg. II. Response of the cytoplasm. *Radiat. Res.* **8,** 248–253.

Whiting, A. R. (1946). Motherless males from irradiated eggs. *Science* **103,** 219–220.

Whiting, A. R. (1949). Androgenesis, a differentiator of cytoplasmic injury induced by x rays in *Habrobracon* eggs. *Biol. Bull. (Woods Hole, Mass.)* **97,** 210–220.

Wilson, W. L. (1950). The effect of roentgen rays on protoplasmic viscosity changes during mitosis. *Protoplasma* **39,** 305–317.

Zirkle, R. D., Bloom, W., and Uretz, R. B. (1955). Use of partial cell irradiation in studies of cell division. *Proc. Int. Conf. Peaceful Uses-At. Energy, 1st, 1955* Vol. 11, pp. 273–282.

CHAPTER 4   From Nonlocalized Toward Localized Nuclear Effects

Many of the topics to be considered in this chapter have a bearing upon some of the matters discussed toward the end of Chapter 3. When a cell begins to divide and the elaborate mitotic structure develops, almost every aspect of the cell changes. The successful completion of cell division within a normal period of time involves considerably more than the functioning of the kinetic mechanism. A separation of longitudinally duplicated parts of chromosomes depends upon the culmination of processes providing such structures.

When the dose of radiation amounts to more than a few hundred R and is delivered between late prophase and anaphase, a chromosomal change occurs which has been termed *stickiness*. By definition, chromosome stickiness is an adherence of chromosome segments by means other than gross chromosomal aberrations. The ultimate expression may be the merging of the entire chromosome complement into a single irregular mass. Subsequently this mass elongates in the direction of the poles, but division may be accomplished only by the cleavage furrow.

Cytologically, the diffuse attachments described as thin chromatin bridges are visibly different from anaphase bridges. Associations can be acute or lined up side-by-side. Some toxic chemicals cause it, and the presence of the mutant gene "sticky" in maize results in its expression in the absence of exogenous agents. Various chromosomal constituents including an RNA surface coating were postulated in earlier molecular explanations, but electron microscopy studies suggest that the alteration is in chromosomal compactness. This would allow the entanglement of tiny fibrils from different chromosomes, and if the fibrils cannot disengage easily, physical exchanges of chromatin might ensue (McGill *et al.*, 1974).

Without regard for the mechanism, clumped metaphases were scored in quantitative experiments with *Tradescantia* microspores (Swanson

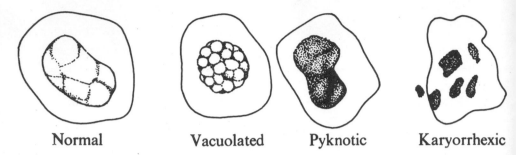

Normal   Vacuolated   Pyknotic   Karyorrhexic

Figure 4.1.   Nuclear changes after irradiation, visible through the light microscope.

and Johnston, 1954). After exposure to 150 R in air, all metaphases showed clumping which persisted for 9 hours. Lower doses resulted in a peak effect 4 hours after irradiation, with regression by the fifth hour. Only a few cells in the group showed the effect after 50 R. For equivalent results, when delivered in a nitrogen atmosphere, the dose had to be increased fourfold.

With mammalian cells, irradiation of dividing cells may have little effect on that division, but does have effect on the next mitosis. Irradiation of HeLa cells in G_1 leads to a variety of changes in cells at the subsequent mitosis, including partial fusion or clumping of chromosomal mass, lagging chromosomes, and loss of regular metaphase plate.

Historically, the earliest recognized morphological change after irradiation was cytolysis following pyknosis of the cell nucleus. The change in state is not immediate but develops during subsequent metabolism wherein catabolic activity predominates. Here too a clumping of chromatin occurs, but often involves cells which normally should be in interphase. Karyorrhexis or nuclear disintegration may follow, and this ultimately results in a scattered group of formless granules (Ellinger, 1941; Bloom, 1948). Figure 4.1 illustrates these phenomena.

Because of these visible alterations, plus the fact that important localized effects (such as chromosome breakage and gene mutation) result from radiation exposure, some investigators have been interested in demonstrating measurable effects upon the prominent chemical components of nuclei and chromosomes. These are nucleoprotein and deoxyribonucleic acid (DNA). A problem in this work is to establish criteria for assaying the degree of alteration. Biophysical studies featuring viscosity tests were favored, before construction of the double helix model stimulated more analytical investigations featuring biochemical techniques.

Viscosity of DNA Systems

The attack can be made along several lines. Nuclear contents may be irradiated *in situ* or after extraction, and various techniques may be used to measure viscosity change. One of the earliest studies was by Sparrow and Rosenfeld (1946) who compared the effects of x radiation on both thymonucleohistone and sodium thymonucleate by using capillary viscometry and streaming birefringence. Changes in both features indicated modification of molecular size and shape, and for equal doses of radiation the loss in viscosity was greater in the nucleate. This, taken as indication of an effect upon the nucleic acids, may have set a whole series of investigations in motion.

A protective effect of histone was believed due to competition for the radicals produced by ionizations in water. Consistent with this are subsequent findings that even a small amount of glucose confers considerable protection to nucleoprotein gels. Doses ten times as large may be needed to reduce rigidity to the equivalent of unprotected systems. On this point, recall that protective effects on enzymes were introduced in Chapter 2 and that the effect has been observed with a variety of organic substances.

A complicating feature soon discovered (Taylor *et al.*, 1947) was a drop in viscosity with aging of DNA dispersions. The drop is accentuated after irradiation and the time that elapses after irradiation is as important as temperature in the interpretation of data. Attempts to elucidate the "after-effect" have led to biophysical studies beyond the scope of this book. Nevertheless, all investigators agree that radiation does alter the viscosity of material extracted from nuclei, and ultracentrifugation sedimentation studies and electron micrographs bear out the hypothesis that the long nucleic acid fibers are broken into short fragments by irradiation. Some such corroborative experiment is desirable since induced cross linkages can also change viscosity.

The torsion pendulum method has been used, as well as the more popular capillary flow procedure, in studying the viscosity of nucleoprotein systems extracted from nuclei. The gel formed from the nuclear contents of chicken erythrocytes, dispersed in an appropriate buffer solution, was significantly changed by a few thousand roentgens of x radiation if the solution were dilute. On the other hand, a tenfold increase in dose did not produce the same effect on a system ten times as concentrated (Figure 4.2). Gels were proportionately less rigid with increased radiation whether nuclei were irradiated while still in the cells or irradiated when isolated prior to dispersion into salt solution. However, direct dose-effect comparison with results from irradiated solutions was not possible.

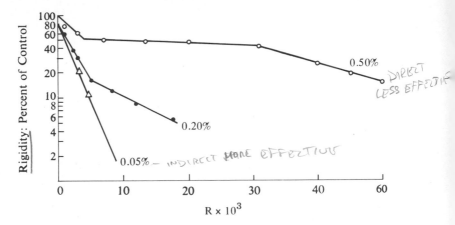

Figure 4.2. Results obtained from irradiation of nucleoprotein gels of different concentrations. Each point is the arithmetic mean of five experiments done on the same batch of nuclei. The curve becomes more complicated with increased concentration. (From Errera, 1947.)

Rats have been employed for *in vivo* experiments in which extracts were studied by capillary viscometry. Twenty-four hours after irradiation of the rodents, changes became demonstrable in structural viscosity, streaming birefringence, and sedimentation constants of thymus extracts. However, released purine bases were detected shortly after treatment (Limperos and Mosher, 1950). Subsequent intense investigation established that the double-helical structure of DNA (Fig. 4.3) is much more sensitive to breakdown than the nucleotide bases. Nevertheless some released bases and nucleosides appeared after doses of 5 krad or more to calf thymus irradiated in O_2-saturated solution (Ward and Kuo, 1976).

The Depolymerization Question

Since no chemical material was lost when "stickiness" was induced, or when viscosity was altered, the changes were postulated to be depolymerization in a decade when "chromatin" was considered a homogeneous chemical substance. Depolymerization implies a separation of a larger unit into smaller like molecules. Whether this is applicable to chromosomal DNA–protein complexes is debatable, and for a time either the DNA or the protein was supposed to depolymerize. Recently, the degree of association between the major chemical constituents has been considered more important. Artificially combining DNA with a protein such as serum albumen produces a system with a

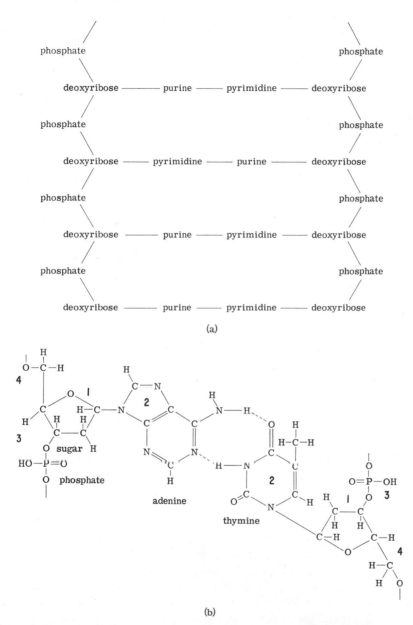

(a)

(b)

Figure 4.3. (a) The ladderlike structure of DNA made of two chains in which sugar and phosphate alternate, and the rungs are comprised of organic bases bonded by hydrogen bonds. The chains coil around each other in helical fashion. (b) Structure of one of the "rungs." Fragments of the ladder will result only if breaks occur at regions 3 or 4. Breaks at 1 and 2 will not shorten the chain. The other common type of rung made up of guanine and cytosine is essentially similar, except that three hydrogen bonds form.

radiosensitivity not exhibited by either component separately (Kaufmann *et al.*, 1955). Furthermore, the stainability of nuclear contents in
animal and plant cells was not altered as expected with depolymerization (Himes, 1950; Kaufmann, 1954). In a *Tradescantia* experiment, radiation doses high enough to markedly reduce DNA viscosity did not
produce a photometrically demonstrable decrease in methyl green
stainability of bud cells (Moses *et al.*, 1951). Once considered a test for
depolymerization, the affinity for methyl green may be a measure of
protein association with DNA. An intranuclear change in this relationship would have to occur to increase the availability of more dye-
binding sites in the DNA. From subsequent studies of gels formed from
isolated nuclei, Dounce (1971) concluded that a major cause of gel
instability is a loss of firm binding of the DNA to residual protein.

Chemical Changes in DNA

Occasionally the labilization of DNA has been reported after whole-
body irradiation (Hagen, 1960), but usually higher organisms have
served merely as a source of extracted nucleic acid which is then irradiated. Ward and Kuo (1976) used calf thymus and *Escherichia coli* DNA
to demonstrate that radiation releases free bases and damaged bases
from the macromolecule treated in aqueous solution with 10 to 50 krads.
The initial attack by OH· radicals appears to be upon the deoxyribose
moiety. Alkaline sucrose gradient centrifugation and uv absorption
studies of Sephadex column eluants were among the methods employed.

The earliest positive investigations required millions of rads to demonstrate freed organic phosphate, liberated bases, titratable acidity
increases, and ammonia (Scholes and Weiss, 1954). Initially the "ionic
yield" ratio was employed, which expressed the number of molecules
changed per number of ionizations as M/N. Now "G values" are preferred, which give the number of molecules damaged per 100 eV. Okada
(1970) provides a sample calculation and Ward (1975) tabulates G-value
yields of base destruction and radiation products. These reviews and
that of Adams (1972) present advances in our understanding of molecular mechanisms but are mainly devoted to experiments with simple
model systems.

Although much less work has been done on model systems, the
determination of strand breaks is currently the major method used to
detect *in vivo* radiation damage to DNA. Tests with deoxynucleotides
indicate the probable site of breakage to be at a sugar phosphate bond.
Breaking bonds in the base or sugar rings would not decrease the

molecular size immediately (Fig. 4.3b). Early investigations with synthetic molecules indicated that the P—O bond is radioresistant whereas a reaction at the P—C bond is more easily obtained (see Bacq and Alexander, 1955). However, a double helix will not fall apart unless two independently and approximately opposite breaks occur, one in each of the two polynucleotide chains. The Bacq and Alexander summary of the complexities of induced cross-linkage and scission proposed that a double break from juxtaposition of single breaks may occur for every 70 random single breaks. Adequate juxtaposition was interpreted as a break in each of two strands less than 5 nucleotides apart. Certainty replaced probability for dense localizations of ions. Main chain scission is expected every time a DNA molecule is traversed by an α particle (600 eV event), and whenever a cluster of ionizations (850 eV) is formed by an otherwise sparsely ionizing radiation. These estimates derive from experiments with DNA from salmon sperm.

Subsequently, several laboratories have determined the ratios of single to double breaks in viral and bacterial DNA but have not speculated about the contribution of single breaks to two-strand ruptures (see Okada, 1970). Freifelder's (1966) ultracentrifugal analysis of x-rayed coliphage T7 and *Pseudomonas* phage B3 demonstrated that the production of one double-strand break per phage led to the interaction of the phage. Single-strand breaks were ineffective and their contribution seemed insignificant. In an earlier study of a series of x-ray doses there was close correlation between the number of broken double-stranded molecules and the percentage of dead T7 phage.

A different approach is to use cell-free protein biosynthesis systems to study base destruction by different types of radiation. Purines and pyrimidines are destroyed by thermal neutrons in proportion to their nitrogen content (Wacker and Chandra, 1969). A neutron dose of 0.5×10^{14} $n/cm^2/sec$ degraded 9% of thymine, 12% of uracil, 57% of guanine, and 75% of the adenine content. Thus adenine-containing code sequences are significantly more sensitive than those containing other bases. The converse was observed after x-irradiation. Cytosine and uracil are more sensitive to x rays than adenine. The electromagnetic ray spectrum in the ultraviolet wavelengths also attacks pyrimidines preferentially.

DNA Synthesis: Tissue Studies

Hevesy (1945) publicized the discovery that tissues containing cells actively synthesizing nucleic acids and associated materials are especially radiosensitive. A large number of papers on the effect of ionizing radiations on DNA synthesis soon appeared. Many authors found that relatively large doses depressed DNA synthesis to less than 50% of the control values (Feinstein and Butler, 1952). Typically, a study of the rate of incorporation of ^{32}P- or ^{14}C-labeled precursors has been the approach. However, usually the specific activities compared have been for DNA separated from bulk tissue, radiated and unirradiated. Thus, the measurements reflect the average behavior of all cells in the tissue, and the number of synthesizing cells can be of great importance. The generally observed inhibition of DNA synthesis after radiation may be a secondary effect due principally to changes in cell populations (Kelly, 1958).

Pelc and Howard (1955) avoided such complications by employing autoradiography. The individual cells of a tissue can be scored in this technique (Figure 4.4). When inorganic ^{32}P is supplied to actively growing tissue such as the root meristem of _Vicia faba_, the radiophosphorus becomes incorporated into newly synthesized DNA. It is detected by autoradiography after the extraction of other P compounds. Cells which have synthesized DNA during the time of ^{32}P treatment are labeled and are distinguishable from other cells. Results could have varied in two different ways: In contrast with unirradiated tissue, (1) fewer photographic grains might develop per cell; or (2) fewer positive cells may be obtained. The former would indicate a reduced amount of DNA synthesized, the latter a reduction in the number of synthesizing cells. Pelc and Howard found the latter.

A threshold is exceeded somewhere between 35 and 70 R. This dose reduces the number of cells which synthesize DNA during the subsequent 12 hours to about two-thirds of the normal value. Higher doses

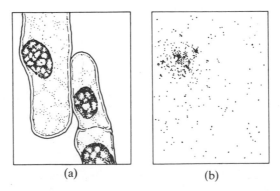

(a)   (b)

Figure 4.4. Squash preparation of meristem of a _Vicia faba_ root given ^{32}P 12 hours previously. (a) As viewed by phase contrast microscope; (b) same field, standard lighting showing photographic grains. Note the nuclear autoradiograph. (Based on photograph courtesy of S. R. Pelc and A. Howard.)

up to the mean lethal dose of about 180 R do not cause any greater effect. Apparently 35–70 R of x radiation is sufficient to prevent synthesis in all cells which are in their sensitive period. Those cells already in synthesis or those not yet in it are unaffected.

Somewhat different results were obtained for the grain count distribution from autoradiographs of thymidine-labeled and synchronized HeLa cells (Hopwood and Tolmach, 1971). Most of the cells synthesized a reduced amount of DNA if the *preceding* generation had been given 500 rads. The reduction was greater in some cells than in others. Those most severely damaged were arrested in mitosis during a subsequent generation.

A full understanding of the situation involves clarification of the interrelationships between different phases in the cell cycle. The synthesis of DNA during its scheduled period is the culmination of a sequence of biochemical activities. During the G_1 period that precedes S, the precursors were formed and the necessary enzymes and proteins were assembled for DNA synthesis. In turn, G_1 depends upon the progress of events in G_2 and the division phases of the mother cell. Therefore although a change in DNA synthesis becomes evident during the S phase, the biochemical damage usually has occurred earlier. High doses have been employed to cause prompt changes in the DNA incorporation of labeled precursors, but cell death results too. In the lethal range of dosage, most tissues of irradiated vertebrates exhibit a decreased uptake of precursors into DNA within the first two hours after exposure (Ord and Stocken, 1961).

When entire organisms are irradiated, complications of interpretation arise from the augmented precursor pools from damaged cells as well as from the diversion of nucleotides to nonutilizable pools. Also our understanding of remote effects in higher organisms is inadequate. Hormonal influences are only part of the problem. Puzzling results occur in animals with two tumors, one of which is irradiated, the other shielded. Although the response is not as impressive in the shielded tumor, why should the formation of tracer-labeled nucleic acid be reduced in both? Blood transfusions from irradiated to nonirradiated animals do not necessarily influence nucleic-acid synthesis in the recipient.

DNA Synthesis: Cell Studies and Molecular Aspects

The effect of radiation on the DNA pathway has drawn the most attention of the three major molecular synthetic processes: DNA, RNA, and protein synthesis. This emphasis reflects the important role that

DNA synthesis plays in the cell and the sensitivity of techniques for measuring damage to the molecule. Since DNA is the stable component of information transmitted through successive cell generations, damage to it will have serious consequences, even result in permanent change. Damage to RNA and protein molecules and to their synthesis will not be as serious since the DNA molecule can still synthesize new, correct RNA and protein molecules. Recent techniques have allowed the isolation of larger intact DNA molecules. Because the size of these molecules presents a larger target for radiation damage then does either RNA or protein, damage to DNA can be measured at much lower doses.

Radiation affects both the structure of DNA and its synthesis. The affects on the structure were shown initially in bacterial cells by the elegant experiments of McGrath and Williams (1966), and in mammalian cells by Lett and co-workers (1967). Both investigations involved the centrifugation of DNA in an alkaline sucrose gradient. The high pH caused a separation of strands to the single-strand state. Any change in the sedimentation rate was related to a change in the size of the DNA molecule. Both groups showed a decrease in the size of DNA with radiation. In the mammalian cell system, this decrease can be seen at 1000 rad or less. If the cells are incubated under normal growth conditions for several hours after irradiation and the DNA then analyzed, the sedimentation rates return to normal (see following text for repair mechanisms). It is important to distinguish between structural integrity and functional soundness: although the DNA may appear as a continuous strand, the correct order of bases may not have been maintained. Thus at first glance one might say that single-strand breaks have no relation to cell survival since they are repaired, but on further inspection the faithfulness of the repair is still questionable.

Concurrent with the early studies of the structure and composition of DNA were studies of the radiation effects on radioactive precursor incorporation into DNA. As early as 1941, Marshak reported radiation-induced disturbance of the ^{32}P uptake of nuclei isolated from mouse livers and lymphomas. A series of studies by Hevesy (1945) and by Holmes (1947) have since focused attention on the matter. They measured the rate of ^{32}P incorporation in rat sarcomas. A few hundred roentgens reduced the rate of DNA formation to half, and 2000 R reduced it to three-quarters the untreated value.

By 1962, Nygaard and Potter could write that "the inhibition of DNA synthesis by ionizing radiation is a well established phenomenon," but had to add that the mechanism was still unknown. Interpretation of experiments has been complicated by the inhibition of mitosis influencing the onset of synthesis as well as by cell deaths. In order to avoid the results reflecting changes in the cell population, these investigators used ^{14}C-labeled thymidine to study DNA synthesis over very early time periods after γ irradiation of the whole animal. Their one-minute exposures to a ^{60}Co source ranged from 125 to 400 rep. C^{14} incorporation into DNA was immediately depressed in dose-dependent fashion for both spleen and small intentine. Subsequently tritiated thymidine has been especially popular for corroborative studies in a variety of cell types.

More recent studies from a variety of mammalian cells *in vitro* and *in vivo* have demonstrated a fairly uniform pattern, a biphasic curve (see Okada, 1970). At doses below 1000 rads, the incorporation decreases rapidly as a function of dose down to approximately 50%. Then the subsequent decrease progresses at a slower rate; in some cases the decrease does not surpass 50% for doses up to 5000 rads.

More detailed studies in several laboratories have revealed that the decrease is time-dependent. Regardless of the dose, the maximum depression occurs at 2–3 hours after radiation; the magnitude of the depression is related to dose, however. Subsequently, the rate in the irradiated cultures surpasses that of the unirradiated ones.

The original explanations for the depression of DNA synthesis were based on target theory considerations: the more sensitive slope was believed due to inactivation of a large target such as that involved in nuclear phosphorylation and the more resistant slope to inactivation of a smaller target such as that responsible for template activity. More recent evidence supports replicon initiation as the sensitive component and reduced chain growth as the resistant one (Hopwood, 1974).

In the attempt to explain molecular events, much of the research has been devoted to microbial systems (Ginosa, 1967). In the relatively simple *E. coli* situation, a replicating point moves along the DNA molecule until it meets a damaged site. Then the process stops unless the bacterium has a repair system functioning, or the ability to reinitiate synthesis at another site.

The eukaryote chromosome is a more complex structure with active and inactive states of DNA attained by strand dispersal and condensation promoted by protein complexing. Nevertheless, the DNA replication of mammalian cells, believed to occur in small replicon units, is conceived as a discontinuous type of replication following the bacterial pattern. Accordingly, the techniques of microbial biochemistry have been applied to investigations of radiation-induced depression of DNA synthesis in cultured cells such as mouse leukemia "L" and human carcinoma HeLa, in ascites tumors *in vivo*, and in regenerating rat liver lobes. Despite vigorous efforts by radiation biochemists, the definitive explanation is not yet available.

From time to time, various investigators have posed objections to the use of labeled precursors such as thymidine as a valid measure of DNA synthesis. Differences in the uptake rates of the various different DNA precursors are quite striking (Walters and Enger, 1976). Also it is possible that degradation and transport changes would influence pool sizes of precursors. Evidence from continuous measurements of DNA content and of DNA replication from density gradient studies has indicated a smaller decrease in DNA synthesis after irradiation. In spite of these objections, x-irradiation does appear to decrease DNA synthesis. No degradation or effects on transport have been noted. The measurements of DNA content are continuous ones and thus are not as sensitive as the pulse measurements with labelled precursor.

Despite a great deal of research, this matter is not settled. The question of whether radiation causes an actual depression in DNA synthesis or whether the depression is artifactual is still a debated point. Saha and Tolmach (1976) have discussed some of the alternatives.

Photoreactivation of Ultraviolet Damage

The most dramatic response in all the experiments on postirradiation amelioration is obtained when exposure to waves in the visible range follows irradiation in the ultraviolet range (Jagger, 1958). In particular, Kelner in 1949 demonstrated that a greater number of actinomycetes cells survived a given ultraviolet dose when they subsequently received visible light. Table 4.1 demonstrates how this unsuspected recovery-promoting agent can increase survival rate as much as 400,000-fold. Variables, such as the duration of visible light, went a long way toward explaining a puzzling degree of variance in previous investigations.

Subsequently the phenomenon which involves DNA repair has been demonstrated in a wide variety of organisms including viruses, bacteria, protozoa, marine invertebrates, insects and terrestrial arthropods, and lower vertebrates (Cook and McGrath, 1967). The necessary photo-reactivating enzymes are easily demonstrated in the tissues of fish, amphibia, birds, and marsupials, but with the exception of cultured human leukocytes (Sutherland, 1974), negative tests have been the rule for mammalian tissues. Usually the activity is not limited to a particular tissue and the enzyme tends to be in the nuclei.

Experiments in cell-free systems established that photoreactivation is accomplished by enzymatic cleavage of pyrimidine dimers, even for uv-induced chromosomal aberrations (Griggs and Bender, 1974). The enzyme, originally obtained by extracting it from yeast, is activated by visible light which serves as a source of energy. Unwanted chemical

TABLE 4.1
Results Typifying Kelner's (1949) Experiments with *Streptomyces griseus*[a]

Illumination time (min)	Viable cells per ml of suspension
0	2–3
2	6–9
4	1,600
10	25,000
20	92,000
30	130,000
40	160,000
50	200,000
60	530,000
145	550,000
173	770,000
240	800,000
Control (unirradiated)	4,200,000

[a] The effect of the duration of visible light from photoflood lamps subsequent to a 1½-min exposure to ultraviolet from a mercury lamp. The temperature remained constant. (From Kelner, 1949.)

bonds between adjacent bases are cleaved to restore the nucleotide sequence to its original form (Setlow, 1968). In other words, killed cells were not brought back to life. Instead, a type of induced change which would otherwise limit a cell population by interfering with the replication of its members has been prevented from doing so. In eukaryotes possessing the system, photoenzymatic repair can prevent uv-induced chromatid-type aberrations from developing.

Excision Repair

Photoreactivation is only one of a number of possible repair systems now known. Other systems operate in the dark. Simultaneously in two laboratories, Oak Ridge (Setlow and Carrier, 1964) and Yale (Boyce and Howard-Flanders, 1964), a second prereplication type of repair was identified. This removes a length of nucleotide chain containing the defective part of the DNA molecule and uses the complementary chain as a template to guide resynthesis. At least five steps are involved: the recognition of localized distortion of the molecule, the incision by an endonuclease specific for base damage, exonuclease removal of a short length from one chain, replacement of the section of nucleotides aided by polymerase, and ligation of the newly inserted bases to the extant part of the DNA molecule. In contrast to photosynthetic repair, excision repair is not specific for pyrimidine dimers. It can operate on other uv-induced defects and those from chemical mutagens as well as respond to some of the lesions caused by ionizing radiations.

Unscheduled DNA synthesis accompanied by nucleotide replacement has been demonstrated for cultured cells from man and many animals. Typically the doses used in such experiments are high, ranging from 5 to 60 krad. The distribution of this capacity in higher plants has been debated. The first positive finding after a long series of negative reports was for cultured wild carrot cells where a limited number of pyrimidine dimers were excised from the DNA of isolated protoplasts (Howland, 1975).

Supporting evidence for the importance of an excision system at the organism level emerged from investigations of the UV-sensitive hereditary disease xeroderma pigmentosum. XP cells are unable to excise UV-induced lesions because the specific endonuclease needed to initiate the repair process does not function.

Other DNA Repair Mechanisms

A process of recombination repair occurs in DNA made after ultraviolet irradiation. It was first observed in excision-negative strains of *E. coli* as smaller molecular strands joining to make long strands when nucleotides were added interstitially. The sequence of events begins with gaps left when replication bypassed dimer sites. Later the replication gaps are filled in by a postreplication process which must use information from a sister chromatid or homolog. The genetic result resembles the consequence of crossing over or gene conversion. The process has now been demonstrated in other microbes, and in cultured *Drosophila* and mammalian cells. Furthermore, in viruses and bacteria, repair involving recombinational events between intact portions of the gene strands occurs as a "multiplicity" reactivation fostered by multiple cell infection or populous cell conditions.

Still another type of repair may use a stretch of genetic information which cannot be copied accurately, or may use no template at all. Although chemically sound DNA may be produced, the repaired segment is likely to differ from the informational content of the original undamaged strand. Accordingly the expression "error-prone" is somewhat appropriate, but "mutagenic repair" is a designation that avoids the implication that wrong information was inserted by mistake rather than as a necessity.

Integrating the Pathways

Diagrams which systematize the alternate modes of repair of DNA damage are beginning to appear. A rational way to organize a complexity of systems was conditioned by a historical sequence of events whereby additional repair pathways were discovered in microbial strains deficient in previously known mechanisms.

In *E. coli* and yeast which possess at least four distinct methods of repair, the channeling of lesions into mutagenic repair pathways was devised to explain the numerous mutator loci. This hypothesis states that lesions in DNA may be repaired by any one of a number of metabolic routes which have evolved. If a repair pathway is blocked by mutation of one of the genes concerned with one of the steps, the lesion may be handled by a different pathway (von Borstel *et al.*, 1976). Successful switching to an alternate path may depend upon whether the block affects the first step or a branching point in a pathway. The published schemes radiate out from the primary lesion without indicating hierarchy or precedence of pathways, but this may be an oversimplification. If not, early divergence may predispose the cell to death when a mutant block occurs at an intermediate step, because the molecular condition attained might not be a suitable substrate for any alternate repair system. On the other hand, an increased mutation rate will occur in viable cells when the substitute pathway is more error-prone than the blocked pathway.

In their *Sacharomyces* scheme, Cox and Game (1974) speculated about the synergism of two mutations in different pathways that use a common substrate and contrasted this with epistatic mutations which occur for different steps in the same pathway. Boyd and Setlow (1976) proposed a scheme for *Drosophila* which includes photorepair and at least three dark-repair pathways. The complementation groups associated with each pathway are indicated on their figure.

Irrevocable Ionization Lesions

Unlike the molecular defects obtained from ultraviolet rays and chemical mutagens, the DNA lesions are not only heterogeneous but also are not well delineated—particularly in eukaryotic organisms. A current presumption is that the integrity of genetic mechanisms is safeguarded by enzymatic repair mechanisms in virtually all organisms. Since excision and postreplication repair systems have been demonstrated in mammalian cells, there is some basis for the premise. However, the excision response occurs at lower levels in cultured tissues than in bacteria (Evans, 1975).

Experimental results are not yet available for making a definitive statement about events in organisms receiving medically or ecologically realistic doses. Mammalian cells are 500 to 1000 times more susceptible to damage induced by ionizing radiation than to that caused by uv (Painter, 1974). At sublethal doses, the yield of chemical products of x- or γ-irradiated DNA molecules is extremely small. Therefore investigations concerned with molecular fragments are performed at doses 10 to 100 times the mammalian lethal doses. Extrapolation then assumes that the products do not differ qualitatively from those formed at lower doses, and only speculation relates these to the chromosomal aberrations responsible for most of the cell-reproductive death. Painter suggests that there are alterations induced in DNA by radiations which the mammalian cell has not encountered frequently in its evolutionary history. His conclusion retains something of the viewpoint of earlier decades: "certain kinds of lesions formed in mammalian DNA by ionizing radiation" "have little" or "no probability of being repaired." The amelioration of damage by dose fractionation in experiments on tissues with a stem cell component has been explained in terms of cell populations rather than by molecular events (von Borstel and St. Amand, 1963).

Concluding Remarks

In this chapter we have presented experiments concerned with the elucidation of a generalized basis of nuclear damage. These efforts naturally followed the demonstration that the nucleus is more radiosensitive than the cytoplasm under the criteria employed (see Chapter 3). Early biophysical and cytological techniques have been supplanted by efforts concentrated on the molecular biochemistry of DNA. Areas of investigation include products of degradation, the synthesis process, strand breakage, and repair mechanisms. Attention is now focused upon a limited number of nucleotides in a single strand of DNA. In this sense, each lesion is localized conceptually. However in practice, since many lesions are under simultaneous consideration at numerous sites which are neither optically visible nor genetically mapped, a corporate aspect of nonlocalization characterizes much of the data. The next four chapters contain accounts of how biological procedures demonstrate the localization of radiation damage and its far-reaching consequences. Modification of tissue damage is considered in Chapter 13.

References

Adams, G. E. (1972). Radiation chemical mechanisms in radiation biology. *Adv. in Radiat. Chem.* **3,** 126–208.

Bacq, Z. M., and Alexander P. (1955). "Fundamentals of Radiobiology," pp. 142–153. Academic Press, New York.

Bloom, W. (1948). "Histopathology of Irradiation," Natl. Nucl. Energy Ser. Div. IV. Vol. 22 I, p. 27. McGraw-Hill, New York.

Boyce, R. P., and Howard-Flanders, P. (1964). The release of uv-induced thymine dimers from DNA in *E. coli* K-12. *Proc. Natl. Acad. Sci. U. S. A.* **51,** 293–300.

Boyd, J. B., and Setlow, R. B. (1976). Characterization of postreplication repair in mutagen sensitive strains of *Drosophila melanogaster*. *Genetics* **84,** 507–526.

Cook, J. S., and McGrath, J. R. (1967). Photoreactivating—enzyme activity in metazoa. *Proc. Natl. Acad. Sci. U. S. A.* **58,** 1359–1365.

Cox, B., and Game, J. (1974). Repair systems in *Saccharomyces*. *Mutat. Res.* **26,** 257–264.

Dounce, A. L. (1971). Nuclear gels and chromosomal structure. *Am. Sci.* **59,** 74–83.

Ellinger, F. (1941). "The Biologic Fundamentals of Radiation Therapy." Am. Elsevier, New York.

Errera, M. (1947). In vitro and in situ action of ionizing radiations on nucleoproteins of the cell nucleus. *Cold Spring Harbor Symp. Quant. Biol.* **12,** 60–63.

Evans, H. J. (1975). Genetic repair. *Genetics* **79,** Suppl., 171–178.

Feinstein, R., and Butler, C. L. (1952). Effect of whole body x radiation on rat intestine and intestinal nucleoprotein. *Proc. Soc. Exp. Biol. Med.* **79,** 181–182.

Freifelder, A. (1966). DNA strand breakage by x-irradiation. *Radiat. Res.* **29,** 329–338.

Ginosa, W. (1967). The effects of ionizing radiation on nucleic acids of bacteriophages and bacterial cells. *Annu. Rev. Nucl. Sci.* **17,** 469–512.

Griggs, H. G., and Bender, M. A. (1974). Photoreactivation of ultraviolet induced chromosomal aberrations. *Science* **179,** 86–88.

Hagen, U. (1960). Labilization of DNA in thymonucleoprotein after whole body irradiation. *Nature (London)* **187,** 1123–1124.

Hevesy, G. (1945). Effect of roentgen rays on cellular division. *Rev. Mod. Phys.* **17,** 102–111.

Himes, H. M. (1950). Studies on the chemical nature of 'sticky' chromosomes. *Genetics* **35,** 670.

Holmes, B. (1947). The inhibition of ribo- and thymo-nucleic acid synthesis in tumor tissue by irradiation with x rays. *Brt. J. Radiol.* **20,** 450–453.

Hopwood, L. E. (1974). Cause of deficient DNA synthesis in generation 1 of x-irradiated HeLa cells. *Radiat. Res.* **58,** 349–360.

Hopwood, L. E., and Tolmach, L. J. (1971). Deficient DNA synthesis and mitotic death in x-irradiated HeLa cells. *Radiat. Res.* **46,** 70–84.

Howland, G. P. (1975). Dark-repair of ultraviolet-induced pyrimidine dimers in the DNA of wild carrot protoplasts. *Nature (London)* **254,** 160–161.

Jagger, J. (1958). Photoreactivation. *Bacteriol. Rev.* **22,** 99–142.

Kaufmann, B. P. (1954). Chromosome aberrations induced in animal cells by ionizing radiations. Part II. *In* "Radiation Biology" (A. Hollaender, ed.), Chapter 9. McGraw-Hill, New York.

Kaufmann, B. P., McDonald, M. R., and Bernstein, M. H. (1955). Cytochemical studies of changes induced in cellular material by ionizing radiation. *Ann. N. Y. Acad. Sci.* **59,** 553–566.

Kelly, L. S. (1958). DNA synthesis in irradiated animals. *Proc. U. N. Int. Conf. Peaceful Uses At. Energy, 2nd, 1958.* Vol. 22, pp. 521–523.

Kelner, A. (1949). Effect of visible light on the recovery of *Streptomyces griseus* conidea from ultraviolet irradiation injury. *Proc. Natl. Acad. Sci. U. S. A.* **35,** 73–79.

Lett, J. T., Caldwell, I., Dean, C. J., and Alexander, P. (1967). Rejoining of x ray induced breaks in the DNA of leukemia cells. *Nature (London)* **214,** 790–792.

Limperos, G., and Mosher, W. A. (1950). Roentgen irradiation of desoxyribosenucleic acid. *Am. J. Roentgenol., Radium Ther. Nucl. Med.* **63,** 681–690.

McGill, M., Pathak, S., and Hsu, T. C. (1974). Effects of ethidium bromide on mitosis and chromosomes: A possible material basis for chromosome stickiness. *Chromosoma* **47,** 157–167.

McGrath, R. A., and Williams, R. W. (1966). Reconstruction in vivo of irradiated E. *coli* DNA, the rejoining of broken pieces. *Nature (London)* **212,** 534–535.

Marshak, A. (1941). P^{32} uptake by nuclei. *J. Gen. Physiol.* **25,** 275–291.

Moses, M. J., DuBow, R., and Sparrow, A. H. (1951). The effect of x rays on desoxypentose nuclei acid in situ. *J. Natl. Cancer Inst.* **12,** 232–233.

Nygaard, O. F., and Potter, R. L. (1962). Effect of radiation on DNA metabolism in various tissues of the rat. *Radiat. Res.* **16,** 243–252.

Okada, S. (1970). "Radiation Biochemistry," Vol. 1, pp. 166–179 and 203–218. Academic Press, New York.

Ord, M. G., and Stocken, L. A. (1961). The biochemical lesion *in vivo* and *in vitro*. *In* "Mechanisms in Radiobiology," M. Errera and A. Forssberg, eds.), Vol. 1, pp. 259–331. Academic Press, New York.

Painter, R. B. (1974). DNA damage and repair in eukaryote cells. *Genetics* **78,** 139–148.

Pelc, S. R., and Howard, A. (1955). Effect of various doses of x rays on the number of cells synthesizing deoxyribosenucleic acid. *Radiat. Res.* **3,** 135–142.

Saha, B. K., and Tolmach, L. J. (1976). Delayed expression of the x-ray-induced depression of DNA synthetic rate in HeLa S3 cells. *Radiat. Res.* **66,** 76–89.

Scholes, G., and Weiss, J. (1954). Chemical action of x rays on nucleic acids and related substances in aqueous systems. *Biochem. J.* **56,** 65–72.

Setlow, R. B. (1968). The photochemistry, photobiology, and repair of polynucleotides. *Prog. Nucleic Acid Res. Mol. Biol.* **8,** 257–295.

Setlow, R. B., and Carrier, W. L. (1964). The disappearance of thymine dimers from DNA. *Proc. Natl. Acad. Sci. U. S. A.* **51,** 226–231.

Sparrow, A. H., and Rosenfeld, F. M. (1946). X-ray induced depolymerization of thymonucleohistone and of sodium thymonucleate. *Science* **104,** 245–246.

Sutherland, B. M. (1974). Photoreactivating enzyme from human leucocytes. *Nature (London)* **248,** 109–112.

Swanson, C. P., and Johnston, A. H. (1954). Radiation-induced pycnosis of chromosomes and its relation to oxygen tension. *Am. Nat.* **88,** 425–430.

Taylor, B., Greenstein, J. P., and Hollaender, A. (1947). The action of x rays on thymus nucleic acid. *Cold Spring Harbor Symp. Quant. Biol.* **12,** 237–246.

von Borstel, R. C., and St. Amand, W. (1963). Stage sensitivity to x-radiation during meiosis and mitosis in the egg of the wasp *Habrobracon*. *In* "Symposium on Repair from Genetic Radiation" (B. Sobels, ed.), pp. 87–100. Pergamon, Oxford.

von Borstel, R. C., Hastings, P. J., and Schroeder, C. (1976). Comparison of replication errors and mutagenic repair as a source of spontaneous mutations. *Abh. Akad. Wiss. DDR, Abt. Math., Naturwiss. Tech.* **9,** 89–93.

Wacker, A., and Chandra, P. (1969). Aspects of modification of nucleic acids in mutational processes. *Mutat. Cell. Process, Ciba Found. Symp., 1969* pp. 171–183

Ward, J. F. (1975). Molecular mechanisms of radiation-induced damage to nucleic acids. *Adv. Radiat. Biol.* **5,** 181–239.

Ward, J. F., and Kuo, I. (1976). Strand breaks, base release, and postirradiation changes in DNA γ-irradiated in dilute O_2-saturated aqueous solution. *Radiat. Res.* **66,** 485–498.

Walters, R. A., and Enger, M. D. (1976). Effects of ionizing radiation on nucleic acid synthesis in mammalian cells. *Adv. Radiat. Biol.* **6,** 1–48.

CHAPTER 5   Localized Effects on Chromosome Structure

The opportunity to view visible evidence of an effect of irradiation has appealed to many investigators. At times papers based upon chromosomal aberration predominated the radiobiological literature. However, in the classic experiments with higher organisms the relationships between the initial events following irradiation and the cytologically visible alterations have not been direct and immediate. The preparation of slides for microscopic examination was delayed until the chromosomes attained the greatest degree of visibility during cell division. If irradiated in metaphase, chromosome damage is usually not immediately apparent.

Recently, new techniques have enabled the rapid visualization of chromosome aberrations by producing premature condensation of the chromosomes in cultured cells. The diffuse strands of an irradiated G_1 nucleus can be changed into compact rods by fusing a mitotic cell with the interphase cell (Waldren and Johnson, 1974).

Traditionally, organisms with a small number of large chromosomes supplied the best material for objectively scored experiments. In plants, preference was shown for the mitotic divisions in root tips or the division figures in developing pollen. Chromosomes of the developing gametes of both sexes have been studied in a variety of animals (Kaufmann, 1954). Somatic tissues studied include the tail tips of amphibian larvae, grasshopper neuroblasts, and dipteran salivary glands. The last has provided exceptional material because of the somatic pairing of giant, banded chromosomes. Corroboration of the results from classic materials is now appearing for the chromosomes of cultured cells, including those from human tissues.

Table 5.1 gives a comparison between the classic results with *Tradescantia* reviewed in Lea's (1947) book and more recent leukocyte studies by Bender and Gooch (1962, 1963). The high value for chromatid deletions in the plant microspores is due to the early investigators classifying achromatic lesions as presumptive breaks. Using the same approach, Chu's group obtained a value of 0.0060 (Chu *et al.*, 1961).

TABLE 5.1

'A Comparison of Aberrations Produced by X Rays in *Tradescantia* Microspores and Cultured Human Leukocytes under Aerobic Conditions[a]

Material	Chromatid deletions per cell per R	Isochromatid deletions per cell per R^2	Chromosome deletions per cell per R	Dicentrics per cell per R^2 $\times$ 10^{-3}
Microspores	0.0073	0.0027	0.0006	0.0052
	$\pm$ 0.0001	$\pm$ 0.0002	$\pm$ 0.0001	$\pm$ 0.0008
Leukocytes	0.0015	0.0015	0.0011	0.0045
	$\pm$ 0.0004	$\pm$ 0.0001	$\pm$ 0.0001	$\pm$ 0.0002

[a] Based on Bender and Gooch (1962, 1963).

Ordinarily the value is lower. A number of different mammalian cells have provided aberration values between 0.0015 and 0.0060 per cell per rad. These include human epitheloid tissue, monkey bone marrow, monkey kidney, hamster fibroblasts, and mouse ascites tumor. Exact agreement is not expected between cells of different species irradiated with different equipment under different conditions. Nevertheless similarities, especially in the last two columns of Table 5.1, argue for an essential similarity of the mechanics of the production of chromosome aberrations for both plant and animal cells. However, as related later in this chapter, chromosome number is an important factor in determining the yield of chromosomal interchanges, and in this aspect quantitative differences between plants and animals are found.

Types of Aberration

Figure 5.1 diagrams various types of chromosomal aberrations (Sax, 1941). The two general classes of aberrations are related to the stage treated, and to the progress of nuclear events by the time of irradiation. That is, chromosomes may respond to irradiation as if they were single strands or double at the time of exposure. This results in chromosome and chromatid aberrations respectively. In each class, two subclasses are recognized on the basis of whether single or double breakage is necessary in their production (Giles, 1954).

In addition to the fragments, bridges, and rings which are scored by microscopic examination of dividing cells, other types of aberrations are produced. The detection of intraarm inversions and symmetrical translocations requires some special consideration, such as the study of

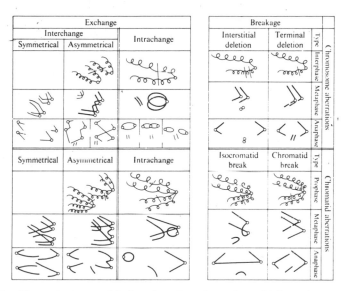

Figure 5.1. The major types of induced nuclear aberration which can be recognized in cytological analysis (after K. Sax and Associates). Other arrangements of exchanged parts may not be recognizable by microscopic examination.

chromosome pairing in heterozygotes. In some investigations, induced structural changes are detected genetically through linkage studies.

Carefully timed exposures enable a demonstration of the transition from chromosome to chromatid types of induced aberration as metaphase is approached (Table 5.2). In the original formulation of the chromosome theory, such results have been taken to indicate the time of functional longitudinal splitting of submicroscopic structures. Subsequently this view has been supported by studies of cultured mammalian cells. Human leukocytes irradiated in G_1 resulted in chromosome aberrations, while an identical exposure of G_2 cells produced chromatic deletions. The change-over was apparent in tests of the S phase (Brewen, 1965).

A chromosome break resulting in a terminal deletion is the simplest type of aberration. Such fragments lack a kinetic element and accordingly lag behind the centric chromosomes during polar movement (Figure 5.2). As shown, acentric fragments usually are not incorporated in the daughter nuclei. If many divisions elapse between irradiation and examination, acentric fragments are not observed. An example is the type of experiment in which *Drosophila* sperm are irradiated and larval salivary glands are studied in the offspring. Note the chromosomal bridge formed as the centric portions move to opposite poles (Figure

TABLE 5.2

Transition from Chromosome to Chromatid Types of Aberration[a]

Irradiated hours before metaphase	Interchanges per 100 cells	
	Chromosome	Chromatid
34	12.0	0.0
33	9.9	0.6
32	9.9	0.0
31	11.1	3.9
30	8.1	4.2
29	5.1	3.3
28	9.9	2.1
27	3.9	5.1
26	0.0	6.6
25	0.0	10.8
23	0.0	17.7

[a] When 160 R of x ray is delivered to pollen grains entering mitosis. (*Tradescantia* data by courtesy of K. Sax.)

5.2). If cell division is to be completed, this bridge must break. However this may set a "breakage–fusion–bridge" cycle in progress which would be evident at subsequent divisions. We shall explore the significance of these events in our discussion of lethal effects.

Quantitative Aspects

If we wish to study how much breakage results from a series of exposures, we soon discover that there are a number of variables which influence the yield. Usually some quantity less than the maximum number of potential breaks is observed. We need to examine the theories in more detail later in the chapter. For the present it will suffice to mention two possibilities: (1) Completion of the breakage process may depend upon additional features; and (2) broken chromosomes may have an ability to reunite.

Quantitative studies of two-break aberrations emphasize the importance not only of the location of breaks but also of the length of time taken to complete the irradiation treatment. In order for two breaks to participate in an aberration they must coexist in time and space. If the ability of one region to participate in an aberration disappears before a second adjacent region is brought to a similar reactive capacity, a

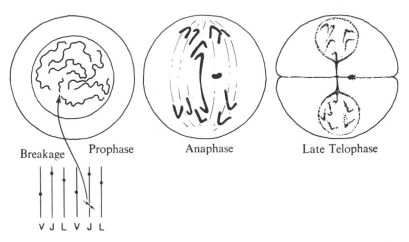

Breakage   Prophase   Anaphase   Late Telophase

V J L V J L

Figure 5.2. Formation of a bridge and fragment with loss of the fragment at subsequent division.

two-break aberration is impossible. It would be simpler, but less exact, to say that if one break heals before a second forms, an aberration involving both is impossible.

The dosage relationships for two-break aberrations will be modified if the irradiation is spread through time by employing irradiation of low intensity (Beatty *et al.*, 1956) or by fractioning the dose. The decreased yield from attenuated or fractionated doses, initially demonstrated in plant experiments, has now been observed in a variety of vertebrate cells including the corneal epithelium of hamsters *in vivo* and cultured human peripheral leukocytes (Okada, 1970).

If the yield is plotted against acute doses of x or gamma rays (Figure 5.3), the frequency of one-break aberrations increases linearly (Carlson, 1941), while the frequency of two-break aberrations tends to increase at a greater rate. The rate may depend on the material. It has approached the square of the dose in *Tradescantia*, but in *Drosophila* it is usually found nearer to the 3/2 power of the dose (Lea, 1947; Sax, 1950; Giles, 1954). Theoretically, the linear increase indicates a probability p that radiation will break a chromosome, and this is proportional to dose. If two independent breaks take part in a chromosome aberration, the probability of both existing simultaneously is represented by $p \times p$ or p^2 (Wolff and Atwood, 1954).

A decrease in the frequency of aberrations when the exposure is spread through time is attributed to restitution. Lesions produced early in the treatment period have had time to "heal" and are not available for

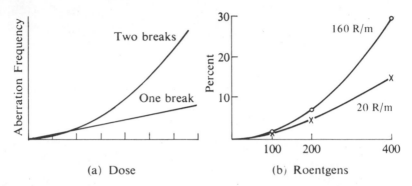

Figure 5.3. The relationship between dosage of electromagnetic ionizing radiations and frequency of chromosome aberrations. (a) At any given intensity, one-break aberrations tend to increase in proportion to dosage while two-break aberrations increase at a greater rate. (b) Contrasts between dose rates. At a higher intensity, the aberration frequency increases to approach the square of the dose, *Tradescantia* results. (Courtesy of K. Sax.)

participation with those caused later in the exposure. Only when additional reactive sites are produced while the first group still persists can rings, dicentries, inversions, and translocations result.

When densely ionizing particles such as neutrons (Giles, 1940, 1943) and α rays (Kotval and Gray, 1947) are used, all aberrations show a linear relation to dose. This has been demonstrated for neutrons of varying energies from experimental installations (Conger and Giles, 1950) as well as those released from nuclear detonations (Kirby-Smith and Swanson, 1954). Apparently these particulate radiations are capable of breaking more than one chromosome during the passage of a single ionizing particle through the nucleus. Hence we should not expect a dose-squared relation.

Since an exchange can occur only if the broken ends have opportunity to come into contact, coexistence in space determines which type of aberration is most probable. Different parts of the same chromosome are obviously in closer regular association than parts of different chromosomes. In organisms other than the Diptera, the various chromosomes lie at random in the nucleus and in the mitotic figure. Even in the Diptera where there is somatic pairing of homologous chromosomes, most of the exchange is between breaks in the same chromosome. The number of interchanges is comparatively small. So far as intraarm versus interarm are concerned, no consistent pattern has been reported. However, intraarm changes are more easily overlooked and there may be unintentional bias in the experimental data.

Whether certain regions of a chromosome are more susceptible to breakage or whether breaks occur at random along a chromosome is controversial. There is no evidence that the initial effects of ionizing radiations are nonrandom. However, it seems likely that restitution is nonrandom due to differences in the intimate physiology of diversified regions of the chromosomes. A tabulation by Sparrow (1951) of reported cases of nonrandom "breakage" of chromosomes by x rays shows diametrically opposed reports from nine different organisms. From the standpoint of mechanics, strains or movement which would interfere with restitution may be expected in association with the centromere. Thus, as suggested by Sax, more breaks recoverable as aberrations might be expected from the centromere region. To complicate interpretations, the parts of chromosomes nearest the centromeres are made up of proximal heterochromatin in the best investigated organism, *Drosophila melanogaster*. When a high proportion of breaks is found in such a region, we cannot tell if the cause is mechanical or biochemical.

The presence or absence of other breaks in other chromosomes of the cell does not seem to affect the occurrence of any specific break. The mathematical approach applies the Poisson formula to an analysis of the relative frequency with which cells are found containing zero, one, two, three, four or more aberrations. Lea's 1947 monograph may be consulted for details. Chi square tests showed satisfactory agreement between experimental and expected frequencies in grasshopper neuroblasts and in *Tradescantia* microspores. In experiments in which *Drosophila* sperm were irradiated and the salivaries examined, a discrepancy was found to be due to aberrations more complicated than four-break exchange.

Differences in Sensitivity between Organisms

There are considerable differences in the doses reported to induce chromosomal aberrations in different organisms. For example, although 24 R of x rays produces breaks in 1% of the chromosomes in *Chortophaga* neuroblasts, about 400 R is required to do likewise in *Drosophila* sperm. In contrast, the relatively massive dose of 20,000 R did not noticeably damage the chromosome of a Holomastigoid protozoan (Sax and Swanson, 1941). Some of the discrepancy may be due to the different techniques used in detecting chromosome change. For plants, Sparrow's group (Sparrow *et al.*, 1952, 1963) has demonstrated that apparent differences may be spurious, provided enough is known to enable calculation of the energy absorbed per chromosome. As yet we do not know enough about chromosome chemistry to speculate whether great differences of intrinsic organization exist at levels higher than the nucleic acid molecule. However, there is one cytological aspect which has attracted attention, ploidy.

The sensitivity of individual chromosomes to radiation does not change in polyploids, but with more chromosomes present the frequency of chromosome breaks *per cell* is higher. Species and strains of cereals have provided readily available material for such a study, although their divergence in genetic background complicates an interpretation of results. In an ideal situation (a mixed population of cells from a single *Tradescantia* bud), Conger and Johnston (1956) found that diploid micropores showed twice as many chromosome aberrations as did haploids.

This type of response may or may not explain the relative radiosensitivity of organisms. In the wasp *Mormoniella*, a doubling of the chromosome complement from n to $2n$ doubles the sensitivity of sperm when dominant lethality in the zygote is the criterion (Mortimer and von Borstel, 1963), but in the wasp *Habrobracon*, differential radiosensitivity between haploids and diploids depends upon the stage of development irradiated when completion of development is scored (Clark and Mitchell, 1952).

In general, when postirradiation *survival* of tissues or organisms is considered, polyploidy per se does not necessarily confer radiosensitivity. Often the reverse has been found for animal tumors and the growth of higher plants (see Chapter 9).

To characterize the cellular response, Figure 5.4 presents results on a yeast experiment (Mortimer, 1958). There is an increase in resistance to x-ray inactivation from haploid to diploid as generally demonstrated.

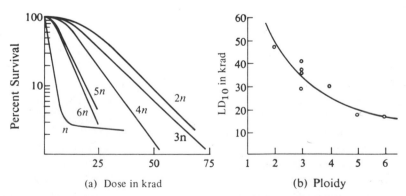

(a) Dose in krad   (b) Ploidy

Figure 5.4.   The relation of radiosensitivity to polyploidy. (a) X-ray survival curves for yeast cultures of a polyploid series. (b) The dose necessary to reduce viability to 10%, plotted against ploidy of yeast cultures. (From Mortimer, 1958.)

This is followed by a progressive decrease in radioresistance, diploid through hexaploid. These results are consistent with the supposition that much of the inactivation of haploid cultures is brought about by recessive changes, whereas higher-ploidy cultures are inactivated chiefly by dominant lethals. In other words, point mutations are contrasted with gross chromosomal aberrations. Results for diploid cultures other than that shown are available. There is some variability of radiation resistance between diploid cultures, which may be explained in part by variations in genetic homozygosity.

Information from animal experiments is limited to observations on only a few organisms which have received most of the research attention. Although the plant species of classic cytology have larger nuclei and more DNA per nucleus, the chromosome damage is greater in human cells receiving equivalent exposures. When yields of x-ray-induced aberrations obtained in the same laboratory were compared, human leukocyte chromosomes were respectively three to five times more sensitive than those from *Tradescantia* pollen or *Vicia* roots. Possibly the higher chromosome number in human cells may be an important factor contributing to the number of interchange events (Evans, 1967b).

Differences in the Sensitivity of Cells during the Division Cycle

In recent years, considerable attention has been given to the changing sensitivity of cells during the course of cell division, especially as provided by evidence of chromosomal damage. A pioneering study was that of Anna R. Whiting (1940), who recognized the unique suitability of the sequential arrangement of insect oocytes for such investigations. Egg counts, which demonstrate that experimental females are depositing as many ova as are controls, provide direct evidence over a wide range of doses that germinal selection is not operating up to a week after irradiation. When division figures were examined in these eggs, chromosome fragments and bridges were found to explain the dominant lethality observed for emryyos (Whiting, 1945a,b). At a given dose, hatchability is much lower for eggs exposed in metaphase of the first meiotic division than for oocytes exposed in prophase.

General acceptance of the vulnerability of metaphase awaited results from plant material, particularly the study of meiotic *Trillium* microspores shown in Figure 5.5 (Sparrow, 1951). We note here that the comparative resistance of metaphase chromosomes to breakage is de-

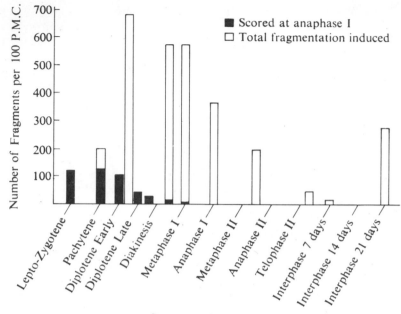

Figure 5.5.   The numbers of chromosome fragments induced by 50 R of x rays at various stages of microsporogenesis in *Trillium*. If breaks are scored only at anaphase I, an erroneous picture is obtained. (Based on data provided by courtesy of A. H. Sparrow.)

ceptive. Aberrations not detectable immediately appear in quantity at the next division, so that at the optimum time for scoring, late prophase and metaphase are most susceptible to nuclear alterations by ionizing radiations. However, stage differences in the frequency of recovered aberrations do not necessarily mean that the chromosome sensitivity is changed at the molecular level. Admittedly there may be differences in coiling, or DNA, or water content, but spatial relationships of chromosomes and parts are changed as well as the facility of breakage repair.

Additional differences between types of cells within an organism will be discussed in the chapters on histopathology.

Modifying Factors

Any factor which promotes restitution of chromosome lesions will decrease the yield of induced aberrations. Conversely, any factor which interferes with restitution will increase the yield. Thus high temperature and chemical inhibitors of mitosis are agents which decrease yield. Low temperature, centrifugation, sonic vibration, and mechanical agitation increase yield. Giles' 1954 review may be consulted as a guide to the literature on modifying factors in plant experiments.

A comprehensive and unified interpretation of the supplementary effects of infrared and ultraviolet on x-ray studies is not possible. Although ultraviolet at 2537 Å itself induces breaks in a growing system, it can reduce the frequency of aberrations induced by x rays, regardless of the order of exposures (Swanson, 1944). This is understandable if one treatment reduces the free radicals produced by the other. However, the two radiations were synergistic in other experiments employing dry pollen grains instead of the growing pollen tubes (Kirby-Smith, 1963). Lesions produced by one radiation might develop into actual breaks when additional energy is provided by another radiation, or uv as well as x rays may damage a chromosome-rejoining mechanism.

Infrared alone is ineffective in producing aberrations. Another difference from ultraviolet is that the interval between infrared and x-ray exposures can be very long without altering the subsequent yield of aberrations. Initially Swanson (1957) suggested that both infrared and x rays might induce metastable states in chromosomes, but subsequently Wolff (1965) demonstrated that cells of different sensitivity can be presented for x-ray treatment by a shift in the mitotic cycle induced by far-red.

The Oxygen Effect

Oxygen is a particularly important modifying factor. Its presence during irradiation has been shown to have special significance, and this discovery changed the interpretation of the effects of modified temperature. Early hypotheses, strongly influenced by the Lea school, emphasized the physical factors of type, dose, and intensity of irradiation in considerations of hereditary damage. New vitality and interest were injected into radiobiology by the studies of Thoday and Read (1947, 1949), who demonstrated that oxygen has a marked effect in increasing the frequency of induced chromosomal aberrations. They had set out to investigate Mottram's report that root tip growth in *Vicia* was less inhibited by irradiation under anaerobic conditions. Not only did they confirm Mottram's findings, but they explained the results on the basis that a decrease in radiosensitivity was accompanied by a parallel decrease in the proportion of cells having chromosomal aberrations (Figure 5.6).

Soon afterward, Giles and Riley (1949), working at Oak Ridge, demonstrated a pronounced effect of oxygen on x-ray-induced rearrangements in *Tradescantia* microspores. Argon and helium were used, as well as nitrogen, to replace the air of the exposure chamber. The quantitative relation shown between the aberration frequency and percentage of oxygen during exposure is given by Figure 5.7. There is a characteristic leveling off when the oxygen tension in air (21%) is reached. Little additional aberration is promoted by oxygen increases up to 100%. Because preradiation and postradiation presence or absence had no effect (Table 5.3), it was concluded that the chief effect was upon the breakage mechanism. Subsequent experiments by others have demonstrated that chromosomes may be broken by oxygen alone when partial pressures greater than that of air are used (Conger and Fairchild, 1952).

On the other hand, whether the initial number of primary events was reduced or whether the reunion of broken chromosome ends was being influenced has been considered an open question by various investigators. The recovery hypothesis is favored in maize experiments when

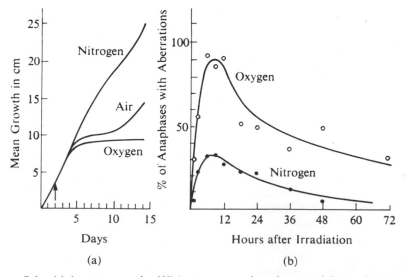

Figure 5.6. (a) Average growth of *Vicia* roots x-rayed on the second day in the presence of gases as shown. (b) The percentage of anaphases with bridges and fragments after x-radiation with 143 R (4 min). Nitrogen or oxygen was bubbled through the water of the exposure chamber. (Based on Thoday and Read, 1947.)

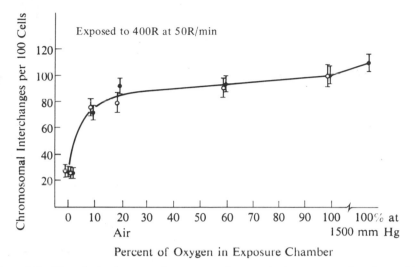

Figure 5.7. The relation between the amount of oxygen in the exposure chamber and the frequency of a type of chromosomal aberration on *Tradescantia* microspores. The actual intracellular oxygen under these conditions is much lower. (Courtesy of N. H. Giles, Jr., and H. P. Riley.)

hypoxia gives differential protection against interstitial and terminal deletions (Schwartz, 1952). It is also supported by the undisturbed sex ratios in ring X chromosome stocks of *Drosophila*. Ring Xs should be lost and the sex ratio disturbed if oxygen favored breakage in these fruit flies (Baker and von Halle, 1955). Also, more than merely a change in the amount of radiation injury is suspected for grasshopper neuroblasts because they do not respond to change in oxygen tension at irradiation as they do to a change in radiation dose.

Regardless of interpretations, the reduction factor can be expressed conveniently by the ratio of the effect in air to the effect in nitrogen, or air/N_2. As shown in Table 5.4, ratios are obtained directly from simple deletion data, but the square root of each frequency must be used to calculate exchange ratios. Different reduction factors are obtained for the various types of aberrations, and the ratio varies with the stage of the cell cycle irradiated. Furthermore, the oxygen effect is associated with sparse ion density. Very little reduction in aberration occurs when heavily ionizing alpha particles are used. The practically zero percentage of reduction may be compared with 59% for Co^{60} γ rays, 48% for 250 kV x rays, and 33% for neutrons. However, the period of time required for exposure must be brief. At dose rates lower than 1 R/min the aberration yield may be higher for the *anoxic* sample (Beatty *et al.*,

TABLE 5.3

Experiments on the Effects of Oxygen in Increasing the Radiosensitivity of *Tradescantia* Chromosomes[a]

Nature of experiment	Pre-treatment conditions	Exposure conditions	Posttreatment conditions	No. cells	Interchanges per cell	Interstitial deletions per cell
Addition after irradiation	Vacuum	Vacuum	Vacuum—10 min	880	0.12 ± 0.01	0.11 ± 0.01
			Within 3 sec; oxygen to 1500 mm Hg—10 min	700	0.09 ± 0.01	0.10 ± 0.01
Removal after irradiation	Oxygen	Oxygen 1500 mm Hg	Oxygen—10 min; 1500 mm Hg	150	0.70 ± 0.07	0.83 ± 0.07
			Evacuation within 25 sec; vacuum—10 min	200	0.72 ± 0.06	0.85 ± 0.07
Addition during irradiation	Vacuum	Vacuum 1st 30 sec; oxygen 2nd 30 sec; (within 3 sec) to 1500 mm Hg	Evacuation within 25 sec; vacuum—10 min	350	0.39 ± 0.03	0.50 ± 0.04
Removal during irradiation	Oxygen	Oxygen 1st 30 sec at 1500 mm Hg; evacuated to 1–2 mm Hg within 25 sec; total time evacuated 30 sec	Oxygen within 3 sec to 1500 mm Hg— 10 min	518	0.61 ± 0.03	0.59 ± 0.03

[a] Buds were given 300 R of 250 kV (15 mm) x rays for 1 min. Acetocarmine smears of microspores at first postmeiotic mitosis were studied. (Based on Giles and Riley, 1950.)

TABLE 5.4

Frequency of Aberration Induced in *Tradescantia* Microspores by Four Qualities of Radiation in Air and in Nitrogen[a]

Radiation	Atmosphere	Aberrations per 100 cells		
		Chromatid deletions	Isochromatid deletions	Exchanges
X ray 50 kVP;	Air	49.3	84.6	35.3
unfiltered	Nitrogen	98.2	15.0	9.5
	Air/N$_2$ ratio	0.50	5.6	1.9
X ray 100 kVP;	Air	66.0	62.5	30.5
1 mm of Al	Nitrogen	79.3	14.0	7.3
	Air/N$_2$ ratio	0.83	3.9	2.0
X ray 250 kVP;	Air	78.0	44.0	28.0
4 mm of Cu	Nitrogen	63.5	16.6	6.0
	Air/N$_2$ ratio	1.25	2.7	2.3
γ Rays	Air	96.2	32.5	26.0
from ^{60}Co;	Nitrogen	50.5	14.0	5.0
1.3–1.3 MeV	Air/N$_2$ ratio	1.9	2.3	2.3

[a] 150 R at 8.9 R/min. (Based on Swanson, 1955.)

1956), probably due to the nonfunctioning of a rejoining system to be discussed below.

Chromosome Structure and Aberration Theory

Precisely what gives rise to a chromosome break is still not known. Ideas on the subject are conditioned by the interim model of submicroscopic structure espoused by the investigator. Despite electron microscopy, the argument of uninemy vs. polynemy of the mitotic chromosome still lingers, and the presence of a core ribbon has not been ruled out. A multistranded structure was suggested by the mass of fibrils seen in EM sections, but a long folded fiber consistent with the appearance of whole-mount preparations would provide a similar aspect when sectioned.

Since electron microscopy has not revealed half- and quarter-chromatids but long multilooped filaments, the so called subchromatid exchanges (Ostergren and Wakonig, 1954) have been interpreted as events in which different segments of the single folded fiber have participated. The term subchromatid reflects the thinking of proponents of the multistranded theory. Genetic tests appear to confirm the folded-fiber model of chromosome structure when lesions spanning only part of the visible chromatid diameter result in exchange affecting the entire axial arrangement of functional genes (Dupraw, 1968).

The original or classical theory of the formation of aberrations was developed by the early 1940s, antedating electron microscopy. Postulating the induction of immediate random breaks and the prompt refusions of a linear structure, long before it had achieved microscopically visible dimensions, was a parsimonious way of explaining a puzzle which was invisible except at metaphase. The breakage-first theory succeeded reasonably well in explaining most of the experimental results obtained by the Sax (1950) group of investigators (Wolff, 1959).

Furthermore, the Sax explanation fits data obtained more recently with cultured mammalian cells. Agreement is excellent between the amount of cell killing and the number of chromosome aberrations. On the average, 1 aberration per cell corresponded to 37% cell survival (Dewey *et al.*, 1971).

However, Revell (1963) and associates decided that certain classes of data such as the relative frequencies of chromatid and isochromatid breaks are explained better by another hypothesis. Instead of aberration starting from outright breaks in two chromatids, this alternate hypothesis postulates activated exchangeable states as the primary radiation damage. Reciprocal interaction between these primary events produces exchanges which may be followed by breakage elsewhere than at the exchange site. Also, failure to complete an exchange between chromosomal segments results in discontinuity, but if not used for exchange, the activated region would gradually transform into a nonexchangeable site.

From Revell's viewpoint (1974), the achromatic lesions or gaps seen by light microscopy are not considered to be true chromatid discontinuities. Evidence from electron microscopy is consistent with this view. Brinkley and Hittelman (1975) state that chromatin threads extending across the "gap" are always demonstrable. Presumably the supposed chromatid breaks Bishop (1942) found as early as 3 min after irradiating grasshopper spermatocytes fall into this category, and cannot be cited as evidence for immediate breakage.

Dose Fractionation Experiments

Both hypotheses assume a primary event of temporary nature which decays unless another is available to react with it. That is, interaction occurs between events which coexist in space and time, but Revell's (1974) interpretation avoids the perplexity of breaks staying open for hours. Two sets of experiments have been performed which provide results of divergent interpretative differences.

On the basis that breaks are produced at the instant of radiation, the pattern of decline in the exchange frequency from dose fractions separated by increasing periods of time would permit an estimate of how long breaks from the first exposure stay open to rejoin with breaks induced by the second exposure. Furthermore, the effectiveness of specific inhibitors during the interfraction period would indicate the type of molecular resynthesis impeded and the molecular pathways involved. Two-dose exposures of *Vicia* seeds were used by Wolff and Luippold (1955) in experiments based on the premise that 4 hr was the maximum effective interfraction period. The increased yield of aberrations was interpreted to indicate nonrejoined breaks when one of the following conditions was used during the interfraction period: low temperature, KCN, CO + darkness, and vacuum + $Na_2S_2O_4$. Furthermore, inhibition of the formation of ATP with dinitrophenol gave persistent lesions whereas supplying ATP decreased the aberration yield. Evidently, cellular respiration and oxidative phosphorylation are somehow involved in modifying the yield of radiation-induced aberrations, but whether it is in repair of broken gene strings is debatable. Wolff (1959) found inhibitors of protein synthesis effective rather than inhibitors of DNA synthesis. This is not consonant with the repair of breakage in strands or fibers of DNA.

On the other hand, if the first event is not breakage, the second event resolved in a fractioned dose experiment cannot be chromatid reunion. Instead, the experiment simply measures the time that primary events stay available to interact with events available later. In Revell's (1963) terminology, pairs of primary events associate in some way to initiate exchange. Also, there may be more stages than first suspected at which recovery may occur.

Evans (1967a,b) confirmed a fall in chromosome aberration yield with an increasing interfraction interval up to 4 hr, not only in *Tradescantia* microspores and *Vicia* root tips, but also with human leukocytes. Then, following earlier work by Lane, Evans found the aberration yield increased again, until with an 8-hr period the yield obtained with a split dose was almost as high as that obtained with the acute unsplit dose. He postulated that the cell's own systems for repairing nucleoprotein strands could elevate the initial radiation damage to a state giving rise to chromosome aberrations. Evans (1967a) proposed a four step scheme in the formation of aberrations: (1) induction of a lesion, (2) its stabilization, (3) later transition to a new unstable state, (4) synthesis or repair. Step 3 could involve excision of the damaged region, much like a process discussed for microorganisms in Chapter 4. Two lesions induced together may interact and produce an aberration at the time of repair, or if two lesions approach each other later in the sequence of events the repair step provides opportunity for misrepair. Evans' fractionation results could be accounted for if new unstable lesions can interact with the unstable product of step 3.

On the other hand, the Sax/Wolff interfraction period was considered adequate for interpreting experiments with cultured mammalian cells. After irradiation a rapid reduction in the number of chromosome fragments occurred within 2 hr (Waldron and Johnson, 1974). A reduction in damage was observed as the time period between dose fractions was increased up to 2 hr, but much of the repair was accomplished within 12 min (Dewey *et al.*, 1972).

Crossing-Over

The phenomenon of an exchange of genetic material in corresponding segments of homologous chromosomes is a normal occurrence during meiotic prophase. Ionizing radiations have not proven effective in modifying the frequency of crossing-over for higher organisms, except in *Drosophila* and other Diptera where there is a tendency to somatic associations in somatic cells. Here again we are dealing with a system of considerable complexity in which the nature of the radiation-induced lesions is in doubt.

Even in *Drosophila* experiments, the results have unusual aspects. Whittinghill (1955) managed to induce interchanges in the male, where they do not occur spontaneously presumably because spermatocytes lack synaptinemal complexes. Further, he observed what seemed to be gonial crossover products. However, not all regions showed an increase. Increases in the proximal regions were accompanied by decreases in the distal regions. This pattern can be explained by a competition for enzymes now believed to mediate the events (Roberts, 1969).

Experiments with complexly marked stocks have led to the conclusion that x-ray-induced recombination is really an interchange process involving the breakage and rejoining of homologues (Williamson *et al.*, 1970a,b). Small duplications and deficiencies provided evidence that the induced breakage was not precisely between homologous loci, and therefore the induced crossover chromosome was really a type of translocation. Roberts' (1969) experiments, in which results for heterochromatic and euchromatic regions of the X chromosome could be compared, indicated that breakage/rejoining explained the "crossovers" in the former. However an additional aspect may be required to explain the euchromatin results, where an induced predisposition persisted through at least one cell division until manifested at the usual time of crossing-over. A special feature of these tests was the irradiation of females containing a crossover-suppressing genotype.

Somatic Crossing-Over

A related topic is the induction of somatic mosaicism in *Drosophila*. An increased incidence of single and twin spots occurs when flies heterozygous for bristle and body-color genes are irradiated during development. Traditionally, such mosaicism has been attributed to somatic crossing-over. Now it should be viewed as another example of a response to chromosomal damage. Stauffer (1972) clearly demonstrated an oxygen effect on the incidence of induced mosaicism. Also, he found evidence for a postirradiation oxygen-dependent system which could repair some of the x-ray-induced chromosome lesions.

Organisms Other Than Diptera

The meager literature on radiation influencing crossing-over in other organisms is interpreted to reflect a general reluctance to publish negative evidence. During the 1930s and 1940s, tests were made with various organisms, especially other types of insects and plants. The data which demonstrated no significant increase in crossing-over in response to irradiation were filed away unpublished.

Concluding Remarks

In this chapter we have presented a survey of radiation effects upon a visible level of cell structure, the chromosome. Ordinarily, these vehicles of inheritance behave regularly and predictably throughout interphase and at cell division. This is fortunate in view of the delicate genic balance in diploid organisms. Loss, displacement, or aberrant chromosome behavior disturbs cell function, often so drastically that the cell is unable to survive. Loss of a cell or, more important, loss of cell progenies which were to be derived from the defunct unit may affect organisms in a variety of ways. Altered morphology, sterility, or even organism mortality may result, depending upon the significance of the cell. More often than not, groups of similar cells show the same kind of radiation effect which makes more probable the occurrence of an obvious alteration at the organ or organism level.

Unfortunately, the definitive explanation of the mechanism of eukaryote chromosomal breakage is still not available. Two theoretical themes have emerged. In one view, the breakage-first theory, discontinuity occurs immediately after irradiation. The alternate theory is that overt breaks develop from subsequent chemical events at activated spots. Experimental evidence is presented for both possibilities.

References

Baker, W. K., and von Halle, E. S. (1955). Evidence on the mechanism of the oxygen effect by use of a ring chromosome. *J. Cell. Comp. Physiol.* **45**, 299–307.

Beatty, A. V., Beatty, J. W., and Collins, C. (1956). Effects of various intensities of x radiation on chromosomal aberrations. *Am. J. Bot.* **43**, 328–332.

Bender, M. A., and Gooch, P. C. (1962). Types and rates of x ray induced chromosome aberrations in human blood irradiated *in vitro. Proc. Natl. Acad. Sci. U.S.A.* **48**, 522–532.

Bender, M. A., and Gooch, P. C. (1963). Chromatid-type aberrations induced by x rays in human leukocyte cultures. *Cytogenetics* **2**, 107–116.

Bishop, D. W. (1942). Cytological demonstration of chromosome breaks soon after x radiation. *Genetics* **27**, 132.

Brewen, J. G. (1965). Cell-cycle and radiosensitivity of the chromosomes of human leukocytes. *Int. J. Radiat. Biol.* **9**, 391–397.

Brinkley, B. R., and Hittelman, W. N. (1975). Ultrastructure of mammalian chromosome aberrations. *Int. Rev. Cytol.* **42**, 49–101.

Carlson, J. G. (1941). An analysis of x ray induced single breaks in neuroblast chromosomes of the grasshopper (*Chortophaga viridifasciata*). *Proc. Natl. Acad. Sci. U.S.A.* **27**, 42–47.

Chu, E. H. Y., Giles, N. H., Jr., and Passano, K. (1961). Types and frequencies of human chromosome aberrations induced by x rays. *Proc. Natl. Acad. Sci. U.S.A.* **47**, 830–839.

Clark, A. M., and Mitchell, C. J. (1952). Effects of x rays upon haploid and diploid embryos of *Habrobracon. Biol. Bull.* **103**, 170–177.

Conger, A. D., and Fairchild, L. M. (1952). The breakage of chromosomal aberrations by oxygen. *Proc. Natl. Acad. Sci. U.S.A.* **38**, 289–299.

Conger, A. D., and Giles, N. H., Jr. (1950). The cytogenetic effects of slow neutrons. *Genetics* **35**, 397–419.

Conger, A. D., and Johnston, A. H. (1950). Polyploidy and radiosensitivity. *Nature (London)* **178**, 271.

Dewey, W. C., Miller, H. H., and Leeper, D. B. (1971). Chromosome aberrations and mortality of x irradiated mammalian cells: Emphasis on repair. *Proc. Natl. Acad. Sci. U.S.A.* **68**, 667–671.

Dupraw, E. J. (1968). "Cell and Molecular Biology." Academic Press, New York.

Evans, H. J. (1967a). Repair and recovery at chromosome and cellular levels: Similarities and differences. *Brookhaven Symp. Biol.* **20**, 111–133.

Evans, H. J. (1967b). Dose-response relations from *in vitro* studies. "Human Radiation Cytogenetics" (H. J. Evans, W. M. Court Brown, and A. S. McLean, eds.), pp. 20–36. North-Holland Publ., Amsterdam.

Giles, N. H., Jr. (1940). The effect of fast neutrons on the chromosomes of *Tradescantia*. *Proc. Natl. Acad. Sci. U.S.A.* **26**, 567–575.

Giles, N. H., Jr. (1943). Comparative studies of the cytogenetical effects of neutrons and x rays. *Genetics* **28**, 398–418.

Giles, N. H., Jr. (1954). Radiation induced chromosome aberrations in *Tradescantia*. *In* "Radiation Biology" (A. Hollaender, ed.), Chapter 10. McGraw-Hill, New York.

Giles, N. H., Jr., and Riley, H. P. (1949). The effect of oxygen on the frequency of x ray-induced chromosomal rearrangements in *Tradescantia* microspores. *Proc. Natl. Acad. Sci. U.S.A.* **35**, 640–646.

Giles, N. H., Jr., and Riley, H. P. (1950). Studies on the mechanism of the oxygen effect on the radiosensitivity of *Tradescantia* microspores. *Proc. Natl. Acad. Sci. U.S.A.* **36**, 337–344.

Kaufmann, B. P. (1954). Chromosome aberrations induced in animal cells by ionizing radiation. *In* "Radiation Biology" (A. Hollaender, ed.), Chapter 9. McGraw-Hill, New York.

Kirby-Smith, J. S. (1963). Effects of combined uv and x radiation on chromosome breakage in *Tradescantia* pollen. *In* "Radiation-Induced Chromosome Aberrations" (S. Wolff, ed.), pp. 203–214. Columbia Univ. Press, New York.

Kirby-Smith, J. S., and Swanson, C. P. (1954). The effects of fast neutrons from a nuclear detonation on chromosome breakage in *Tradescantia*. *Science* **119**, 42–45.

Kotval, J. P., and Gray, L. H. (1947). Structural changes produced in microspores of *Tradescantia* by alpha radiation. *J. Genet.* **48**, 135–154.

Lea, D. E. (1947). "Actions of Radiations on Living Cells," Chapters 6 and 7. Cambridge Univ. Press, London and New York.

Mortimer, R. K. (1958). Radiobiological and genetic studies on a polyploid series (haploid to hexaploid) of *Saccharomyces cerevisiae*. *Radiat. Res.* **9**, 312–326.

Mortimer, R. K., and von Borstel, R. C. (1963). Radiation-induced dominant lethality in haploid and diploid sperm of the wasp *Mormoniella*. *Genetics* **48**, 1545–1549.

Okada, S. (1970). "Radiation Biochemistry," Vol. I. Academic Press, New York.

Ostergren, G., and Wakonig, T. (1954). True or apparent subchromatid breakage and the induction of labile states in cytological chromosome loci. *Bot. Not.* **4**, 357–375.

Revell, S. H. (1963). Chromatid aberrations—the generalized theory. *In* "Radiation-Induced Chromosome Aberrations" (S. Wolff, ed.), pp. 41–86. Columbia Univ. Press, New York.

Revell, S. H. (1974). The breakage-and-reunion theory for chromosomal aberrations induced by ionizing radiations: A short history. *Adv. Radiat. Biol.* **4**, 367–416.

Roberts, P. A. (1969). Some components of x ray induced crossing over in females of *Drosophila melanogaster*. *Genetics* **63**, 387–404.

Sax, K. (1941). Types and frequencies of chromosomal aberrations induced by x rays. *Cold Spring Harbor Symp. Quant. Biol.* **9**, 93–101.

Sax, K. (1950). The effects of x rays on chromosome structure. *J. Cell. Comp. Physiol.* **35**, Suppl. 1, 71–82.

Sax, K., and Swanson, C. P. (1941). Differential sensitivity of cells to x ray. *Am. J. Bot.* **28**, 52–59.

Schwartz, D. (1952). The effect of oxygen concentration on x-ray induced chromosome breakage in maize. *Proc. Natl. Acad. Sci. U.S.A.* **38**, 490–494.

Sparrow, A. H. (1951). Radiation sensitivity of cells during mitotic and meiotic cycles with emphasis on possible cytochemical changes. *Ann. N.Y. Acad. Sci.* **51,** 1508–1540.

Sparrow, A. H., Moses, M. J., and Dubow, R. J. (1952). Relationships between ionizing radiation, chromosome breakage and certain other nuclear disturbances. *Exp. Cell Res., Suppl. 2,* **3,** 255–267.

Sparrow, A. H., Schairer, L. A., and Sparrow, R. C. (1963). Relationship between nuclear volumes, chromosome numbers and relative radiosensitivities. *Science* **141,** 163–166.

Stauffer, H. H. (1972). The effect of oxygen on the frequency of somatic recombination in *Drosophila melanogaster. Genetics* **72,** 277–291.

Swanson, C. P. (1944). X-ray and ultraviolet studies on pollen tube chromosomes. I. The effect of ultraviolet on x-ray induced chromosomal aberrations. *Genetics* **29,** 61–68.

Swanson, C. P. (1955). The oxygen effect on chromosome breakage. *J. Cell. Comp. Physiol.* **45,** Suppl. 2, 285–298.

Swanson, C. P. (1957). "Cytology and Cytogenetics." Prentice-Hall, Englewood Cliffs, New Jersey.

Thoday, J. M., and Read, J. M. (1947). Effect of oxygen on the frequency of chromosome aberrations produced by x rays. *Nature (London)* **160,** 608.

Thoday, J. M., and Read, J. M. (1949). Effect of oxygen on the frequency of chromosome aberrations produced by alpha-rays. *Nature (London)* **163,** 133–134.

Waldren, C. A., and Johnson, R. T. (1974). Analysis of interphase chromosome damage by means of premature chromosome condensation after x- and ultraviolet irradiation. *Proc. Natl. Acad. Sci. U.S.A.* **71,** 1137–41.

Whiting, A. R. (1940). Sensitivity to x rays of different meiotic stages in unlaid eggs of *Habrobracon. J. Exp. Zool.* **83,** 249–269.

Whiting, A. R. (1945a). Effects of x rays on hatchability and on chromosomes of *Habrobracon* eggs treated in first meiotic prophase and metaphase. *Am. Nat.* **79,** 193–227.

Whiting, A. R. (1945b). Dominant lethality and correlated chromosome effect in *Habrobracon* eggs x rayed in diplotene and in late metaphase I. *Biol. Bull. (Woods Hole, Mass.)* **89,** 61–71.

Whittinghill, M. (1955). Crossover variability and induced crossing over. *J. Cell. Comp. Physiol.* **45,** Suppl. 2 189–220.

Williamson, J. H., Parker, D. R., and Manchester, W. G. (1970a). X-ray induced recombination in the fourth chromosome of *Drosophila melanogaster* females. I. Kinetics and brood patterns. *Mutat. Res.* **9,** 287–297.

Williamson, J. H., Parker, D. R., and Manchester, W. G. (1970b). II. Segregational properties of recombinant fourth chromosomes. *Mutat. Res.* **9,** 299–306.

Wolff, S. (1959). Interpretation of induced chromosome breakage and rejoining. *Radiat. Res., Suppl.* **1,** 453–462.

Wolff, S. (1965). Radiation effects as measured by chromosome damage. *In* "Cellular Radiation Biology," pp. 167–179. Williams & Wilkins, Baltimore, Maryland.

Wolff, S., and Atwood K. C. (1954). Independent x-ray effects on chromosome breakage and reunion. *Proc. Natl. Acad. Sci. U.S.A.* **40,** 187–192.

Wolff, S., and Luippold, H. E. (1955). Metabolism and chromosome break rejoining. *Science* **122,** 231–232.

CHAPTER 6   Response of the Single Cell

The two previous chapters have described the effects of ionizing radiation on the various structures in the cell. Later chapters will be devoted to radiation effects in tissues. The study of the cell occupies an important middle position. It allows for the selection of the subcellular events that are relevant to the survival of the cell: i.e., those that occur in the dose range where cells are killed and under the biochemical conditions that exist in the cell. Also, the study of cell sensitivity recorded for various physiological conditions is useful in predicting the response of certain tissues in which these conditions exist.

An important advancement in the understanding of the nature and of the severity of radiation damage to mammalian cells was accomplished by the introduction of several techniques to measure the survival of single cells. These techniques provided the opportunity, for the first time, to quantify the biological effects of radiation on a cellular basis. Previously, the biological effects of radiation were recorded on a more qualitative basis such as reddening of the skin or necrosis of tissue. The introduction of these techniques also hastened the understanding of the effects of various biological, chemical, and physical modifications on the survival of cells to radiation.

These techniques are limited to dividing or potentially dividing cells. Although this limitation may seem severe, the dividing cells of an organism are important because they comprise the stem-cell compartment and are more sensitive than the differentiated cells. In whole-body exposure to radiation, the ability of the stem cells to divide determines the life or death status of the individual. In addition, the dividing cells are the ones of interest in the treatment of mammalian tumors with radiation.

A further limitation of this chapter restricts the discussion to mammalian cells only. Since human cells respond generally like most other mammalian cells, much of the effort in the study of single cell response, involving mammalian cells, is directed toward human clinical application. Techniques for studying the response of single cells from other organisms such as plants and invertebrates are a more recent development. In some organisms such as insects, dividing cells constitute a less significant fraction of the tissue. Finally, the mammalian cell plays an important role in radiation biology not only in the study of the lethal response but also in such areas as mutagenesis and carcinogenesis.

In Vitro Studies of Cell Survival

Survival of cells after radiation is defined as their ability to undergo unlimited proliferation. In practice, this ability is measured as the formation of a colony from a single cell. These techniques are divided conveniently into the survival of cells to irradiation measured either *in vitro* or *in vivo*. Remarkably, the initial investigations of both were conducted at the same time with very similar results.

The *in vitro* determination was made possible by advances in cell culture techniques to allow for the growth of single cells. The colony formation assay was accomplished by Puck and Marcus for mammalian cells in 1956. The technique has not changed much since that time. Single cells are plated into a plate or flask containing a cell culture medium including a serum fraction. Different series of replicate plates are treated with a particular radiation dose. The survival is measured by scoring the number of single cells that develop colonies. Since some unirradiated cells fail to form colonies, a correction has to be made in terms of the plating efficiency. Thus survival is calculated by:

$$S = \frac{\text{number of colonies formed}}{\text{number of single cells plated} \times (PE)c}$$

where $(PE)c$ is the number of colonies formed per number of single cells plated without irradiation. A simplified example showing only one plate for control and 500 rad is given in Figure 6.1. In practice, it is difficult to obtain pure single-cell populations so a correction is made generally for higher multiplicities (average number of cells per group at the time of irradiation).

The initial results of Puck and Marcus with HeLa cells have been verified by scores of investigators using an equal number of cell types *in vitro*. All the survival curves share certain basic characteristics. At low doses up to 200 rad, the slope of the curve is zero or near zero. After a certain point then survival decreases exponentially with a linear increase in dose (Figure 6.2).

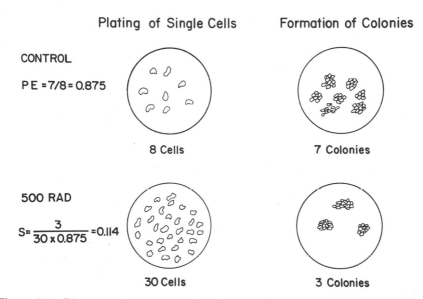

Figure 6.1. Diagrammatic representation of colony-forming assay *in vitro*. In reality, only colonies with more than 50 cells are scored as viable.

The shape and parameters of the curve are obtained from target theory (see Chapter 2). The slope of the exponential portion of the curve is given in terms of D_0, the dose to give an average of one hit per target and thereby to reduce survival to 0.37 of any survival level on the exponential portion of the curve. The shoulder region of the curve at low doses suggests that the cells have the ability to accumulate sublethal damage before additional radiation causes the sublethal damage to become lethal. In terms of target theory, the shoulder region is indicative of either several targets in the cell which must be inactivated or target(s) which must be hit several times to kill the cell. The exponential portion of the curve can be extrapolated to zero dose to obtain the extrapolation number n. Puck and Marcus found the extrapolation number equal to 2. From target theory, this extrapolation would imply the existence of two targets. However, subsequent work has shown this number to be highly variable.

Another useful term to describe the shape of survival curve is D_q, the dose in rad where the exponential portion of the curve intercepts 100% survival. D_q is a convenient number since it measures the shoulder width in rad, not a unitless number like the extrapolation number n. The importance of this term will be demonstrated in the section on

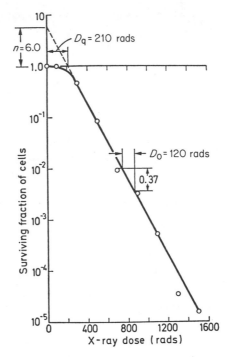

Figure 6.2. Dose response survival curve for Chinese hamster (CHO) cells irradiated with 220 kV x rays. (From Tolmach and Hopwood, 1974; courtesy of authors and Springer Verlag.)

repair of sublethal damage. Most D_q values are in the range of 50–250 rads for acute doses of x irradiation to well-oxygenated cells. The three parameters are related from derivation of multitarget theory:

$$D_q = D_0 \ln n$$

A comparison of many cell lines from different species shows little variation in these parameters, even between those of normal and of tumor cells (see Okada, 1969). The variation seen for D_0 values (70–200 rad) among different cell types is similar to the variation seen for one cell type among different laboratories. This uniformity in the sensitivity of different cell types to irradiation differs from their sensitivity to chemicals where the specificity is more cell-type dependent in comparison with that produced from the random nature of irradiation.

In a comparison with other organisms, mammalian cells seem far more sensitive. However in terms of target theory, the size of the nucleus or the amount of DNA would necessitate a much smaller dose.

The disparity between the actual D_0 and that predicted by target theory is greatest for mammalian cells and decreases as one examines simpler organisms. One obvious suggestion is that the entire nucleus is not involved in lethal damage. Much effort has been devoted to delineating the critical target(s) whose inactivation is lethal to the cell.

In Vivo Studies

In contrast to the singular mode of determining cell survival to irradiation *in vitro*, the ascertainment of cell survival *in vivo* to irradiation is as complex as the variety of cells being measured. A technique for measuring the survival of tumor cells was developed by Hewitt and Wilson in 1959. At the same time, Till and McCulloch published a report for the survival of normal bone-marrow cells. More recently, Withers has developed a system for measuring the survival of two important normal cell types, the stem cells of the skin and jejunum. Techniques are also being developed to measure the survival of normal tissue such as bone, muscle, and cartilage, but these are not a direct measure of single-cell survival.

Hewitt and Wilson (1959) utilized the ability of leukemia cells to form tumors as the measure of unlimited proliferation. Lymphocytic leukemia cells were isolated and a cell suspension prepared. A range of cell numbers was injected into the peritoneal cavity of mice and the number of mice developing tumors was recorded. A single unirradiated cell was usually not enough to form a tumor in all animals. The number of cells required to produce tumors in 50% of the hosts is called the TD_{50}. Hewitt and Wilson (1961) found a TD_{50} of two cells for lymphocytic leukemia and 85 for a solid sarcoma. Several conditions are responsible for the lack of complete cellular tumorigenicity: trauma to the cell in the isolation and injection, contamination of tumor cells with normal cells, a certain amount of death associated with a growing population of cells, and different degrees of tumorigenicity and differentiation. The importance of the host's immune response generated against certain tumor cells is indicated by the change in the TD_{50} for hosts at different ages during which the immune capability varies.

The radiation sensitivity of cells was determined by irradiating them before or after isolation from the donor and injecting an appropriate number into the host. Naturally as the radiation dose increases, the number of cells injected must also increase to maintain the necessary number of viable tumor cells. Survival is determined for each dose from the relationship:

$$S = \frac{\text{TD}_{50} \text{ of control}}{\text{TD}_{50} \text{ of irradiated dose}}$$

Since the TD_{50} value is best obtained by injecting a range of cells that will produce both a low and a high fraction of animals with tumors, the *in vivo* method obviously requires greater time and expense than the *in vitro* one. The first survival determination of Hewitt and Wilson and the subsequent ones confirmed the validity of the in vitro methods: the survival parameters were within the range of the early *in vitro* ones (D_0 of 150 rad for leukemic cells).

Even though the *in vitro* determination of cell survival by Puck and Marcus agreed with the *in vivo* determination by Hewitt and Wilson, both these investigations involved tumor cells. The spleen colony assay of McCulloch and Till (1960) provided the first measure of non-tumor-cell survival.

In their initial experiments, they utilized the ability of nucleated isologous bone-marrow cells to rescue lethally irradiated hosts. About 10^6 bone-marrow cells were required to rescue 50% of the hosts irradiated with 950 rad; fewer cells rescued fewer hosts. To determine radiation survival, 10^6 cells were irradiated with a given dose. Since there were fewer cells remaining to rescue the host, the fraction of surviving hosts decreased. This surviving fraction of hosts could be related to the number of unirradiated bone-marrow cells to produce equivalent rescue. For example, the rescue of 5% of the hosts required 8.5×10^4 unirradiated cells and 10^6 irradiated ones. Thus the surviving fraction of bone marrow cells would be $8.5 \times 10^4/10^6$ or 0.085. In this manner, Till and McCulloch generated a survival curve with an average D_0 of 105 rad for two strains of mice.

Because the actual data obtained by this technique were highly variable, Till and McCulloch (1961) introduced a modification in which the survival of nucleated bone-marrow cells was measured as the ability to form nodules in the spleen of lethally irradiated hosts. The hosts were sacrificed on the tenth or eleventh day and the number of nodules in the spleen quantified. About 10^4 bone-marrow cells were required to produce one nodule which consisted of erythroblasts, granulocytes and megakaryocytes. The large number of bone-marrow cells necessary to form one nodule was attributed to two factors: some cells were differentiated to the extent that the limited number of divisions were not enough to form nodules, and not all cells found their way to the spleen. As the irradiation dose was increased, larger numbers of cells were injected to maintain the numbers of nodules per spleen between 5 and 20. Survival for a given irradiation dose was calculated as:

$$S = \frac{\text{nodules}_x \text{ per cells}_x}{\text{nodules}_c \text{ per cells}_c}$$

For a 500-rad dose typical numbers were:

$$S = \frac{10/10^6}{10/10^5} = 0.10$$

With this technique, Till and McCulloch obtained survival curves with a D_0 of 115 rad and extrapolation number of 2. The survival of the bone-marrow cells did not vary significantly when the irradiation was performed under several conditions: before isolation from the donor, after isolation in the test tube, or after transplantation into the host (McCulloch and Till, 1962).

A more recent innovation in the measurement of normal cell response was introduced by Withers for stem cells of the skin and jejunum. This technique involves the use of irradiation to reduce the dividing stem cell population to a number which is small enough to allow the discernment of a nodule evolving from a single stem cell after 10 to 20 days postirradiation. In the skin assay (Withers, 1967), a ring of defined size is protected with a lead or steel shield. The size of the center circle determines the magnitude of the test dose: the smaller areas (smallest was 398 microns in diameter) will contain the fewer stem cells and can be used to produce a few nodules for low radiation doses. The larger areas (maximum of 1.2 cm) will contain more stem cells and therefore can be used to measure survival for higher doses. Since the density of stem cells in even the smallest area is too great to permit the determination of the number in the unirradiated tissue, the ordinate of the survival curve does not measure absolute survival. Instead the number of surviving cells per cm^2 is recorded; thus, the D_0, not the extrapolation number (n), can be determined. For the skin assay, the D_0 was 135 rad. Using a similar technique for the jejunum in which the jejunum was exteriorized and a test segment produced by sterilizing cells on both sides (Figure 6.3), Withers and Elkind (1969) recorded a D_0 of 97 rad. Again, these values for cells from normal tissue irradiated and assayed *in vivo* were in agreement with the values obtained from other *in vitro* and *in vivo* techniques.

Dependence on Radiation Quality

The Relative Biological Effectiveness (RBE) for different forms of radiation and Oxygen Enhancement Ratio (OER) for different oxygen

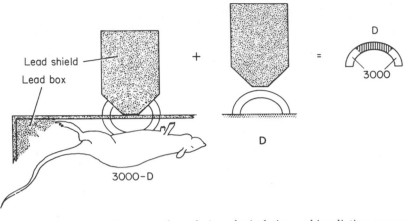

Figure 6.3. A diagram illustrating the technique for isolating and irradiating a segment of mouse jejunum. (From Withers and Elkind, 1969; courtesy of authors and Academic Press, Inc.)

concentrations and their dependence on Linear Energy Transfer (LET) are closely related in that the indirect action of radiation is involved in the understanding of each. As the density of ionization increases (given in terms of keV/μm for the loss of energy per unit distance), the radicals formed from the ionization of water (H$\cdot$,OH$\cdot$) increase their concentration to the extent that they recombine with themselves before they can recombine with oxygen or biologically significant molecules. This also means the contribution from indirect action decreases and the importance of direct action increases. The absence of indirect action lessens the multihit type of interactions, where two hits combine to form a lethal event. Thus the cell cannot accumulate sublethal damage at higher LET, and radiation becomes more effective since the shoulder region of the survival curve disappears. In addition, target theory predicts that if multiple hits per target are necessary to inactivate that target, the RBE should increase to a point where the number of hits per target is optimal and then decrease as a result of the overkill phenomenon (Figure 6.4). Experimentally, this prediction is verified for mammalian cells.

Relative Biological Effectiveness (RBE)

Although the term RBE can be applied to a variety of radiobiological endpoints, its definition and method of determination remain constant. The RBE is given as a ratio of doses from different radiation sources to produce a common effect. Since x rays were discovered first and were

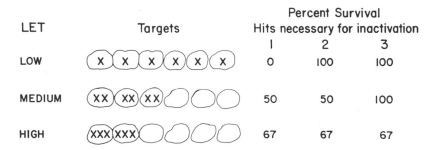

LET	Targets	Percent Survival Hits necessary for inactivation		
		1	2	3
LOW	X X X X X X	0	100	100
MEDIUM	XX XX XX	50	50	100
HIGH	XXX XXX	67	67	67

Figure 6.4. A diagram demonstrating the interaction of radiations of different LET values with several targets. Note that if two hits per target are necessary for its inactivation, the survival is higher for high LET compared to medium LET.

most readily available, they were used as the basis for comparison. This selection turned out to be fortuitous since the RBE is relatively constant in the x- and γ-ray region. RBE is determined from the following equation:

RBE = absorbed dose (rad) from 250 kV x rays to produce a certain effect/absorbed dose (rad) from another radiation to produce the same effect

It is also important to note that the absorbed dose is used and thus the differential penetration properties of various energies do not influence the RBE calculation.

A typical RBE calculation for neutron irradiation is shown in Figure 6.5. Notice that the ratio of doses for a common effect, not the ratio of effects for common doses, is used in the calculation. The latter will produce a quite different result than the former. An examination of the individual survival curves will show a major loss of the shoulder with the higher-LET irradiation..Thus the value of RBE must change with survival level, from a high value at high survival to a low value at low survival.

The RBE can be measured for several endpoints: survival of cells, chromosomal aberrations, mutations, etc. Although the actual curves for the responses as a function of the dose may vary in shape, the pattern for RBE variations with LET is quite similar for the various endpoints.

When a constant endpoint such as a particular survival level is selected for a variety of radiation types, the relationship in Figure 6.6 is formed. The RBE increases with LET to a certain point (~ 100 keV/μm) and then decreases abruptly. Based on target theory, this pattern can be explained by the necessity of inactivating one or more targets several

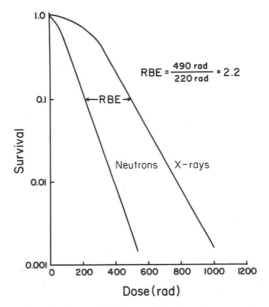

Figure 6.5. A typical survival curve for the inactivation of mammalian cells by neutrons and x rays. The RBE value is defined for a particular survival level.

times. The more densely ionizing radiation is more effective to a certain point, beyond which the energy is wasted and the RBE decreases (Figure 6.4). The relationship in tissue is even more complex with charged particles, since the LET varies with the depth of penetration (Raju *et al.*, 1976).

The term RBE is related to the term Quality Factor (QF) used in health physics for protection standards in that both attempt to equalize the various forms of radiation. However the RBE does so for a biological endpoint; it varies tremendously depending on the endpoint and the radiation conditions. On the other hand, QF is assigned a number based on physical considerations.

Oxygen Effect

The term *oxygen effect* refers to the increased sensitivity of cells to radiation in the presence of oxygen. Since most systems in the presence of low concentrations of O_2 respond to radiation as though they are fully oxygenated (Figure 5.7) and since higher-LET radiations result in increased sensitivity whether O_2 is present or not, perhaps the effect could more properly be called the hypoxic effect.

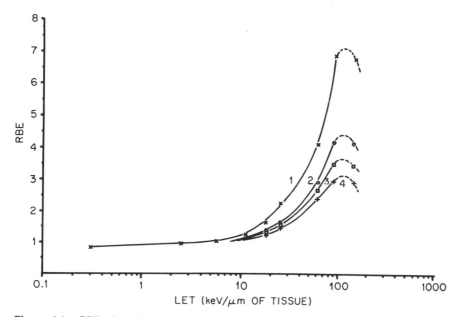

Figure 6.6. RBE values for survival of human cells to irradiations of different LET values produced from α particles, deutrons, x rays and β particles. The different curves correspond to different survival levels with curve 1 being the highest. (From Barendsen *et al.*, 1963; courtesy of authors and Academic Press, Inc.)

In any case, for low-LET irradiation the biological effect is greatest when O_2 is present. Although the shapes of the survival curves in the presence and absence of O_2 differ in some reports, most show a similarity of shape under both conditions. If the extrapolation numbers are identical, the radiation dose on the abscissa of the hypoxic curve can be divided by a constant number, the OER, to make it coincide with the oxic curve (Figure 6.7). Therefore O_2 is said to be dose-modifying and the OER does not vary with the endpoint. OER is defined as the ratio of doses under two O_2 conditions, one of which is usually fully oxygenated or anoxic.

As mentioned earlier, the OER varies with LET. Since oxygen affects the indirect action and the indirect action becomes minimal at high LET, the OER then equals 1; i.e., the sensitivity is independent of the O_2 concentration.

The increased sensitivity of cells in the presence of oxygen occurs at such low concentrations in mammalian cells that the instances where decreased sensitivity results from hypoxia are limited. While certain tissues such as skin may contain some hypoxic cells, the prime example

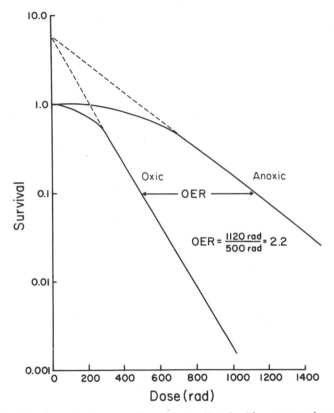

Figure 6.7. The survival of mammalian cells irradiated with x rays under anoxic and oxic conditions. If the curves have the same extrapolation number, the OER value is constant for any survival level.

of hypoxia appears in cells from regions of tumors distant from a capillary. Since the growth of the tumor is rapid and somewhat disorganized with respect to the blood supply, certain sections of the tumor become hypoxic as the tumor grows. The distance from the region of hypoxic cells to the capillary was estimated by Thomlinson and Gray (1955) to be 100 μm based on the diffusion and the utilization of oxygen. The appearance of necrotic cells (presumably a result of hypoxia) at this distance from capillaries in histological sections seems to confirm their estimate. However, the chronically hypoxic cells which become necrotic are of little concern in a radiobiological sense; the hypoxic cells which remain clonogenic are more important. Using a transplantable mouse lymphosarcoma and the TD_{50} assay, Powers and Tolmach (1963) first demonstrated the existence of clonogenic hypoxic cells in a biphasic survival curve (Figure 6.8). The ratio of the D_0 values for the two slopes was 2.5 and the more resistant slope extrapolated to 1%. They concluded that the more resistant population represented the hypoxic fraction of 1%. The existence of hypoxic cells in human tumors is suggested from the experimental animal tumor results and from the histology of human tumors.

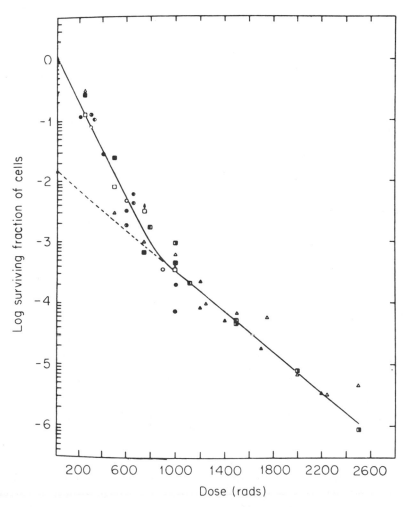

Figure 6.8. The x-ray survival curve for mouse lymphosarcoma cells irradiated *in vivo*. The biphasic curve results from populations of cells with different oxygen levels. (From Powers and Tolmach, 1963; courtesy of authors and MacMillan Journals Ltd.)

Repair of Sublethal Damage

The shape of the survival curve for low-LET irradiation (shoulder region followed by exponential portion) suggested to some radiobiologists that not all the lesions at low doses led to lethality. Apparently the cells accumulated "sublethal" damage until the targets became saturated, and then any further dosage was lethal. This hypothesis agreed well with multitarget theory, which predicted a shoulder region as the radiation dose led to inactivation of a number of targets until the lethal limit was surpassed.

If some of the sublethal lesions could be repaired before additional ones caused lethality, survival would be enhanced. The repair of sublethal damage was demonstrated by Elkind and Sutton (1959) with split dose experiments. After administering a dose of approximately 500 rad to V79 cells, they gave a series of doses at various times after the first dose (Figure 6.9). By 18 hr the shoulder of the survival curve had returned almost to its original value. If complete repair was accomplished, the survival from the two doses would be the product of the survival from each dose ($0.095 \times 0.082 = 0.0078$). If no repair took place, the survival for the two doses would be equal to that produced from the sum of the two doses on the single dose survival curve (0.00186). A plot of survival versus time between two constant doses reveals the extent and kinetics of repair. The majority of the sublethal damage is repaired in a few hours. The dip in the curve at 4 to 5 hr is a result of redistribution of cells in the cell cycle (see later section). The repair of sublethal damage has been demonstrated for almost all mammalian cells subjected to low-LET irradiation.

An advantageous situation in the radiation treatment of tumors would be to have greater or faster repair of sublethal damage in normal cells compared to tumor cells. Unfortunately although some normal cells appear to provide substantial sublethal repair, the situation is not universal enough to exploit it (Withers, 1975).

Inhibition of Sublethal Damage Repair

As the LET of the radiation increases, the shoulder region diminishes. More of the damage is caused by direct single-hit mechanisms. Thus if sublethal damage does not exist, fractionation of the dose should not lead to increased survival. Barendsen (1962) showed that fractionation of two doses of alpha particles by 12 hr did not produce survival different from that of a single dose.

For low-LET irradiation, various chemical and physical agents can inhibit both the accumulation and repair of sublethal damage. The former is demonstrated by the elimination of the shoulder region on the survival curve for single dose irradiation and the latter by the elimination of increased survival when the agent is present during the time between the doses. Many agents present at the time of irradiation produce a certain amount of killing which reduces survival to a point equivalent to the exponential portion of the curve. Thus when irradiation is given in the presence of the agent, the absence of a shoulder region on the radiation survival curve does not necessarily imply an inhibition in the accumulation of radiation sublethal lesions but more possibly an additive or synergistic effect between the lesions produced by the two agents.

The more easily interpreted experiments involve the use of various agents between doses. The work of Elkind (Elkind et al., 1967) and others has demonstrated the resistance of sublethal repair to inhibition. Inhibitors of DNA and protein synthesis do not prevent repair. Actinomycin D does inhibit but its action appears to be independent of its effect on RNA synthesis and more related to its binding to DNA. The weight of this evidence suggests that the repair of sublethal damage can be attributed to some preexisting repair molecules acting upon the DNA damage.

Another interesting situation is the influence of oxygen concentration on both the accumulation and repair of sublethal damage. The former has been discussed in a previous section: most reports indicate the ability to accumulate sublethal damage in the absence of oxygen. The concentration of oxygen needed to inhibit repair might be quite different than that needed to affect survival of cells to a single dose. The latter involves a chemical effect: enough O_2 enhances the production of radical products. The former may involve a biochemical enzymatic reaction: a low enough oxygen level may inhibit repair enzymes. Indeed drastic measures have been required to produce levels of hypoxia low enough to show inhibition of repair of sublethal damage: either multiple changes of ultrapure gases (Koch et al., 1973) or the respiration of O_2 by cells in a closed system (Hall et al., 1974). Both methods produce O_2 concentrations lower than that required to show the oxygen effect. Koch's work best demonstrates this difference since he has used well-defined oxygen concentrations. For moderately hypoxic cells (0.2 μM O_2) and extremely hypoxic cells (<0.025 μM O_2) an OER of 3.0 was obtained for both concentrations. However, the moderately hypoxic cells were slowed only minimally in their repair of sublethal damage while the extremely hypoxic cells showed no recovery (Koch et al.,

1973). Thus in fractionated doses, the absence of O_2 works in both directions: it protects the cells during irradiation and sensitizes them by inhibiting repair between doses.

In addition to the oxygen concentration affecting survival during fractionated doses, the converse is also true for cells in tumors: survival during fractionated doses affects the oxygen concentration. Although the oxygen concentration *per se* is not measured, the fraction of cells with low enough oxygen to appear hypoxic is recorded by the Powers and Tolmach method (1963). Since the oxygenated cells are more sensitive, an initial dose should preferentially kill them and thereby increase the fraction of hypoxic cells. In fact, the fraction of hypoxic cells in experimental tumors remains rather constant with fractionated doses (Van Putten and Kallman, 1968); thus reoxygenation must occur between doses. The effect of radiation in killing cells and in reducing oxygen metabolism in the remaining cells provides the opportunity for the hypoxic cells to acquire enough oxygen to respond to subsequent doses as oxygenated cells.

Low Dose Rate

A logical extension of fractionation investigations leads to the study of low dose-rate irradiation. Low dose-rate irradiation (typically less than 50 rad/min down to 0.2 rad/min) can be thought of as many small fractionated doses separated by short times. This consideration is valid only if the repair of sublethal damage can occur while the irradiation is continuous. A somewhat intermediate situation appears to be the case. As the dose rate is decreased, higher survival results as if the exponential portion of the survival curve were composed of minishoulders. The initial investigations of Bedford and Hall (1963) with HeLa cells showed an increase in the D_0 value for doses from 100 rad/min to 1 rad/min, and a decrease in the extrapolation number to 1.0 at 1 rad/min. Below 1 rad/min, no further increase in survival occurred. The absence of further repair probably results from a high-LET component of low-LET irradiation; i.e., there is a certain probability that several sparsely ionizing events will occur close enough in time and space to be lethal before any repair can take place (Kellerer and Rossi, 1972). More recent investigations have shown that the ability to repair sublethal damage during continuous low dose-rate irradiation may vary (Fu *et al.*, 1975). Indeed, the response of bone-marrow stem cells changes very little with dose rate.

Potentially Lethal Damage

Finally, one other area that must be considered in any discussion of repair of radiation damage is the phenomenon of repair of "potentially lethal" damage. The fixation and repair of this damage depend on the metabolic state of the cell before and after irradiation (Phillips and Tolmach, 1966). Such conditions as temperature changes, inhibition of DNA, RNA, and protein synthesis, and density inhibition of growth will influence survival compared to a "normal" exponential cell state. Some conditions such as 20°C postirradiation incubation favor repair over fixation and thus increase survival; others such as inhibition of DNA synthesis favor fixation over repair. The relationship between sublethal and potentially lethal damage is not too difficult to understand operationally. The study of sublethal damage repair involves fraction-ated doses and is evidenced by change in the shoulder region while the study of potentially lethal damage involves a single dose and modified metabolism and a change predominantly in slope. On a molecular level, the relationship between the two lesions is not at all clear (Winans *et al.*, 1972).

Cell Cycle

Since the discovery of the cell cycle by Howard and Pelc (1953) and the demonstration of a means to synchronize cells at a certain point in the cycle by Terasima and Tolmach (1961), much effort has been ex-pended in determining the variation of sensitivity to irradiation during the cell cycle and the cause of the variation. The cell cycle of rapidly dividing cells contains four phases: M, G_1, S, G_2. Mitoses can be deter-mined visually by the rounding process, formation of metaphase plate, and cytokinesis; S phase is located by the replication of DNA as shown by labeled precursor uptake. Although G_1 and G_2 initially stood for "Gap" 1 and 2, which implies absence of any activity, it is now appar-ent that tremendous activity proceeds in preparation for S and M phases. Although the variation in radiation sensitivity during the cell cycle is not totally consistent among different cell types, a general pattern emerges: The most sensitive phases are M and the G_1/S transi-tion; the most resistant is late S phase (Figure 6.10). For cells with long G_1 phases, an additional resistant peak appears in mid G_1 phase.

An explanation for the variation of sensitivity during the cell cycle is still elusive. Several processes show a cell cycle variation consistent with a mechanism for cell killing: repair of single strand breaks, and protection by intracellular nonprotein sulfhydryl compounds are two prominent ones.

Although attempts have been made to exploit cell cycle differences between normal and tumor cells in cancer therapy and to enhance differences by synchronization, the importance of cell cycle differences is exemplified in multiple dose exposures, including mixtures of radiation and chemotherapeutic agents. The initial dose kills preferentially the more sensitive cells in the cycle and leaves the more resistant cells. As these more resistant cells progress through the cell cycle before the

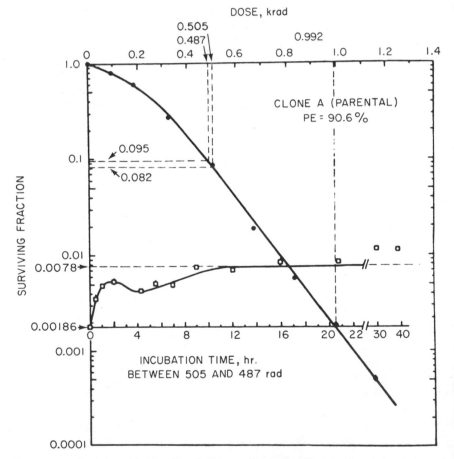

Figure 6.9. Recovery of x-irradiated Chinese hamster cells as a function of time of incubation at 37°C between two doses. (From Elkind and Sutton, 1959; courtesy of authors and MacMillan Journals Ltd.)

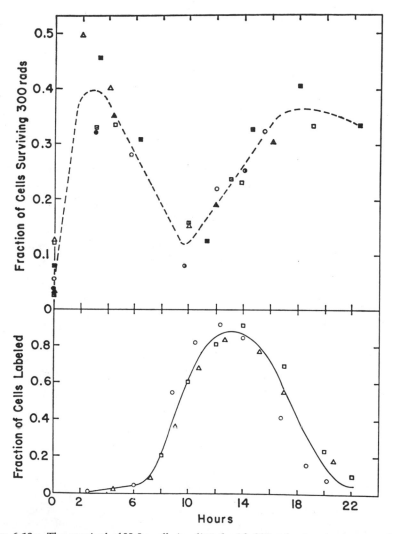

Figure 6.10. The survival of HeLa cells irradiated with 300 rads at various stages of the cell cycle. The lower curve, showing the fraction of cells labeled with the DNA precursor ³H-thymidine, shows the corresponding stages of the cell cycle following mitotic synchronization. (From Terasima and Tolmach, 1963; courtesy of authors and the Rockefeller University Press.)

next dose, in a few hours they must go into a more sensitive phase: e.g., late S into M phase. Thus a second dose of irradiation at that time will be more lethal than it would be to the initial asynchronous population. This "induced synchrony" explains the dip in survival when two radiation doses are separated by 4 to 6 hr (Figure 6.9). An even more complicated situation is the use of two agents with different cell cycle age responses.

Concluding Remarks

This chapter describes some of the recent efforts to understand radiation effects on a cellular level. The alterations in cell survival caused by changes in the physical, chemical, and biological environment have been outlined in a singular fashion. However, the cell is usually in an environment that has several of these factors existing simultaneously. For instance, the RBE for high LET irradiation can be calculated for fractionated doses or for hypoxic conditions in addition to single well-oxygenated exposures. Likewise, the cell cycle variation decreases with LET. Several texts are addressed more specifically to these problems (e.g., Hall, 1978).

Hopefully a better understanding of the interaction of these factors will lead to their manipulation to obtain better therapeutic results and less environmental hazards. The present knowledge is quite important in the explanation of the response of tissues and whole organisms to be described in later chapters.

References

Barendsen, G. W. (1962). Dose survival curves of human cells in tissue culture irradiated with alpha-, beta-, 20 kVx-, and 200 kVx-radiation. *Nature (London)* **193**, 1153–1155.

Barendsen, G. W., Walter, H. M. D., Fowler, J. F., and Bewley, D. K. (1963). Effects of different ionizing radiations on human cells in tissue culture. III. Experiments with cyclotron-accelerated alpha-particles and deuterons. *Radiat. Res.* **18**, 106–119.

Bedford, J. S., and Hall, E. J. (1963). Survival of HeLa cells cultured *in vitro* and exposed to protracted gamma irradiation. *Int. J. Radiat. Biol.* **7**, 377–383.

Elkind, M. M., and Sutton, H. (1959). X-ray damage and recovery in mammalian cells in culture. *Nature (London)* **184**, 1293–1295.

Elkind, M. M., Moses, W. B., and Sutton-Gilbert, H. (1967). Radiation response of mammalian cells grown in culture. VI. Protein, DNA and RNA inhibition during repair of x-ray damage. *Radiat. Res.* **31**, 156–173.

Fu, K. F., Phillips, T. L., Kane, L. J., and Smith, V. (1975). Tumor and normal tissue response in irradiation *in vivo*: Variation with decreasing dose rates. *Radiology* **114**, 709–716.

Hall, E. J. (1978). "Radiobiology for the Radiologist," 2d ed. Harper, New York.

Hall, E. J., Lehnert, S., and Roizin-Towle, L. (1974). Split-dose experiments with hypoxic cells. *Radiology* **112**, 425–430.

Hewitt, H. B., and Wilson, C. W. (1959). A survival curve for mammalian cells irradiated *in vivo*. *Nature (London)* **183**, 1060–1061.

Hewitt, H. B., and Wilson, C. W. (1961). Survival curves for tumor cells irradiated *in vivo*. *Ann. N.Y. Acad. Sci.* **95**, 818–827.

Howard, A., and Pelc, S. R. (1953). Synthesis of deoxyribonucleic acid in normal and irradiated cells and its relation to chromosome breakage. *Heredity, Suppl.* **6**, 261–273.

Kellerer, A. M., and Rossi, H. H. (1972). The theory of dual radiation action. *Curr. Top. Radiat. Res. Q.* **8**, 85–158.

Koch, C. J., Kruuv, J., and Frey, H. E. (1973). Variation in radiation response of mammalian cells as a function of oxygen tension. *Radiat. Res.* **53**, 33–42.

McCulloch, E. A., and Till, J. E. (1960). The radiation sensitivity of normal bone marrow cells, determined by quantitative marrow transplantation into irradiated mice. *Radiat. Res.* **13**, 115–125.

McCulloch, E. A., and Till, J. E. (1962). The sensitivity of cells from normal mouse bone marrow to gamma radiation *in vitro* and *in vivo*. *Radiat. Res.* **16**, 822–832.

Okada, S. (1969). "Radiation Biochemistry," Vol. 1, pp. 265–268. Academic Press, New York.

Phillips, R. A., and Tolmach, L. J. (1966). Repair of potentially lethal damage in x-irradiated HeLa cells. *Radiat. Res.* **29**, 413–432.

Powers, W. E., and Tolmach, L. J. (1963). A multicomponent x-ray survival curve for mouse lymphosarcoma cells irradiated *in vivo*. *Nature (London)* **197**, 710–711.

Puck, T. T., and Marcus, P. I. (1956). Action of x-rays on mammalian cells. *J. Exp. Med.* **103**, 653–666.

Raju, M. R., Blakely, E., Howard, J., Lyman, J. T., Kalofonos, D. P., Martins, B., and Yong, C. H. (1976). Human cell survival as a function of depth for a high-energy neon ion beam. *Radiat. Res.* **65**, 191–194.

Terasima, T., and Tolmach, L. J. (1961). Changes in x-ray sensitivity of HeLa cells during the division cycle. *Nature (London)* **190**, 1210–1211.

Terasima, T., and Tolmach, L. J. (1963). Variations in several responses of HeLa cells to x-irradiation during the division cycle. *Biophys. J.* **3**, 11–33.

Thomlinson, R. H., and Gray, L. H. (1955). The histological structure of some human lung cancers and the possible implications for radiotherapy. *Br. J. Cancer* **9**, 539–549.

Till, J. E., and McCulloch, E. A. (1961). A direct measurement of the radiation sensitivity of normal mouse bone marrow cells. *Radiat. Res.* **14**, 213–222.

Tolmach, L. J., and Hopwood, L. E. (1974). Radiation research: Survival kinetics. *Handb. Exp. Pharmakol.* **38**, 489–506.

Van Putten, L. M., and Kallman, R. F. (1968). Oxygenation status of a transplantable tumor during fractionated radiotherapy. *J. Natl. Cancer Inst.* **40**, 441–451.

Winans, L. F., Dewey, W. C., and Dettor, C. M. (1972). Repair of sublethal and potentially lethal x-ray damage in synchronous Chinese hamster cells. *Radiat. Res.* **52**, 333–351.

Withers, H. R. (1967). The dose-survival relationship for irradiation of epithelial cells of mouse skin. *Br. J. Radiol.* **40**, 187–194.

Withers, H. R. (1975). Lethal and sublethal cellular injury in multifraction irradiation. *Eur. J. Cancer* **11**, 581–583.

Withers, H. R., and Elkind, M. M. (1969). Radiosensitivity and fractionation response of crypt cells of mouse jejunum. *Radiat. Res.* **38**, 598–613.

CHAPTER 7   Localized Effects on
Genetic Loci

The experiments on chromosomal aberration have provided us with visible evidence that radiations can destroy organized structures of biological importance. Now attention is turned to events at a submicroscopic level. However, the seemingly simple term "gene mutation" poses semantic difficulties.

Both words have meant various things to different people. "Gene" has been used to refer to a unit of function, or to a unit of recombination, or to the smallest portion of the genetic code which can undergo detectable permanent change. When originally proposed in 1900 by de Vries, "mutation" had the inclusive meaning of all changes in the hereditary material capable of altering the individual phenotype, whether or not chromosomal aberration is involved. Subsequently, a much more restricted meaning has usually been implied, expressed in the term "point mutation." In this chapter we will consider this restricted sense.

In the narrow sense, mutation now refers to an alteration in the genetic code which can be localized to as small a change as a single nucleotide of the base sequence of a DNA molecule. Or it may involve an addition or subtraction of nucleotides. These base sequences (taken three at a time) specify the amino acid arrangements of the structural and functional proteins, which in turn determine the activities of cells and characteristics of organisms. Although defining mutation in the sense of the "structural" gene is consistent with the focus of the classic radiation experiments in eukaryotes, it oversimplifies the DNA content. Additional nucleotide sequences serve as controlling elements, specifiers of types of RNA, and spacers. Little is known about radiation damage to these regions of the DNA strands.

Historical

Attempts to induce genetic change were made early in the history of genetics. At some time or other every conceivable environmental influence or combination of modifications has been used. Quite likely the wing mutations obtained in 1911 after radium exposures of *Drosophila* by Morgan were of the induced type. However, the members of the Morgan group were well aware of the importance of genetic purity of the material used for such studies and were reluctant to accept any isolated example of heritable change as a case of induced mutation.

It was not until Muller published his x-ray studies in 1927 that a way to obtain repeatable results was presented. In addition to laboratory organisms, which provided large numbers of offspring in a short time, special techniques were required which eliminated human inadequacies in observation and kept the amount of work within feasible limits. This involved studying the lethal changes induced for all the loci of a chromosome. Compared with what would be involved in the study of induced change for a single locus, labor is reduced by a factor corresponding to the number of vulnerable loci on the chromosome, that is, in the order of hundreds. Instead of several million observations, several thousand may suffice. Furthermore, it seems reasonable to expect that the most common types of gene changes would be those likely to disturb development so drastically that mutant individuals die.

Stadler's convincing studies with plants (1928), which have certain advantages of their own, closely followed Muller's success with *Drosophila*. Subsequently, both lethal and visible point mutations have been induced by ionizing radiations in practically every type of living organism. It will be more orderly to consider these experiments by type of organism rather than in chronological order.

Microorganism Techniques

The majority of induced point mutations are recessive to the standard or wild-type condition. This is a major problem complicating the design of experiments with higher diploid organisms, but requiring no consideration with microorganisms in which the vegetative stage is haploid. Haploids with only one member of each pair of chromosomes have no place to carry alleles which would hinder or hide the expression of induced recessive mutations.

With viruses the characteristic damage to, or reaction by, the host is studied rather than the morphology of the organism itself. The shape, size, and appearance of the area of a bacterial plate cleared by bacteriophage is one example. Another is the application of plant virus to leaves of its specific host in order to assess the lesions produced. A popular approach has been to irradiate a strain in which the unchanged virus does not give local necrotic lesions. If lesions occur they imply a mutation to virulence. The lesions can be cut out to isolate the strain and test the permanence of change. With certain animal viruses the skin reaction after inoculation may be studied. With viruses lacking such an effect, a limit-dilution technique is employed along with inoculation into chick embyros.

Investigations with bacteria are somewhat more direct. Irradiated bacteria may be plated out and differences sought in size, color, and texture of the colony. Ability to grow in a particular medium is in itself useful even though growth may be normal, for by this approach loss of biosynthetic capacity can be detected for mutant strains. Isolates which fail to grow on the simplest (or minimal) media used by the standard type are suspected to be mutant. The addition of substances such as amino acids and vitamins to the basic medium enables the identification of what is necessary for growth. Further investigation of the related compounds in the metabolic scheme makes it possible to identify which specific link in a biosynthetic chain has been broken. Other ingenious techniques include the replica plate method in which velvet cloth pressed to the surface of a culture plate is used to produce replicas of the original on different selective media. The results from such research have been of as much interest to biochemists as to radiobiologists. Other traits such as antigenic makeup of the bacterium or susceptibility to phage have also been studied, but the appeal which results in intensive investigation has not been as great.

Experiments with Fungi

Production of enormous numbers of offspring within hours has a recognized advantage when relatively rare events like mutation are to be studied. However, the cytology of viral and bacterial reproduction is not exactly like that of higher organisms. We must turn to the fungi if we want an orthodox meiotic process as well as the advantages of microorganisms. *Neurospora crassa* has been the type used especially for mutagenic studies. Biochemical as well as morphological traits occur, yet each meiotic product can be identified, isolated, and studied. Since ascospores retain their exact order in the ascus, it is possible to determine from their positions the lineage of each and to assess whether heterozygous loci separated at the first or second meiotic division, or during mitosis in the ascus. This involves micromanipulation whereby ascospores are isolated and grown individually to determine their genetic constitution. Not only are genetic loci mapped but the kinetochore position is also demonstrated.

Neurospora was the original organism studied by a minimal medium technique. The wild type has simple requirements: water, sugar, salts, and the vitamin biotin. All other requirements can be produced by the organism itself unless it has mutated. For example, consider the study of one of the best-known series of gene controlled reactions, that leading to the synthesis of arginine. A number of mutant strains, which fail to grow unless the amino acid arginine or related compounds have been added to the basic medium, can be obtained by irradiation. Of seven strains used by Srb and Horowitz (1944), one grew only on arginine, two required either arginine or citrulline, and four grew on arginine, citrulline, or ornithine. As shown in Figure 7.1, such results can be

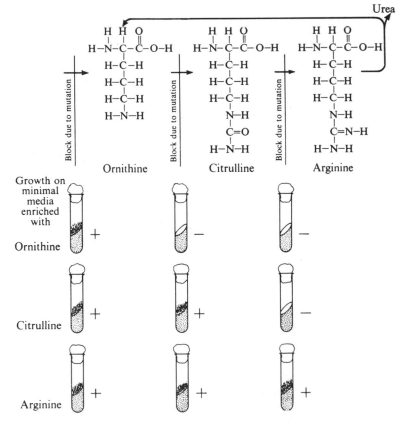

Figure 7.1. The ornithine cycle in *Neurospora*, based upon nutritional requirements of mutant strains. (Diagrammatic interpretation of the experiments of A. M. Srb and N. H. Horowitz, 1944.)

organized on the basis of genetic control of a series of stepwise reactions by which substances are synthesized in the organism. In well-investigated cases, an enzyme which represents the intermediate agency between the gene and the end product has been identified for early reactions. Such results led Beadle (1945) to popularize a one-gene–one-enzyme hypothesis, which was later modified to a one-primary-action hypothesis (Horowitz and Leupold, 1951) and finally refined to one-cistron–one-polypeptide specificity. Subsequently, de Serres (1958, 1964) studied the different types of alterations in the gene complex of the adenine-3 region. This along with other research revealed situations in which more than one gene may be involved in determining the translational product of gene action.

Mammalian Cell Culture Techniques

The principles employed for the detection and isolation of nutritionally deficient mutants in microbiology have been adapted to investigations with mammalian cell cultures. A heterogeneous cell population is placed on limiting medium in which nutritionally deficient types cannot grow, and an agent is applied which kills only the dividing cells (Kau and Puck, 1968). By this and related techniques, a variety of clones differing from the ancestral cell lines in biochemical abilities have been isolated (Chu *et al.*, 1969). However the emphasis has been on the chemical mutagens and the approach has not yet been fully exploited for radiation research.

Specific locus tests are being developed. The X-linked hypoxanthine-guanine phosphoribosyltransferase (*HGPRT*) locus of Chinese hamster cells, and the autosomal thymidine kinase (*TK*) locus of mouse lymphoma cells lend themselves to the detection and quantification of both forward and backward mutations.

Higher Organism Techniques

Except in cases like Hymenoptera where one sex is parthenogenetically produced and haploid, higher organisms, being diploid or even polyploid, pose more difficult technical problems for the investigator. In some forms self-fertilization is an advantage, although it has been employed routinely only in plants. With this ultimate degree of inbreeding, the problem becomes one of merely growing an F_2 of suitable size after irradiating seeds or flowers. In this way induced damage at all loci is under investigation.

With self-sterile or dioecious plants more elaborate means must be adopted, although the irradiation of pollen is a convenience so far as treatment is concerned. A method favored by Stadler (1928) was the detection of "A losses" in F_1 progenies produced by a cross aa by AA, the pollen of the male parent being x-rayed just before pollination. This approach is concerned with specific loci (Figure 7.2), and availability of the recessive allele is a necessity. Nevertheless in mice, Russell (1951) has used a stock with recessive alleles at seven loci, and one of the *Drosophila* stocks used by Fryer and Gowen (1942) included 12 recessives. Subsequently, Muller and associates developed the Maxy stock with 14 recessive loci and the Jynd stock with 15 recessive loci on the X chromosome (Muller and Oster, 1963). However, because of their incorporated inversions and marker genes the *Drosophila* stocks are even more complicated. In order to appreciate the traditional experimental approach in these insects we shall have to give them detailed attention.

Drosophila Techniques

Because the Y chromosome of flies carries nothing to hide expression of genetic determiners on the X chromosome, single generation experiments can be performed in which the mother is irradiated and her sons examined for alterations in sex-linked traits. Or alternately, and more elegantly, males are irradiated and mated to females from attached-X stock. In this case the sons get their Y chromosomes from the mother and the treated X from the father. However, it is easy to overlook a single mutant fly among a large group of male offspring, especially when the more drastic changes have been lethal and only flies with subtle modifications have survived.

Methods like Muller's *ClB* technique, diagrammed in Figure 7.3, give more reliable results to the average observer, although an additional generation is required. A sex-linked visible mutation will be shared by a group of males, whereas a sex-linked lethal would eliminate the group. Human error is reduced to a minimum by this approach which involves a stock incorporating suppression of crossing over (*C*), a recessive lethal (*l*), and a marker gene (*B*). These features enable the investigator to select for use the particular flies among the F_1 offspring which carry a treated X chromosome in heterozygous condition, yet he need not be concerned about viable gametes containing untreated chromosome regions obtained by crossover exchange with the homologous X.

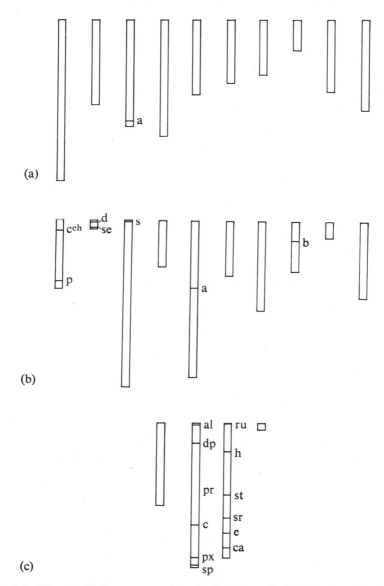

Figure 7.2. The specific locus approach to the detection of lethals involves the mainte-nance of stocks which can be employed in test crosses to reveal changes from the dominant form. Thus, only a very limited number of loci are studied and nothing is revealed concerning the response of thousands of other loci which occupy the blank areas of our diagrams of chromosomes. The gametic complement is diagrammed for corn and flies. Shown for the mouse are the best investigated linkage groups corresponding to 10 of the 20 pairs of mouse chromosomes. (a) Corn chromosomes with the *A* locus carrying the recessive allele (Stadler, 1954). (b) Mouse chromosomes with seven loci carrying recessive alleles (Russell, 1951). (c) Fly chromosomes with 12 loci carrying recessive alleles. (Fryer and Gowen, 1942.)

121

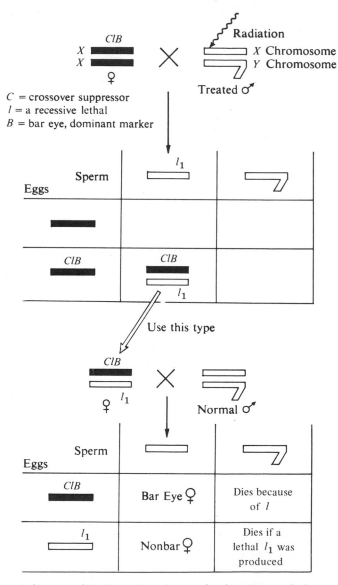

Figure 7.3. A diagram of Muller's *ClB* technique for detecting sex-linked recessive lethal mutations. Only the sex chromosomes are shown, but all loci on the X not influenced by the Y material are investigated.

Also the recessive lethal (*l*) routinely kills half the males in the generation to be scored. The other half die if a new lethal (l_1, l_2, l_3, . . . , l_n) is
induced at some other locus on the X chromosome exposed. In many
laboratories the Muller-5 technique has supplanted the *ClB* method.
The *Basc* stock, a designation referring to its content, is used. *B* again
stands for the dominant marker Bar eyes, *a* refers to a recessive apricot,
and *sc* represents a long inversion associated with changes in the scute
locus. In addition there is a moderate-sized inversion included within
the long one, all of which guard against the occurrence of crossover
offspring.

A scheme such as that developed by Child in the Amherst laboratory
(Figure 7.4) is necessary to study recessive mutation frequency in auto-
somes (Plough, 1941). This method involves a stock containing dominant markers for each chromosome and a crossover reducer in one
member of each pair. When mated to an irradiated stock, one exposed
chromosome of each pair can be isolated (generation 1), duplicated
(generation 2), and then brought into offspring from each parent (generation 3) to render loci homozygous. The absence of either or both the
homozygous classes among these offspring indicates the presence of a
lethal in either or both chromosomes. Unlike the X chromosome, which
is free of lethals in adult males, autosome experiments require stocks
which have been rendered free of lethals by a preliminary series of
matings. The typical stock carries accumulated autosomal lethals in
heterozygous condition.

Results from *Drosophila* Experiments

Muller detailed his classic x-ray experiments to the Sixth International Congress of Genetics in 1932. We can grasp the essential principles
from a simple tabulation:

X ray	Chromosomes tested	Lethals obtained	Proportion
None	6016	5	8.3×10^{-4}
24 min	741	59	796.2×10^{-4}
48 min	1177	143	1214.9×10^{-4}

The differences between the control and experimental values are too
large to be explained by chance. Therefore, lethal mutants are more
frequent in the progeny of flies exposed to x rays, and accordingly we

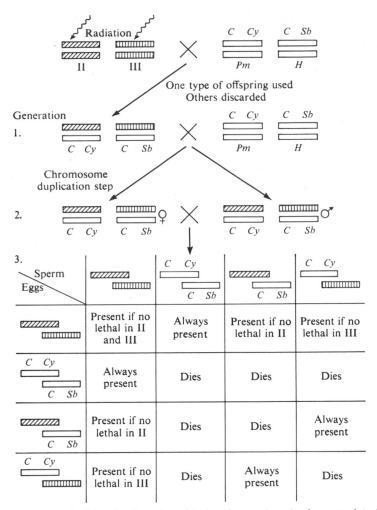

Figure 7.4. A method for the detection of induced mutations in the second and third chromosomes of *Drosophila*. It involves deriving flies homozygous for these chromosomes. *C* represents incorporated crossover suppression; the other symbols refer to dominant marker genes, lethal when homozygous.

concede x rays to be mutagenic. Note too that the higher the dose, the greater the mutational effect.

In the years following the original demonstration, much effort has been put into quantitative experiments (Timofeeff-Ressovsky, 1934). For a considerable period there was hope that this means would reveal the nature of the hypothetical gene unit, based in part upon determining the volume within which ionization causes genic change. More recently, as problems associated with the Atomic Age became apparent, quantitative studies have been performed for their own sake.

Experiments ranging over three decades, by a host of investigators, are interpreted to show (a) direct proportionality between the amount of radiation and the frequency of induced mutation; (b) no threshold below which irradiation is ineffective in producing mutations; and (c) effectiveness independent of the time required for delivery of a particular dose (Congress of the U.S., 1957). Let us consider each point in more detail.

Quantitative Aspects

Figure 7.5 presents data from two significant pioneering papers which revealed how induced genetic lethality increases in relation to

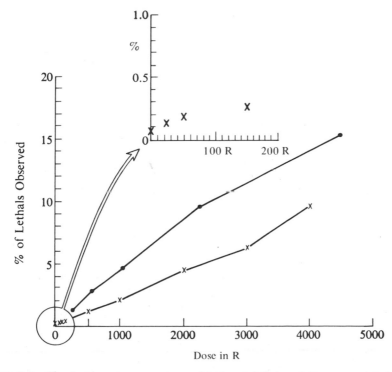

Figure 7.5. The increase in percentage of induced lethal mutations associated with increases in the x-ray dose delivered to male *Drosophila*. The dots plot Oliver's 1930 data obtained by *ClB* tests. The crosses represent values obtained by Spencer and Stern in 1948 using the Muller 5 technique and a stock chosen for its low control mutation rate.

radiation dose. Every increase in amount of radiation to which a chromosome is exposed results in a corresponding increase in mutation rate. Oliver's (1930) investigation was performed at Muller's suggestion. Years later, Spencer and Stern (1948) designed their experiments to test the validity of the linear roentgen dose per mutation frequency relation at low dosage. Until the latter paper, the lowest dose which had been considered was around 400 R. Experiments at low doses are laborious to perform and difficult to interpret because of "spontaneous" mutation which may occur in the absence of intentional radiation exposure. Recent utilization of tremendous sample sizes in bacterial experiments has enabled the study of doses amounting to only a few roentgen. Even with raw data the relationship is roughly linear. It may be improved by correcting for such things as the scoring of two or more lethals as a single lethal.

The study of point mutations following acute exposure to higher doses is complicated by the appreciable yield of chromosomal aberrations, of which many types are deleterious, even dominantly lethal. To minimize two-break phenomena and to allow the recovery of recessive lethals, a low dose rate may be necessary (Figure 7.6). Even at moderate doses, subtle types of lethals are demonstrable for which the yield

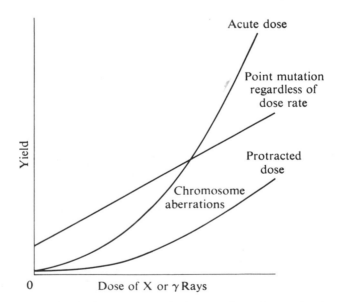

Figure 7.6. Generalized scheme showing both gross aberrations and point mutations. Note how the differences in the slopes of the lines complicate the study of point mutations at high dosages.

increases more rapidly than a linear plot. Edington's Y-suppressed lethals are an example in Drosophila (Edington et al., 1962). If these are taken together with the orthodox point lethals, the frequency–dose relation of total lethals deviates significantly from linearity.

On the time factor, Patterson (1931) and Timofeeff-Ressovsky and Zimmer (1935) found that fractionated doses separated by intervals of days or weeks produced sex-linked lethals in Drosophila sperm at the same frequency as did the same total dose applied in one treatment. For example, 3600 R delivered in 15 min produced 54 sex linked lethals for 493 chromosomes tested, while the same dose delivered in six 5-min exposures at 24-hr intervals produced 47 lethals for 423 chromosomes. There is no significant difference between the two percentages, 10.91 ± 1.40 and 11.10 ± 1.52 respectively.

Visible Mutations

Many visible mutations were obtained as a by-product of quantitative experiments on the induction of lethals. In phenotype, they resembled mutants previously known from their spontaneous occurrence. Also, the distribution along the chromosome was much like that obtained for lethals. Thus it seemed legitimate to use lethal mutation as an index of gene mutation in general and to assume the principles established in the one case to be applicable to the other.

In general, adequate published data on visible mutations are meager, and such "data as are found are characterized by large numbers of observations and small numbers of recorded mutations" (Fryer and Gowen, 1942). Even Lea (see Chapter 2), who was intent upon demonstrating the major criteria whereby target effect is recognized, admitted that statistically adequate experiments were not available on wavelength and intensity. This left him only the dose-proportional effect curves. Observations on flies and related insects of the order Diptera far exceed those for other animals. Next best investigated have been the Hymenoptera, while scattered reports of a few visible mutations have appeared for Lepidoptera and Orthoptera. No one has really ascertained whether the rates of induced mutation based on fly and wasp research are typical of the class Insecta (Grosch, 1974).

Figure 7.7 shows some of the more obvious and interesting morphological mutants. Many other changes are known, ranging into the imperceptible changes of dimension and structural geometry. It is here that criteria are difficult to specify, and vary notoriously from observer to observer. In addition, pigmentation and other physiological differ-

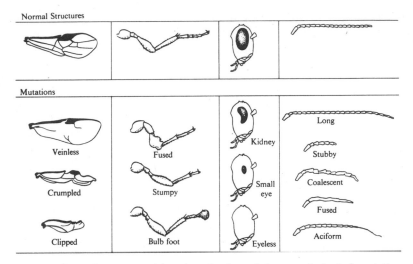

Figure 7.7. Normal structures (above) and a few of the morphological mutations obtained by irradiating the wasp *Habrobracon*. Except for the antennae, which are constructed differently, similar inherited alterations are found in *Drosophila* and other insects.

ences have been studied. If all the possible types of variation in an organism were known and objective means of determining them were available, the frequency of occurrence of visible mutation might be obtained with accuracy. This has not been possible even in *Drosophila*, genetically the most exhaustively studied organism.

The most accurate data are obtained by measuring the frequency of appearance of a specific mutant character which can be clearly distinguished from the norm. In the use of such methods, the diversity of mutation rate at different loci has been shown. Each locus apparently has its own characteristic mutability. Comparison of the frequency of change at different loci has been taken as a measure of the relative mutability of the loci compared. The process is localized in occurrence. Only one member of an allelic pair at a time is influenced and this occurs at a submicroscopic site and does not even influence adjacent regions of the genetic map.

Particular loci may turn out to be both complex and highly mutable. One such case occurs in the small wasp *Mormoniella*, where a surprisingly large number of eye-color changes have been induced, but body-color and morphological changes are rare (Whiting, 1954, 1958, 1961). No such mutability has been demonstrable for the eye colors of another wasp, *Habrobracon*, which was even more intensely investigated. If techniques were available for investigating chromosomal structure in as fine detail as can be done with Diptera salivary gland chromosomes, perhaps in this one species of Hymenoptera an unusual and unstable arrangement of the chromosomal material might be revealed.

Mouse Experiments

Significant differences in the responses of insects and mammals were revealed by the specific locus method in which irradiated wild-type mice were mated to animals homozygous for seven (Oak Ridge) or six (Harwell) autosomal recessive visibles. The offspring were examined for mutations at the loci. The original Oak Ridge experiments employed males mated after their period of temporary sterility. Therefore any mutations recovered were those which had occurred in spermatogonia. The per-locus-induced mutation rate, so keenly desired as a cross reference point between flies and a mammal, turned out to be considerably higher than in flies (Table 7.1). Even when special experiments provided information about the mutation rate in fly spermatogonia, the mouse rate proved to be significantly higher. Additional experiments performed at Harwell, in which an inbreeding scheme was employed to detect recessive changes at all loci, confirmed a higher mutation rate for mice than for flies. Also, repeated tests of 600 R of either x or γ rays given as acute doses yielded frequencies of about 13 mutations per locus per 10^5 gametes. However, there are exceptions to Russell's (1965) mutational yield. In a six-loci test of 615 R (90 R/min), Lyon and Morris (1966) obtained only 4.70 mutations per locus per 10^5 gametes, but five of the six loci differed from those of the Oak Ridge strain. Differences in mutability have been demonstrated even among the seven loci of the Russell test strain. The spotting locus (S) accounted for 41% while the short ear (Se) locus provided only 1% of the mutations obtained.

Whether the loci studied are representative of the entire gene complement remains an open question (Searle, 1974). Since mutation rate serves as a basis for calculations of doubling dose and permissible doses, uncertainty has forced prestigious committees to estimate ranges instead of specific values (see Chapter 8).

Another difference from fly data was a significant departure from linearity for point mutation at higher doses given to mice (Figure 7.8). Also, when irradiation was extended over longer periods of time, the mutation rate was lower for spermatogonia than for spermatozoa. Gonial mutation frequencies were about half those for postmeiotic cells. The yield from a 9 R/min x-ray exposure was significantly lower than that from 90 R/min, but reducing the dose rate to 0.009 R/min or below did

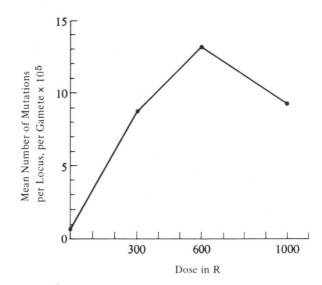

Figure 7.8. Mutation rates at seven specific loci in the mouse due to x rays delivered at 90 R/min. Subsequent research using gamma-ray doses down to a few roentgens per week have provided points which lie much lower. (Courtesy of W. L. Russell.)

not further lower the mutation rate. In explanation, a dose-rate-dependent repair process has been postulated.

High doses given at a high dose rate can cause a selective elimination of the more mutationally sensitive cells in the spermatogonial population. However, the number of cells killed at 0.8 R/min and 90 R/min is nearly identical and does not explain the dose-rate effect. Furthermore, disruption of the cell population does not explain the low mutation rate from protracted doses in female mice where all germ cells are nonmitotic oocytes, and continued fertility provides no evidence for extensive killing. The interpretation of fractionation experiments may be more complicated than protracted dose tests (Russell, 1962). Dose fractionation may increase the mutation yield if fractions are synchronized to coincide with a mutationally sensitive stage of the spermatogonial population's cell cycle. Generally, these effects are characteristic of the more sparsely ionizing radiations. Dose rate has a minimum influence with neutrons and other high LET situations.

Female Mice and Insects

The irradiation of male mice follows the traditional design of *Drosophila* experiments, but in mammals it is the female in which gametes are differentiated prior to sexual maturity. In the mouse, all germ cells develop to dictyate oocytes shortly after birth, and are arrested in this stage until only 12 hr before ovulation. When the interval between radiation exposure and conception is short, an appreciable number of mutations are recovered after acute doses that yield none if more than seven weeks elapse. After chronic exposures, even to fast neutrons, mutation frequencies are little above the spontaneous level. Accordingly differences in mutation rates from those of the male germ line exist, which reflect morphological differences and attendant divergence in physiological abilities between sperm and egg precursors.

The nonlinearity of dose-effect curves and altered mutation frequencies in dose-rate experiments is well established for female insects. In this case, more research has been done with wasps and silkworm moths than with flies, because of the inconvenience of collecting eggs from the latter. Oocytes are continuously differentiating during adulthood, and although cell selection plays a more important role in insect experiments, the histological structure of the insect ovary (Chapter 12) simplifies determining the fate of each cell type. An inclusive range from interphase stem cells to meiotic oocytes provides contrasts in nuclear structure and cytoplasmic capability reflected in distinct differences in the frequency of mutations recovered after a radiation exposure.

Cultured Cells

The development of recent techniques, many derived from microorganism procedures, has allowed the study of mutation in somatic mammalian cells *in vitro*. Three classes of mutants have been obtained: auxotrophic, temperature sensitive, and drug resistant. Although the other two are more valuable in the study of biochemical pathways, only the drug-resistant class has lent itself to quantification. Drug-resistant mutants fall into two groups, those resistant to (1) nucleotide base analogues such as 8-azaguanine, 6-thioguanine, and 2,6-diaminopurine and (2) to metabolic inhibitors such as γ-amanitine, puromycin, and ouabain. Those resistant to the analogues can usually be attributed to the absence of a particular enzyme.

The *in vitro* system allows quantitative study of the induction of mutations under a variety of conditions that are impossible or most difficult to achieve *in vivo* (dose rates, LET, modifying agents). This type of research is in its early stages. Table 7.1 provides a comparison between x-ray-induced mutation frequencies in six different mammalian cell lines and those obtained by the specific locus approach in mice and flies. Methods for studying mutation rates at specific loci have been

TABLE 7.1

Mutation Frequencies Induced by Acute X-Ray Doses of 1000 rad or Less for a Variety of *in Vitro* Selection Systems and for the Specific Locus Method with Mouse and Fly Spermatogonia

Cells	Selection technique	Mutations per rad	Reference
Mouse L5178Y	Alanine auxotrophy to prototrophy	3×10^{-7}	Suzuki and Okada, 1976
Mouse L5178Y	6-Thioguanine resistance	$1–3 \times 10^{-7}$	Knapp and Simons, 1975
Chinese hamster V79	8-Azaguanine resistance	$4–18 \times 10^{-7}$	Chu, 1971
Chinese hamster CHO	8-Azaguanine resistance	$1–8 \times 10^{-7}$	Carver et al., 1976
Human fibroblasts	8-Azaguanine resistance	2.2×10^{-7}	Albertini and DeMars, 1973
Human lung fibroblasts	6-Thioguanine resistance	3×10^{-7}	Thacker and Cox, 1975
Mouse spermatogonia	Specific locus	2.5×10^{-7}	Russell, 1951
Drosophila spermatogonia	Specific locus	0.1×10^{-7}	Alexander, 1954

developed, but to date for only two loci: the hamster *HGPRT* and the mouse *TK* loci. Respectively the mutation rates found in exploratory experiments were 1×10^{-6} per R and 5×10^{-7} per R.

Forward and Reverse Mutations

There are several unanswered questions about the process of mutation. Until we know more about the physics and biochemistry of the matter they will remain unanswerable. Attempts to resolve the situation by experiments in genetics have led to debate. Whether mutation induced by radiation is the same as that obtained "spontaneously" is of fundamental importance. As Stadler (1954) pointed out, we are inclined to assume that some of the mutation detected in radiation experiments must be qualitative changes in the genes concerned because we believe that qualitatively altered genes have arisen in the course of evolution. Our tendency is to expect "true gene mutations" to be included in the unclassified residue of a radiation mutation experiment.

Stadler (1954) found no dominant mutations in the x-ray progenies of barley and maize in the course of experiments in which many hundreds of recessive mutations were detected. Although early experiments with *Drosophila* showed reversals from the recessive to the wild type dominant condition at selected loci, several investigators including Kaufmann, Demerec, and LeFevre (1950) have been unable to repeat such results. Extreme precautions were taken against contamination. LeFevre (1950) for example, would allow in his laboratory no stock which might provide contamination with genes for the traits under investigation.

Despite numerous reports on ionizing radiation mutagenesis in bacteria, insights into molecular mechanisms have come from experiments with ultraviolet and chemical mutagens. Thus a convincing demonstration of true reversion in chemically treated *E. coli* by Yanofsky's group does not settle the question for ionizing radiation (Yanofsky *et al.*, 1966), although it proved that an amino acid characteristic of a mutant polypeptide can be replaced by the original kind. Frame shift studies are also a feature of research in chemical mutagenesis.

Furthermore, changes in the DNA strands of prokaryotic viruses and bacteria are no assurance that a comparable event occurs in the chromosomes of eukaryotes. For this we have to turn to fungi which share microbial advantages in highly efficient screening techniques for enormous samples. In *Neurospora crassa*, Malling and de Serres (1967) used chemical mutagens, which induce base-pair transitions, to revert a number of x-ray-induced mutations of the 33ad-3B locus. This provided a clear positive demonstration that x rays are able to produce some "true" mutations. Earlier, linkage tests on purple adenine mutants had indicated that x rays induced reversions in some of the x-ray-induced mutants.

In the late 1970s, reassessment of the mutation process is in vogue. Of major concern is the relative importance of molecular repair mechanisms for phenotypic reversions, and of misrepair in the events leading to a heritable mutation. Repair processes are covered in Chapter 4. Conceivably, radiation damage to an individual nucleotide or small region of DNA might be premutational, and if faultlessly repaired would not become a mutation. Conversely, if the repair is faulty a nucleotide sequence different from the original may be built into the molecule. Thus although a mutation results it should not be equated to the induced lesion.

The simplest hypothesis to explain results in *Neurospora* is that x irradiation promotes reverse mutational change to a condition genetically and biochemically equivalent to the original wild-type condition. However, it is necessary to carefully distinguish between reverse mutation and suppressor mutation. With methionine-less strains, Giles (1951) found most reversions to be suppressor-mutations, but with purple adenine mutants de Serres (1958) obtained reversions operationally definable as reverse mutations. A further complication is that reappraisal of much mutation data becomes necessary if excision–reactivation mechanisms function in higher organisms.

Applications to Plant Breeding

Stadler's (1928, 1954) experimental results made him pessimistic about the practical value of induced mutations, and this apparently deterred American workers for many years. The Swedish view was more optimistic: Even though loss of chromosomal material may occur, this may be progressive in agricultural plants which have retained primitive unnecessary structure or contain repetitious gene material. As early as 1928, Swedish investigators were considering the potential economic usefulness of radiation-induced mutations. Led by Nilsson-Ehle, within a few years they had obtained and tested the first of a series of erectoides mutants in barley (Gustafsson, 1951). These are characterized by dense ears, stiff straw, and other less obvious morphological characteristics associated with improved fertility. Some are earlier, able to utilize high-N dressing, and have high protein, and good baking and malting properties. Many are associated with chromosomal rearrangement, and the word mutation is applicable only in the broad sense; but some have arisen entirely free from any detectable chromosomal rearrangement and are classifiable as mutations in the strict sense. By 1968, 181 erectoides mutants at 26 loci had been analyzed from 685 cases. They are of particular interest to agriculture when they outyield the mother strain in comparative and competitive trials. Other European laboratories launched investigations with other crop plants including oats, wheat, flax, peas, soybeans, mustard, rape, lupine, and rye, which ultimately provided more than 100 varieties of induced-mutated crop plants. In Asia, perhaps most important in the context of future world food resources are the research programs aimed at improving rice. Already mutants conferring improved cooking qualities and disease resistances have been identified. In Japan, progress has been made toward increasing the protein content and redistributing the protein in the rice kernel.

Italian geneticists have used x rays and neutrons to improve *durum* wheat in a number of respects. By 1974, four mutant lines were released as new varieties. All had improved yield and lodging resistance. Increased adaptability is characteristic of some lines which have performed well on extensive trials in 20 countries of Asia, Africa, and Europe.

Practically every one of the United States and most of the Provinces of Canada have had applied projects in radiation mutation on useful and ornamental plants. However, this did not come about until Konzak (1954) induced stem rust resistance in oats, and Gregory (1956) increased the yield of peanuts by using radiation. Gregory's comprehensive experiment involved 975,000 X_2 plants from which it was possible to select types not only superior in yield, but also better adapted to mechanical harvesting and resistant to a serious leaf-spot disease. Please note the scale of this type of investigation, which required 64 acres to grow nearly 1 million plants. In general the experience of Konzak and others with various crops indicates that success is more likely with distinct characters such as disease resistance than for improved yield and quality. Even in a vegetatively propagated crop where stolons were irradiated, wilt-resistant strains of peppermint were developed within a decade from a starter population of 100,000 plants by Murray (1969). A significant aspect of this solution to a serious commercial problem is that conventional hybridization techniques had failed.

Obviously there is merit in increasing genetic variability in a cultivated species beyond what is available in nature, especially in crops where variability is restricted. But it takes expertise in selection procedures to sort out the useful mutations from the great majority of de-leterious changes. Representative reports from the enormous technical literature on mutational plant breeding are published by the International Atomic Energy Agency in Vienna. These include a symposium series such as that in 1969 on Induced Mutations in Plants, study groups proceedings such as the 1970 Induced Mutations and Plant Improvement, technical reports (notably No. 119, Manual in Mutation Breeding), and various panel proceedings. Crop plant characters that can be improved by mutation breeding include yield, growth habit, lodging resistance, disease and pest resistance, shattering and shedding resistance, and tolerance to extreme temperatures, drought, and salinity.

Concluding Remarks

Chapter 4 discussed induced changes in the important DNA molecules which carry the encoded genetic information. In the present chapter our concern has been gene expression: that is, whether all the structural genes still specify and direct formation of the normal product after exposure to radiation. This implies that transcription and translation of the information occurs, but afterward we must be able to recognize the presence of the gene product or its influence by some test.

As summarized early in the chapter, procedures to reveal induced mutations (usually recessive) were developed in a wide variety of organisms before the significance of DNA was established. Of most concern to humans were the results of animal experiments, initially with insects and in recent years with mammals. In particular, mouse experiments revealed that the so-called principles determined by scoring the offspring of irradiated male insects do not hold when germ cell stages other than mature sperm are exposed. The cytological fact that mammals experience a continual spermatogenesis during reproductive life is no longer ignored when localized point mutations are considered. Because of quantitative differences in the responses of various classes of spermatogonia and spermatocytes, or even among the phases of oocytes, it is not possible to generalize and assign a specific mutation rate to a specific dose of radiation. Mitotic phase, cell type, sex, and species influence the proportion of mutations recovered (Wolstenholme and O'Connor, 1969). Dose rate is now known to be important in cells with functional repair mechanisms. An open question, especially for higher organisms, is the contribution of the error-prone mechanisms of Chapter 4 to the "visible" mutations obtained in classic experiments.

In a qualitative sense, the classic position is still valid: no genetically permissible or safe amount of ionizing radiation is known. Some point mutations will probably result from any exposure. Also, the deleterious nature of newly induced mutations is firmly established. However when special agricultural types are required for the artificial conditions of mass cultivation, adaptable rare individual plants can be selected from large samples of useless mutant types. Examples are given in the above chapter. The consequences of mutation for natural and experimental populations are considered in Chapter 8.

References

Albertini, R. J., and DeMars, R. (1973). Detection and quantification of x-ray-induced mutation in cultured, diploid human fibroblasts. *Mutat. Res.* **18**, 199–224.

Alexander, M. L. (1954). Mutation rates at specific autosomal loci in the mature and immature germ cells of *Drosophila melanogaster*. *Genetics* **39**, 409–428.

Beadle, G. W. (1945). The genetic control of biochemical reactions. *Harvey Lect.* **40**, 179–194.

Carver, J. H., Dewey, W. C., and Hopwood, L. E. (1976). X-ray induced mutants resistant to 8-azaguanine. II. Cell cycle response. *Mutat. Res.* **34**, 465–480.

Chu, E. H. Y. (1971). Mammalian cell genetics. III. Characterization of x-ray-induced forward mutations in Chinese hamster cell cultures. *Mutat. Res.* **11**, 23–24.

Chu, E. H. Y., Brimer, P., Jacobson, K. B., and Merriam, E. V. (1969). Mammalian cell genetics. I. Selection and characterization of mutations auxotrophic for L-glutamine or resistant to 8-azaguanine in Chinese hamster cells in vitro. *Genetics* **62**, 359–377.

Congress of the U.S. (1957). Hearings before the special subcommittee on radiation of the Joint Committee on Atomic Energy. U.S. Govt. Printing Office, Washington, D.C.

de Serres, F. J. (1958). Studies with purple adenine mutants in *Neurospora*. III. Reversion of x-ray induced mutations. *Genetics* **43**, 187–206.

de Serres, F. J. (1964). Mutagenesis and chromosome structure. *Oak Ridge Symp., 1964* pp. 33–42.

Edington, C. W., Epler, J. L., and Regan, J. D. (1962). The frequencey–dose relation of x-ray induced Y-suppressed lethals in *Drosophila*. *Genetics* **47**, 397–406.

Fryer, H. C., and Gowen, J. W. (1942). Analysis of data on x-ray induced visible gene mutations in *Drosophila melanogaster*. *Genetics* **27**, 212–227.

Giles, N. H., Jr. (1951). Studies on the mechanism of reversion in biochemical mutants of *Neurospora crassa*. *Cold Spring Harbor Symp. Quant. Biol.* **16**, 283–313.

Gregory, W. C. (1956). Induction of useful mutations in the peanut. *Brookhaven Symp. Biol.* **9**, 177–190.

Grosch, D. S. (1974). Environmental Aspects: Radiation. *In* "The Physiology of Insecta" (M. Rockstein, ed.), 2nd ed., Chapter 3, pp. 85–126. Academic Press, New York.

Gustafsson, A. (1951). Mutations, environment and evolution. *Cold Spring Harbor Symp. Quant. Biol.* **16**, 263–282.

Horowitz, N. H. and Leupold, J. (1951). Some recent studies bearing upon the one-gene–one-enzyme hypothesis. *Cold Spring Harbor Symp. Quant. Biol.* **16**, 65–74.

Kao, F.-T., and Puck, T. T. (1968). Genetics of somatic mammalian cells. VII. Induction and isolation of nutritional mutants in Chinese hamster cells. *Proc. Natl. Acad. Sci. U.S.A.* **60**, 1275–1281.

Knapp, A. G. A. C., and Simons, J. W. I. M. (1975). A mutational assay system for L5178Y mouse lymphoma cells, using hypoxanthine-guanine-phosphoribosyl-transferase (HGPRT)-deficiency as marker. *Mutat. Res.* **30**, 97–110.

Konzak, C. F. (1954). Stem rust resistance in oats induced by nuclear radiation. *Agronomy J.* **46**, 538–540.

LeFevre, G., Jr. (1950). X ray induced genetic effects in germinal and somatic tissue of *Drosophila melanogaster. Am. Nat.* **84**, 341–365.

Lyon, M. F., and Morris, T. (1966). Mutation rates at a new set of specific loci in the mouse. *Genet. Res.* **7**, 12–17.

Malling, H. V., and de Serres, F. J. (1967). Identification of the spectrum of x ray induced intragenic alterations at the molecular level in *Neurospora crassa. Radiat. Res.* **31**, 637–638.

Morgan, T. H. (1911). The origin of nine wing mutations in *Drosophila. Science* **33**, 496–499.

Muller, H. J. (1927). Artificial transmutation of the gene. *Science* **66**, 84–87.

Muller, H. J., and Oster, I. I. (1963). Some mutational techniques in *Drosophila. In* "Symposium on Methodology in Basic Genetics" (W. J. Burdette, ed.), pp. 249–278. Holden-Day, San Francisco, California.

Murray, M. J. (1969). Successful use of irradiation breeding to obtain *Verticillium*-resistant strains of peppermint. *IAEA/FAO Symp. Induced Mutat. Plants, 1969* pp. 345–371.

Oliver, C. P. (1930). The effect of varying the duration of x-ray treatment upon the frequency of mutation. *Science* **71**, 44–46.

Patterson, J. T. (1931). Continuous versus interrupted irradiation and the rate of mutation in *Drosophila. Biol. Bull. (Woods Hole, Mass.)* **61**, 133–138.

Plough, H. H. (1941). Spontaneous mutability in *Drosophila. Cold Spring Harbor Symp.* **9**, 127–193.

Russell, W. L. (1951). X-ray-induced mutations in mice. *Cold Spring Harbor Symposia on Quantitative Biology* **16**, 327–336.

Russell, W. L. (1962). An augmenting effect of dose fractionation on radiation induced mutation rate in mice. *Proc. Natl. Acad. Sci. U.S.A.* **48**, 1724–1726.

Russell, W. L. (1965). Studies in mammalian radiation genetics. *Nucleonics* **25**, No. 1, 53–56.

Searle, A. G. (1974). Mutation induction in mice. *Adv. Radiat. Biol.* **4**, 131–207.

Spencer, W. P., and Stern, C. (1948). Experiments to test the validity of the linear R-dose/mutation frequency relation in *Drosophila* at low dosage. *Genetics* **33**, 43–71.

Srb, A. M., and Horowitz, N. H. (1944). The ornithine cycle in *Neurospora* and its genetic control. *J. Biol. Chem.* **154**, 129–139.

Stadler, L. J. (1928). Mutations in barley induced by x rays and radium. *Science* **68**, 186–187.

Stadler, L. J. (1954). The gene. *Science* **120**, 811–819.

Suzuki, N., and Okada, S. (1976). Isolation of nutrient deficient mutants and quantitative mutation assay by reversion of alanine-requiring L5178Y cells. *Mutat. Res.* **34**, 489–506.

Thacker, J., and Cox, R. (1975). Mutation induction and inactivation in mammalian cells exposed to ionising radiation. *Nature (London)* **258**, 429–431.

Timofeeff-Ressovsky, N. W. (1934). The experimental production of mutations. *Biol. Rev. Cambridge Philos. Soc.* **9**, 411–457.

Timofeeff-Ressovsky, N. W., and Zimmer, K. G. (1935). Strahlengenetische Zeitfaktorversuche an *Drosophila melanogaster*. *Strahlentherapie* **53**, 134–138.

Whiting, P. W. (1954). Comparable mutant eye colors in *Mormiella* and *Pachycrepoideus* (Hymenoptera: Pteromalidae). *Evolution* **8**, 135–147.

Whiting, P. W. (1958). *Mormoniella* and the nature of the gene. *Proc. Int. Congr. Entomol., 10th, 1956* Vol. 2, pp. 857–866.

Whiting, P. W. (1961). Eye-color mutations from mutant stocks in *Mormoniella*. *J. Hered.* **52**, 247–249.

Wolstenholme, G. E. W., and O'Connor, eds. (1969). "Mutation as Cellular Process." Churchill, London (contains W. L. Russell's review of the mutation process in mice, plus papers and discussion by 25 other specialists).

Yanofsky, C., Ito, J., and Horn, V. (1966). Amino acid replacements and the genetic code. *Cold Spring Harbor Symp. Quant. Biol.* **31**, 151–162.

CHAPTER 8   Consequences of Mutation

Muller focused the attention of the scientific world on the human implications of induced mutation in his Nobel prize acceptance speech and his Sigma Xi National Lectureship (1950). In essence, we are the custodians of the germ plasm of the future, and we should recognize that it is a genetic disadvantage to increase the mutational load by any means. A recessive lethal change may be half responsible for the death of an individual seventy generations after its production. With origin in a common ancestor, such a change may be entirely responsible for death of a descendant (Figure 8.1). Or if merely detrimental, it may hamper a variable, or perhaps a considerable number of descendants until it finally kills. This is known as the "try-and-try-again" or the "genetic-murder-will-out" viewpoint.

This view is based partly upon data obtained from early American genealogies which represent the centuries before radiation hazards, and modern medicine. The proportion of children dying before the age of 21 was higher for consanguinous matings than for unrelated parents: about 17% of the progeny from first cousin marriages, 15% of those from other cousins, and 12% in the case of unrelated parents. It leads to speculation concerning mutational damage in populations. An unexposed population to some degree has reached a balance between the spontaneous input of mutations and elimination by selection. If the balance is changed by an additional input of induced mutation, selection will tend to reduce the total number of mutants and reach another equilibrium. Death of an individual carrier is the price of such reduction of mutants. The period required for elimination depends on the genetic nature of the mutant. With recessives the course of events will be slow, perhaps taking not less than thirty generations, and sometimes many more. Even when a short generation time of twenty years is considered, 20 × 30 = 600 years. What does the year 2580 mean to us? Or put another way, how would we regard ancestors in 1380 whose decisions could reflect on our health or how we live today?

With these convenient figures as a basis, let us further consider the

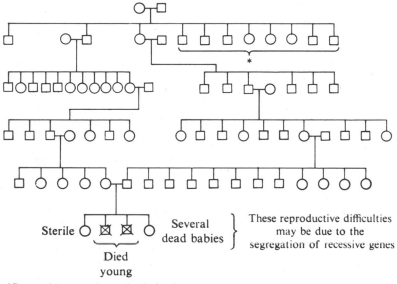

Sterile

Died
young

Several
dead babies

}

These reproductive difficulties
may be due to the
segregation of recessive genes

*Descendants not shown for lack of space

Figure 8.1. A pedigree showing a type of consanguineous marriage quite common in U.S. history. The individuals were not aware that they shared great-great-grandparents. Except for the first son killed in an Indian raid, offspring of the original sire were very prolific and in large measure populated one of the counties of Pennsylvania. Under such circumstances, the replicates of a single recessive gene which have come down through a century or more are brought together in homozygous state.

probability of common ancestry which can bring about a zygotic meeting of two doses of a recessive gene. The number of ancestors for any person is 2^n, n being the number of generations under consideration. Two to the thirtieth power (2^{30}) amounts to more than one thousand million ancestors, a figure which exceeds the population of the world a few hundred years ago. This is also a figure exceeding the present and predicted future population of the United States, and even of the continent of North America for the next several generations. Shared ancestors, or consanguinity, is inevitable under such circumstances.

By simplifying assumptions, it is possible to establish the probability of numbers of offspring affected by a certain dose given to all prospective parents of a population. Thus a 10 R acute dose to the gonad region of each parent has been calculated (Stern, 1973) to cause about 1.6 abnormal children in 10,000. When this is applied to the 3 million births annually in the U.S., as many as 480 affected children would be expected each year. But this is only the first generation. On the bright side is the evidence that chronic exposure at low dose reduces the number.

Mather (1952) voiced concern in slightly different terms by pointing out that the conduct and course of human society is affected by a relatively small section of the community. This group, the leaders in thought, invention, and organization are likely to comprise one tail of a continuous distribution of ability. In such a scheme, a small mutagenic effect, lowering the average, might also shift the whole distribution or otherwise reduce the number of individuals exceeding a certain standard in the tail (Figure 8.2).

General public apprehension has been sharpened by atomic weapons testing. In the United States, the National Academy of Science–National Research Council has issued studied reports to the public (1956, 1960, 1972). Hearings before the joint congressional committee on

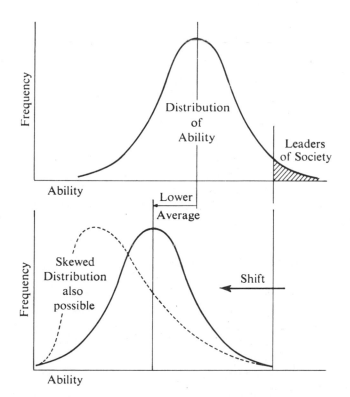

Figure 8.2.   Frequency distributions of members of populations differing in abilities of invention, organization, interpretation, and so on. The intelligence quotients of a large, unselected sample of people actually shows such a bell-shaped "normal" distribution. The lower drawing shows how decreasing the average might seriously reduce the number of individuals exceeding a certain standard in the tail. (Suggested in a lecture by Mather, 1952.)

radiation have also been published. Concern was expressed not only about environmental contamination from testing and the occupational hazards of workers in atomic installations, but also about medical exposures to radiation.

A survey by Sonnenblick (1955) in the metropolitan Middle Atlantic area had produced disquieting evidence that operators and owners were unfamiliar with the x ray output of their generators. Fortunately legislators, manufacturers, and radiologists are taking a socially conscientious view of the types of equipment meriting approval. In addition to legislation and built-in cut-offs, every radiologist can ask himself "Am I doing this examination with the least necessary radiation, especially to the sex cells?" (Newell, 1957).

Doubling Dose

In 1956, the Federal Radiation Council excluded medical radiation from their considerations and proposed 5 R as the 30-year limit for the average individual's exposure. This amounts to about 0.17 R/yr or 170 milliroentgens which is reasonably lower than estimated *doubling doses.* By definition, the doubling dose is the amount of radiation required to produce a mutation rate equal to that which occurs spontaneously.

If mouse mutation rates apply to man, the doubling dose is probably between 30 and 80 R, perhaps 40 R from acute exposure, while the chronic dose may be four times larger. The 1972 MRC Biological Effects of Ionizing Radiation (B.E.I.R.) report gives background on these matters.

Genetically Significant Dose (GSD)

The GSD established by the International Commission on Radiological Protection (I.C.R.P.) in 1956 was adopted in 1964 by the U.S. Public Health Service for their studies of the nation's population dose from x rays. It is an attempt to estimate the exposure relevant to mutation production by calculating an index of the radiation *received* by the genetic pool that determines the progeny of a given population. The algebraic expression is

$$\text{GSD} = \frac{\Sigma \, D_i \, \hat{N}_i \, P_i}{\Sigma \, N_i \, P_i}$$

where D_i = the average gonad dose to persons of age i who receive x-ray examinations

$\hat{N}_i$ = the number of persons in the population of age i who receive x-ray examinations

P_i = the expected future number of children for a person of age i

N_i = the number of persons in the population of age i

The approach takes the product of the gonad dose received by the person examined and the expected future number of children; then sums them by age group for all individuals of a population who receive x-ray examinations. The data used in the formula were obtained by interviews of representative samples from all regions of the United States. Followup radiation-facility inspections provided technical data.

The GSD for 1964 was calculated to be 17 mrem per person per year for a 1976 report (FDA 76-8034) which supersedes all estimates of earlier publications. By the next national study in 1970, despite an increase in procedures performed, the exposure from diagnostic radiation was only 10 mrem per year. The GSD from therapeutic radiation was much less, only about 5 mrem per year. Gonadal radiation from dental radiology was negligible. These amounts from man-made radiation are added to the natural background radiation, which contributes about 90 mrem per year.

Data from Humans

Even if it were not morally reprehensible, we do not have the time to demonstrate by controlled experiments that when irradiated, man reacts similarly to other sexually reproducing animals. We cannot spare the years it would take. Instead we study data gathered from human groups that have received exceptional exposure to radiation. Unfortunately no clear statistically significant results have emerged.

An analysis of questionnaires returned by radiologists suggested trends, but the sample may be biased. Persons with offspring responded more readily. Also a greater proportion of radiologists (74%) than of controls (53.8%) answered. The 5461 radiologists reported 14% abortions and stillbirths in comparison with 12% in families of 4484 physicians not working with radiations. Among the live births were 6% congenital malformations and 5% respectively. These differences and the fewer live sons born to exposed fathers are not necessarily caused by gene mutations.

Over 70,000 births were recorded during 1948–1953 to parents exposed in Hiroshima and Nagasaki. Although most induced mutations would appear as recessives recombining in later generations, one might expect to see some first generation effects as a result of dominant mutations, sex-linked recessives in sons of irradiated mothers, and autosomal mutations in zygotes with preexisting recessives at particular loci. As indicators of these possibilities, the Atomic Bomb Casualty Commission chose five effects (Neel and Schull, 1956). Radiation was expected to increase the rate of stillbirths, infantile deaths, and malformations. It was expected to decrease weight at birth and alter sex ratio. A decrease in males from maternal exposure and a small increase from paternal exposure were conceivable. Attempts were made to divide the parents into several dose exposure groups with appropriate controls. However, there were no statistically significant changes demonstrable at the 90% probability level. In mutagenesis studies the size of the groups is very important. Possibly the "sample" was too small, but it is the only one of appreciable size available. On the basis of this qualification we must conclude that clear evidence of radiation-induced mutations in man does not exist.

Irradiated Natural Populations of *Drosophila*

There is really nothing to equal the analytical work done on flies. We need to turn to them for information from populations. However with a hundred or more fertilized eggs per pair of flies, there is a margin of reproductive effectiveness much greater than that possible for man.

The reproductive capacity of *Drosophila ananassae*, the dominant species from the Marshall and Eastern Caroline islands, has been studied in an attempt to determine the effects of direct and fallout radiation produced by testing atomic devices (Stone and Wilson, 1959). An advantage of island populations is that they are isolated units. Collections were made every summer for four years (Stone *et al.*, 1962). By a series of crossbreeding and inbreeding tests, the evolutionary fitness of populations was assayed by measuring fecundity and development of offspring to adulthood.

The fly populations have managed to return to normal reproductive performance, presumably through the operation of natural selection (Figure 8.3). Periods required for this type of recovery were 26 generations for Rongerik flies, 40 generations for Rongelap, and 106–161 generations for Bikini. Bikini organisms received direct irradiation and fallout; those on Rongelap and Rongerik received only fallout. Although special attempts in detection were made, the number of previously undescribed chromosomal rearrangements was low, and the load of

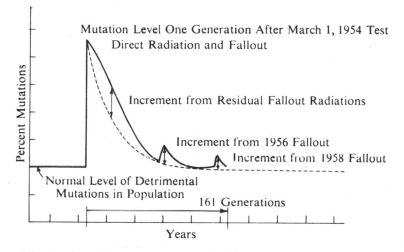

Figure 8.3. A schematic representation of the effect of radiation from thermonuclear explosions on the genetic load of adverse mutations in Bikini populations of the fly *Drosophila ananassae*. Rongelap and Rongerik populations had a similar but smaller increase in mutations. (Based upon Stone and Wilson, 1959.)

visible mutations from the test area was no greater than that from control areas.

Controversy among Geneticists?

From time to time news publications and broadcasts mention disagreements among geneticists concerning the dangers of genetic damage due to radiation exposure. Actually there is no disagreement about irradiation inducing mutations in humans as well as in any other living organism. Nor does any professional geneticist doubt that the typical mutation is harmful in the duplex condition of a homozygote. The difference of opinion concerns several technical matters which are still among the unsolved problems.

One of the most important unsolved and controversial problems of modern population genetics is whether mutant heterozygotes are ever completely identical with standard or "normal" homozygotes. If a mutant gene incapacitates heterozygotes, its equilibrium frequency in the population is lower and the genetic damage produced is higher. On the other hand, heterozygotes might be more fit than standard homozygotes even though the homozygous condition of the mutant gene results in incapacitation or death. This would be an ambivalent situation with mutants impairing fitness when homozygous, but improving it for heterozygous carriers. On such a basis the sweeping statement that mutations are harmful does not hold.

Laboratory Studies with *Drosophila* Populations

Experiments have not yet resolved the controversy. Dobzhansky (1966) and others have revealed that natural populations carry a surprisingly large number of deleterious situations concealed in heterozygous condition. Some lethal genes have been maintained against selection in Japanese populations of *Drosophila* generation after generation. However, flies heterozygous for persistent lethals appear to have the advantage over those heterozygous for newly arisen lethals (Watanabe and Oshima, 1970).

Wallace, a Dobzhansky associate, obtained data from radiation experiments which can be interpreted from the ambivalent view (Wallace and Dobzhansky, 1959). This is, the presence of many deleterious or lethal genes in a population does not mean that the average individual is necessarily less viable or fit. Also an increase in the frequency of such genes over a period of time does not necessarily result in a decrease in the average viability of the population. The mutational load carried may be far smaller than the segregational load.

Wallace (1956) compared the accumulation of second chromosome lethals in control populations with those descended from *D. melanogaster* given sizable acute doses of x radiation and with those given chronic gamma radiation (Figure 8.4). The original parental flies of each population carried second chromosomes that were free of lethals, semilethals, and detectable subvitals.

One population received continuous gamma radiation totaling 2000 R per generation throughout life. This resulted in an accumulation of lethals of 6% per generation as determined by diagnostic crosses using a stock with marker genes and cross over suppressors. Nevertheless in over twenty generations during which the exposure continued, the average viability did not decrease significantly. Thirty generations after a single large x-ray exposure, an irradiated population differed from controls in having a higher frequency of chromosomes with various deleterious effects including lethals, semilethals, and subvitals. These same chromosomes when carried by individuals in random heterozygous combinations resulted in higher viabilities than did those of the control population. High relative adaptive values (Figure 8.5) might

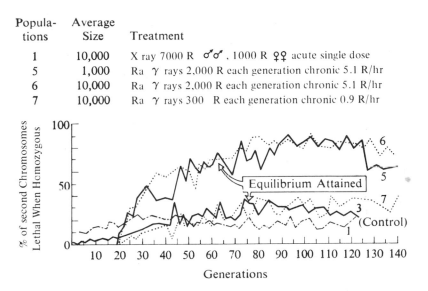

Popula-tions	Average Size	Treatment
1	10,000	X ray 7000 R ♂♂ , 1000 R ♀♀ acute single dose
5	1,000	Ra γ rays 2,000 R each generation chronic 5.1 R/hr
6	10,000	Ra γ rays 2,000 R each generation chronic 5.1 R/hr
7	10,000	Ra γ rays 300 R each generation chronic 0.9 R/hr

Figure 8.4. The frequencies of second-chromosome lethals in five experimental populations as determined by samples taken periodically for nearly 150 generations. (Based on Wallace, 1956.)

exist not merely in spite of but because of the original treatment. Genes or deleterious chromosomes might be retained within populations as a result of selective properties exhibited in heterozygous individuals. By 1956, Wallace's populations had been followed for nearly 150 generations.

The negative side of the debate was initiated by Muller and Falk (1961) who designed experiments that avoided pairing the investigated chromosomes with homologues carrying inversions and marker genes during the testing procedure. After Wallace's (1963) criticisms, Falk (1967) modified his approach but still found lower fitness for irradiated chromosomes. Furthermore, Carson (1964) failed to obtain a sustained increase in fitness despite the increased genetic variance in his irradiated populations of D. melanogaster.

On the other hand Ayala (1968) demonstrated a rapid increase well above the control level in populations derived from x-rayed adults of the sibling species Drosophila serrata and D. birchii. The improvement in productivity indicative of efficient food utilization occurred after an initial 6-week period of low population size during which the carriers of deleterious mutations were eliminated. To obtain such results, certain conditions may need to be met. Most important is to shift the irradiated population to an environment quite different from that to which the

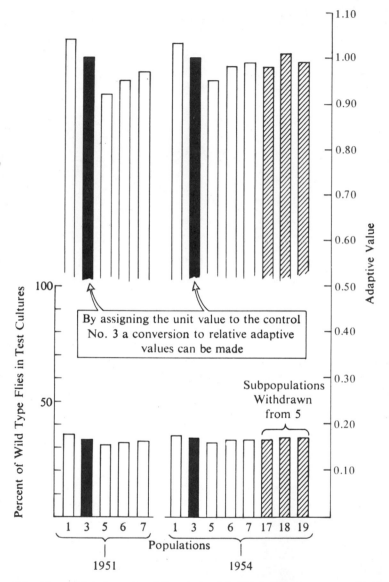

Figure 8.5. Consolidated results of the study of individuals heterozygous for random combinations of the populations described in Figure 8.4. Wild-type offspring should segregate to make up one-third of the total flies in the test used. Deviations from this are ascribed to genes carried by the chromosomes rendered heterozygous by the technique employed. The subpopulations withdrawn from number 5 after 4 years received no radiation subsequently. (Based on Wallace, 1956.)

ancestral strain had become adapted. In other words, a situation in which natural selection is operative must be provided.

Over the years most of the experiments have been run under standard carefully controlled environmental conditions with emphasis placed on the genetic background and derivation of stocks for special testing. Simmons' (1976) paper cites references for the two different schools of thought which express sharp disagreement about the heterozygous effects of irradiated chromosomes on fly viability. In his experiments no beneficial effects were observed for nondrastic mutations. Significant deleterious heterozygous effects occurred with chromosomes drastic when homozygous.

A possible resolution of the decades-old debate, was offered by Mukai's (1969) studies which showed that new mutants were overdominant only under restricted conditions. Mukai defined as polygenes all mutations that slightly alter the viabilities of homozygotes. Thus a major gene controlling a qualitative trait like eye color could influence viability polygenically. Regardless of whether they were spontaneous or induced newly arisen polygenes proved detrimental when heterozygous in heterozygous background but slightly beneficial in an otherwise homozygous genetic background. Experiments placing the limit at 8 to 11 heterozygous loci on a *Drosophila* chromosome have given rise to the Optimum Heterozygosity Hypothesis (Mukai, 1969). Viability was the main consideration. Subsequently, protein variations detectable by electrophoresis and other techniques have entered the discussion. If all fitness components are included in estimating the effective number of overdominant loci, the number of polymorphic loci maintained by heterosis may be much greater (Tracey and Ayala, 1974).

Mammal Populations

A natural deermouse population studied by Blair (1958) in central Texas maintained itself over a number of years despite 500 R given to each male of each generation. Decreased litter size attributable to induced dominant lethals was considered to be obvious evidence of genetic damage. Subsequently the rodents in other enclosed areas have been studied, usually after exposure to chronic γ rays from ^{60}Co or ^{137}Cs sources. Thus dose levels which decrease population size within a few years were demonstrated for pocket mice in the Mohave desert, and for cotton rats in the Savannah River reservation. Nevertheless, the cotton rat population of a radioactive disposal area in Oak Ridge did not differ significantly from control levels. This type of information which appears in the proceedings of the symposia on Radioecology feature the census approach rather than an analysis of components of reproductive fitness.

The genetics literature now carries reports on long-term studies of laboratory and farm populations of mammals. Green's (1968) review cites 10 different experiments in as many different laboratories with one generation exposed to radiation, and seven experiments with one exposure in each of several successive generations. In addition, five separate laboratories investigated populations of mice or rats exposed continuously for several generations.

Despite ample confirmation of induced genetic or chromosomal changes leading to zygotic death or sterility, attempts to measure the effects of presumptive new mutations on the fitness of heterozygotes have been unsuccessful. For example, Spalding et al. (1969) treated the male line with 200 rem per generation for 45 generations of mice, hoping to demonstrate the effects of an accumulated genetic load by alterations of the growth rates and life-time survival curves. No significant differences between the irradiated and control strains were demonstrable.

Other Organisms

Grosch (1966) found individual reproductive performance to be well below that of equivalent controls in Artemia strains derived from ancestors reared in radioisotope-containing seawater. In cultures followed up to 32 generations, the standing crop data obtained from a population census did not reflect the radiation-induced genetic damage, provided the reproductive capability of the adults was adequate to compensate for reduced fecundity and the death of immature stages. Furthermore, although a population of irradiated ancestry might achieve numerical equivalence to control cultures, total reproductive capability might be involved in achieving and maintaining the population size. Then a relatively small additional amount of radiation can set off a trend to extinction.

Fecundity, of critical importance for the survival of Artemia, is also important in another Branchiopod. Continuous γ radiation from a ^{60}Co source was used to deliver doses up to 75 R/hr to populations of Daphnia, the parthenogenetic freshwater flea (Marshall, 1962). The intrinsic rate of increase in populations decreased continuously as a nonlinear function of the dose rate, chiefly due to a falling birth rate. In turn, this was traced to reduced fecundity rather than to prenatal mortality. Also consistent with these results were observations on important soil insects. Collembola exposed to continuous beta rays from ^{90}Sr and ^{90}Y proved more vulnerable to decreased fecundity and fertility than to changes in other components of fitness (Styron, 1971).

We will consider radiation effects on plant communities in a later chapter on radioecology. Here we briefly note that the European successes in radiation plant breeding have been based in part on the use of heterozygotes that are superior to standard types.

In homozygous state, the induced mutants, some of which are associated with chromosome aberration, can be detrimental, often lethal. Also, although usually not induced by radiations, the superiority of heterozygotes has been the basis of the great hybrid corn program of the United States. However, an important point must be made that the strategies of man and nature differ. The monoculture ecosystems of modern agriculture are managed artificial situations, not natural communities.

The variability, polymorphism, and heterosis of natural populations may or may not be explained by a multitude of loci with over-dominant alleles. In order to view these matters in their proper perspective, we must realize that the actual situation in which genetic action occurs is not one in which units are acting independently. Harmonious action of the entire hereditary endowment is necessary for successful completion of development and for meeting the crises of day-to-day survival.

Concluding Remarks

Chapter 7 presented evidence that induced localized gene changes are deleterious when a homozygous condition is attained. The present chapter indicates that although a certain amount of homozygosity may be expected to emerge in populations, the heterozygous state conceivably could be utilitarian. However, there is controversy on this point.

Evidently it is important to distinguish between the individual organism and populations of organisms. The fate of individuals and the fate of a population are two different things. Without questioning the survival of our population, we pay an annual predictable price in individuals while satisfying our desire for rapid transportation. We can enjoy the advantages of atomic energy without paying an equivalent price if we maintain adequate regulations and safeguards, and if we learn enough about the establishment of genetic equilibria in gene pools to predict radiation effects upon human populations. The situation has been summed up by Wallace's group (Annual Report 1954–

1955 Biol. Lab. Cold Spring Harbor). "There is only one morally defensible position one can take regarding the exposure of persons to radiations: No exposure without justification. Negative arguments that irradiation has no genetic effect or that the effect consists merely of a few deleterious mutations are indefensible since they are based on a callous indifference to the health and happiness of other persons." From this stated philosophy it becomes apparent that even geneticists who are convinced about overdominance are reluctant to have individuals from a human population pay a price for a new population equilibrium.

Furthermore, the mouse studies indicate that recessive mutations can be measured in large populations. A main concern is that such mutations induced by radiation may accumulate along with those from other agents to reach a critical level some time in the future. In man, the situation differs from that in experimental animals because many individuals with mutations can be kept alive to procreate by medical control of the physical condition caused by mutations.

References

Ayala, F. J. (1968). Genotype, environment, and population numbers. *Science* **162**, 1453–1459.

Blair, W. F. (1958). Effects of x-irradiation on a natural population of the deer mouse. *Ecology* **39**, 113–118.

Carson, H. L. (1964). Population size and genetic load in irradiated populations of *Drosophila melanogaster*. *Genetics* **49**, 521–528.

Dobzhansky, T. (1966). Genetics of natural populations, the coadapted system of chromosomal variants in a population of *Drosophila pseudoobscura*. 37th paper of a series. *Genetics* **53**, 843–854.

Falk, R. (1967). Fitness of heterozygotes for irradiated chromosomes in *Drosophila, Mutat. Res.* **4**, 805–819.

Green, E. L. (1968). Genetic effects of radiation on mammalian populations. *Annu. Rev. Genet.* **2**, 87–120.

Grosch, D. S. (1966). The reproductive capacity of *Artemia* subjected to successive contaminations with radiophosphorus. *Biol. Bull. (Woods Hole, Mass.)* **131**, 261–271.

Marshall, J. S. (1962). The effects of continuous gamma radiation on the intrinsic rate of natural increase of *Daphnia pulex. Ecology* **43**, 598–607.

Mather, K. (1952). The long term genetical hazard of atomic energy. *In* "Biological Hazards of Atomic Energy" (A. Haddow ed.), pp. 57–66. Oxford Univ. Press (Clarendon), London and New York.

Mukai, T. (1969). The genetic structure of natural populations of *Drosophila melanogaster*. VI. Further studies on the optimum heterozygosity hypothesis. *Genetics* **61**, 479–495.

Muller, H. J. (1950). Radiation damage to genetic material. *Am. Sci.* **38**, 33–59 and 399–425.

Muller, H. J. and Falk, R. (1961). Are induced mutations in Drosophila overdominant? *Genetics* **46**, 727–735 and 737–757.

National Academy of Science–National Research Council (1956). Summ. Rep. "The Biological Effects of Atomic Radiation," NAS–NRC, Washington, D.C.

National Academy of Science–National Research Council (1972). "The Effects on Populations of Exposure to Low Levels of Ionizing Radiation," B.E.I.R. Rep. NAS–NRC, Washington, D.C.

Neel, J. V., and Schull, W. J. (1956). The effect of exposure to the atomic bombs on pregnancy termination in Hiroshima and Nagasaki. NAS–NRC Publ. 461.

Newell, R. R. (1957). Genetic aspects of radiation hygiene. *X-ray News* **29**, No. 10. General Electric Co.

Simmons, M. J. (1976). Heterozygous effects of irradiated chromosomes on viability in *Drosophila melanogaster*. *Genetics* **84**, 353–374.

Sonnenblick, B. P. (1955). On some aspects of the problem of human radiation protection. *J. Newark Beth Isr. Hosp.* **6**, 31–42.

Spalding, J. F., Brooks, M. R., and Tietjen, G. L. (1969). Lifetime body weights and mortality distributions of mice with 10 to 35 generations of ancestral x-ray exposure. *Genetics* **63**, 897–906.

Stern, C. (1973). "Principles of Human Genetics," 3rd ed. Freeman, San Francisco, California.

Stone, W. S., and Wilson, F. D. (1959). Genetic studies of irradiated natural populations of *Drosophila*. IV. 1958 Tests. Univ. Texas Publ. 5914, 223–233.

Stone, W. S., Wheeler, M. R., and Wilson, F. D. (1962). Genetic studies of irradiated natural populations of *Drosophila*. V. Summary and discussion of tests of populations collected in the Pacific Proving Ground from 1955 to 1959. Univ. Texas Publ. 6205, 1–54.

Styron, C. E. (1971). Effects of beta and gamma radiation on a population of springtails, *Sinella curviseta*. *Radiat. Res.* **48**, 53–62.

Tracey, M. L., and Ayala, F. J. (1974). Genetic load in natural populations: Is it compatible with the hypothesis that many polymorphisms are maintained by natural selection? *Genetics* **77**, 569–589.

Wallace, B. (1956). Studies on irradiated populations of *Drosophila melanogaster*. *J. Genet.* **54**, 280–293.

Wallace, B. (1963). Further data on the overdominance of induced mutation. *Genetics* **48**, 633–651.

Wallace, B. and Dobzhansky, T. (1959). *Radiation, Genes and Man*. Holt, New York.

Watanabe, T. K., and Oshima, C. (1970). Persistence of lethal genes in Japanese natural populations of *Drosophila melanogaster*. *Genetics* **64**, 93–106.

PART III

TISSUES AND ORGANS

The preceding chapters have presented radiation influences upon components of the structural unit of eukaryote life, the cell. Virtually any cell-based phenomenon which man has been able to measure may be modified by radiation, but there are great differences in the amount of radiation required. From necessity these matters were discussed one by one, but a variety of disturbances varying in degree may be induced simultaneously. However, relative radiosensitivities place limitations upon the significance of cell disturbances to the welfare of an organism or its progeny, although incidental deviations may contribute to the quantitative level of damage.

Delayed division, a radiosensitive phenomenon, may be reflected in delayed development, but by its very nature does not pose an insurmountable obstacle. Chromosomal aberrations are more critical. Direct evidence is available from experiments like Conger's.[1] By scoring bridges and fragments as well as the time course of mitotic inhibition in irradiated ascites tumors, he demonstrated the significance of chromosomal aberrations. "Even with generous allowance," division

[1] A. D. Conger, Radiation effects on ascites tumor chromosomes. *Ann. N.Y. Acad. Sci.* **63,** 929–936 (1956).

delay could account for no more than one-third of the decrease in tumor growth.

Other kinds of studies also point to chromosomal effects as the source of diverse types of tissue change. These changes which dominate cell fate not only explain histopathology, but they also may underlie radiation sickness and aging effects. Expressly convincing evidence of the importance of chromosome aberrations in cell destiny was obtained in population survival studies with cultured cells. Here, as in the diploid organisms from which they were obtained, recessive changes at the genic level would not be revealed in the absence of a technique to produce homozygosity. At the organism level, results cited below for higher plants gave the first indications that the DNA content of the chromosomes is a particular feature determining radiosensitivity.

CHAPTER 9   Plant Morphology

To date, the best evidence concerning the significance of chromosomal aberrations in the structure and fate of the exposed generation of organisms has come from botanical investigations. In order to understand how radiation-induced changes can be brought about we must appreciate that roots, shoot tips, and other locations in higher plants contain actively dividing cells in localized regions called meristems. Growth, differentiation, and development result from the normal activities of meristematic tissue. Cell-death attributable to loss or unbalance of genetic material has serious consequences. Sparrow and his associates have found that after irradiation there occurs a reduction in the number of cells per meristem, and this reduction varies directly with the proportion of cells showing chromosome damage. Chromosomal size and DNA content are important as contributing factors.

An explanation with predictive utility has come only through searching at the cellular and subcellular level within individual tissues. Descriptive efforts based on external examination of stunted and dwarfed plants, or misshapen and mottled organs, provided little information concerning the basic causes. Furthermore, the observations were often published as aspects incidental to the main subject, typically an investigation of mutation rate. Thus, the biological effects described resulted from acute exposure of some particular part of the plant after germination. These historical x-ray and radium experiments have been conveniently reviewed by Johnson (1936) and by Gager (1936) in the Duggar volumes (1936).

Less attention was given to radiation effects on developing plant embryos, but the general pattern of response resembled that of the mammalian embryo. The embryo is more radiosensitive than the differentiated plant, and induced anomalies are stage-specific, in that the period for induction of a particular abnormality is restricted to a limited period of time during embryonic development (Mericle and Mericle, 1961).

Field Experiments

In recent years, attention has turned to chronic exposures to [60]Co
gamma rays throughout development. Sparrow and Singleton (1953)
installed a γ-ray source in a Brookhaven field like the one depicted in
Figure 9.1. A quantity of several hundred curies of such an isotope is
potentially dangerous and strict safety precautions were observed. The
field was located in an isolated area and fenced to exclude casual visitors
or animals. At all points the fence was far enough from the source to
prevent overexposure of personnel. The single point of entry was locked
with ingenious safety mechanisms which prevented personnel from
entering the field without first lowering the source. Suggestions toward
improving the prototype installation have merely added the erection of

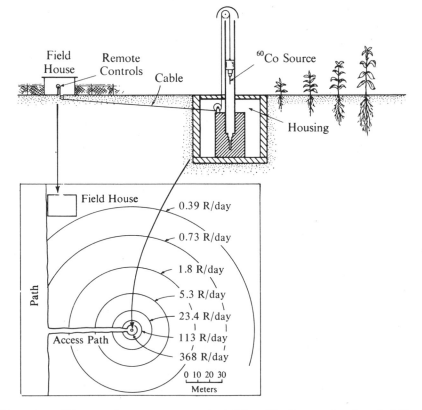

Figure 9.1. Diagram of a gamma source installation like the one developed at Brookhaven National Laboratories by A. H. Sparrow and W. R. Singleton.

an outer fence at a distance where a full day's exposure does not exceed the permissible dose, as indicated on the frequent warning signs. More than 300 species of plants have been exposed at Brookhaven, where the source in the cultivated field was finally stepped up to 3160 Ci, and a small supplemental source was installed in a greenhouse. In addition, a fallout-decay simulator was constructed, with telescoping steel shields which can be lowered to decrease the exposure rate over a predetermined period of time (Sparrow, 1966). Many of the simpler field units are now used in the research stations of America and other continents.

Growth inhibition in a dose related pattern is most striking in a cultivated field containing a particular variety of plant. Close to the source, dwarfing is severe when the radiation dose is high enough to inhibit proliferation of nearly all the meristematic cells. Table 9.1, which gives the tolerance of 31 different plants to chronic gamma irradiation, indicates a 200-fold difference between the least tolerant and most tolerant species investigated. Interestingly enough, the more sensitive plants were those favored by cytologists because of their large chromosomes, *Tradescantia*, *Lilium*, and *Vicia*.

Measurements of metaphase chromosomes seemed too tedious and time-consuming to apply to adequate samples of plants from a large number of species. Therefore the simpler and more efficient method of recording interphase nuclear volume was adopted, after establishing its relationship to chromosome size. Dividing the meristematic nuclear volume by the number of chromosomes provided an average interphase chromosome volume. This index multiplied by the average number of ionizations (1.77 for γ rays) produced per cubic micron per roentgen, and by 32.5 eV per ion pair gave the "energy absorbed per chromosome per R" (Sparrow's 1962 terminology).

$$\frac{v}{2n} \times 1.77 \times 32.5 = \text{electronvolts absorbed per chromosome per roentgen}$$

For higher plants, seemingly different lethal-exposure doses often were resolved into similar amounts of energy absorbed per chromosome. For example, the lethal exposure is 0.8 kR for *Lilium longifolium* but it is 20 kR for *Sedum oryzifolium*. The energy absorbed per chromosome at lethal exposure is 2400 keV and 2480 keV respectively.

The calculation of chromosome volume provides an estimate of DNA per chromosome because these parameters are directly proportional. In turn, a proportionality of DNA to the lethal dose of radiation has been established (Figure 9.2). However in extending investigations of cellu-

TABLE 9.1

The Tolerance of 31 Plants to Chronic γ Irradiation[a]

Plant	Minimum exposure (weeks)	Effect at indicated dose rate[b] (roentgens per day)	
		Mild	Severe[c]
Lilium longiflorum	15	20(?)	30
Tradescantia paludosa	15	20	40
Tradescantia ohiensis	15	35	65
Vicia faba	15	60	90
Impatiens sp.	18	60	90
Coleus blumei	13	100	240
Melilotus officinalis	14	100	240
Nicotiana rustica	15	100	300
Phytolacca americana	15	100	350
Datura stramonium	7	110	360
Gossypium hirsuium	15	110	250
Dahlia (hybrid)	10	110	275
Althea rosea	12	120	250
Luzula purpurea	10	125	300
Chrysanthemum (hybrid)	18	140	250
Canna generalis	18	180	350
Lactuca sativa	7	180	600
Chenopodium album	15	250	450
Antirrhinum majus	18	250	400
Lycopersicon esculentum	15	250	400
Xanthium sp.	15	250	500
Solanum tuberosum	10	300	600
Petunia hybrida	10	300	700
Celosia cristata	18	300	750
Lupinus albus	12	400	—
Kalanchoe daigremontiana	12	400	800
Allium cepa	18	400	800
Linum usitatissimum[d]	10	600	1100
Digitaria (crabgrass)	12	1000	1800
Brassica oleracea (broccoli)	10	1400	2500
Gladiolus (hybrid)	8	1400	6000

[a] From Sparrow and Christensen (1953).

[b] Dose rate is in roentgens per 24-hr day; however, the actual dosage per day averaged about 90% of the dose rate shown.

[c] This dose rate is not necessarily the lowest rate which will produce a severe effect.

[d] Data supplied by C. Konzak.

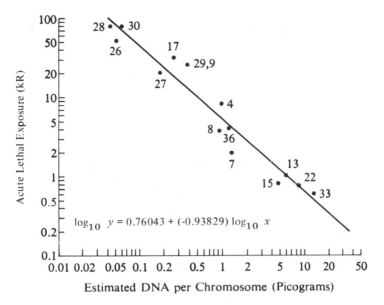

Figure 9.2. Relationship between mean DNA values per chromosome and radiosensitivity in 15 species of plants. (Courtesy of A. H. Sparrow.)

lar radiosensitivity to organisms other than plants, Sparrow and associates (Sparrow *et al.*, 1967; Underbrink *et al.*, 1968) found that DNA content allowed classification into only four groups, while chromosome volumes enabled the recognition of eight "radiotaxa." When 37%-survival doses were plotted against chromosome volumes, eight regression lines were obtained with slopes not significantly different from −1. There were 120 diverse organisms represented by viruses, bacteria, yeasts, protozoa, and cells from bird, amphibian, and mammalian normal and cancerous tissues.

A radiotaxon does not necessarily coincide with other classical taxonomical systems. Determining factors seem to involve some unidentified but inherent similarity in chromosome makeup. Different species may possess different ratios between the structural genes and control and spacer DNA. Also, within a radiotaxon, factors contributing to differences in radiosensitivities may be associated with chromosome structural differences involving DNA: nucleic acid strand arrangements, associated protein, constitutive heterochromatin. Nonchromosomal features may also play a role. These could include the average time between divisions and the amounts of protective chemical substances present naturally.

Specific Anomalies

Both in the older literature and recently, a number of histological and morphological changes have been reported for plants which have been exposed to radiation. Gunckel and associates (1954) have presented many striking photographs of somatic malformations, often similar to those mentioned in Johnson's (1936) review.

One of the most characteristic stem responses is death of the shoot apex, accompanied by failure of the internodes to elongate. Another common effect is fasciation, perhaps formed by the fusion of numerous buds in close proximity. In one experiment, over 12% of the snapdragons given 240–350 R/day showed fasciation, in contrast to zero incidence in thousands of unirradiated plants of the same variety. Localized stem swellings and twistings, as well as tumor-like growths, are induced. In some cases large numbers of aerial roots develop from local stem swellings (Figure 9.3). Stem dichotomy and altered phylotaxis may occur after extended chronic irradiation.

Along with the stem responses, most irradiated plants produce leaf anomalies. These include dwarfing, thickening, altered shape and texture, puckering, abnormal curvatures, marginal curling, distorted venation, fusions, and mosaic-like color changes (Figure 9.4). Some of these responses lend themselves to histological analysis. For example, thickening of tomato leaves can be traced to increased height of palisade

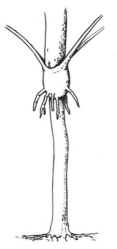

Figure 9.3. Stem swelling and adventitious root production in an irradiated *Xanthium* stem. X-ray dose = 3000 R. Note the irradiated stem section at the base failed to enlarge, while above it the stem enlarged and a number of roots formed. (Based on Gunckel and Sparrow, 1954.)

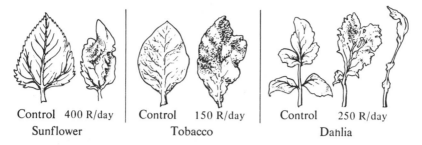

Control 400 R/day	Control 150 R/day	Control 250 R/day
Sunflower	Tobacco	Dahlia

Figure 9.4. Leaf abnormalities from chronic irradiation. (Based on photographs by courtesy of J. E. Gunckel and A. H. Sparrow.)

cells and thick spongy mesophyll. There is a quantitative relationship between these features and dosage.

Flowering is greatly retarded in the gamma field, and abscission of buds occurs at higher dosages. When flowers develop at moderate doses, the form and number of flower parts are modified (Figure 9.5). Increases may occur in numbers of petals and stamens. Double and open ovaries, and multiple or fused styles are additional induced abnormalities. These changes are not heritable, and unlike somatic mutations, cannot be propagated even if they appeal to human fancy or promise some advantage.

A biologically interesting case of apparent advantage is the suppression of crown-gall formation in tomatoes receiving gamma rays at dosage rates above 5 R/hr. The causative bacteria after exposure totaling 50,000 R delivered at 80 R/hr were quite capable of producing galls on nonirradiated plants but not on plants surviving 30,000 R. Before we jump to the conclusion that we should raise tomatoes in gamma fields to avoid disease, let us consider the appearance of the plants. Decreased

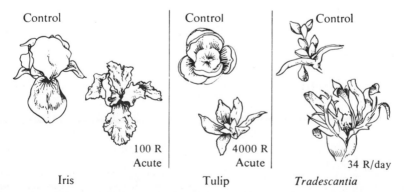

Figure 9.5. Abnormal flower parts following irradiation. (Based on photographs by courtesy of J. E. Gunckel and A. H. Sparrow.)

terminal growth, new growth lacking central parenchyma, under-developed leaf laminae, and very poor root development is the price paid by the plants. Gall suppression is related to damage in the host, which traces in turn to decreases in cell division and cell enlargement.

In all these cases it is important to realize that radiation is really causing damage, although extra structures occur or parts are caused to grow in unusual positions. The delicate balance of development has been disrupted and normal control mechanisms have been disturbed or destroyed. For example, in production of aerial roots the site appears to be one of a phloem block beyond which downward transport cannot occur. Accumulation of organic materials above this area can explain both the swelling and an induction of roots from the swollen region.

Plant Hormones

A disturbed balance in the hormones that control cellular activity may contribute to some of the aberrations in plant morphology. Three groups interact to produce controlled growth and structural differentia-tion. They are the auxins, giberellins, and cytokinins.

Indoleacetic acid (IAA), the most common naturally occurring auxin, possesses the capacity to stimulate plant-cell elongation among its com-plex and multiple effects. Formed IAA withstands inactivation, and cell elongation is not particularly radiosensitive. Target theory predicts little effect for 100 R on relatively small molecules like IAA. On the other hand, IAA synthesis in the mung bean seedling is one of the most radiosensitive biochemical reactions known (Gordon, 1957). Doses under 100 R alter auxin production by blocking the oxidative conver-sion of indoleacetaldehyde to the acid. Aldehyde accumulates behind the block. Unfortunately, the investigation is unfinished. Other inves-tigators could not find equally sensitive "Gordon auxin systems" in other kinds of plants. Because much of the IAA synthesis occurs in terminal buds of the shoot and in young leaves, the bean auxin response may be a secondary process derived from primary nuclear damage.

A different recurrent hypothesis needs to be mentioned: by destroy-ing an inhibitor (alternatively a degredation mechanism), irradiation could cause abnormal amounts of a physiologically active substance which could stimulate plant growth. Reproducible experimental results are uncommon. Much remains to be done in the radiation research of plant hormones.

Tumor Induction

A response to irradiation which involves cell proliferation without differentiation is the initiation of tumors. The delicate balance between differential growth and neoplasia has been upset. This has been demonstrated in a number of different species as well as in tumor-prone *Nicotiana* hybrids (Smith, 1972). Other plants showing the response include peas, beans, ferns, snapdragon, *Crepis* and *Arabidopsis*. An inhibition of tumor development has also been reported.

The importance of a hereditary component has not been established in most cases, but in genetically predisposed *Nicotiana* hybrids, ionizing radiation accelerates tumor initiation. An increased number of plants with tumors is accompanied by an increase in the amount of tumor tissue per plant. Within weeks, low doses induced stem tumors in all the hybrids. Above 300 R/day, 50% of the top wet weight became tumor tissue.

All types of ionizing radiations are effective in a dose-dependent pattern overriding the age-dependent frequency of incidence. Neutrons not only were more effective than x rays, but neutron effect curves were exponential. The yield curves for x rays had a pronounced shoulder associated with no visible consequences of the lowest doses (under 10 R). A unique feature of the tumor formation dose-response curve was that cell lethality predominated at doses above that causing 100% tumorous plants. At higher doses, tumors became progressively less frequent.

Mosaicism

Chromosome aberrations and gene mutations in somatic tissues can cause sectoring or variegation patterns, but such changes are not passed on to the offspring by sexual reproduction. Somatic mutations occur in animals as well as in plants but their presence is more obvious in plant foliage and flower petals. Also, several types of mosaicism are known for kernels of corn. Early examples of induced variegated flowers were obtained in carnations, dahlias, hyacinths, snapdragons, and tulips.

A standard approach is to expose immature plants from a strain heterozygous for alleles determining flower color and observe the changes from the dominant form. Sand and Smith (1973) have used a hybrid *Nicotiana* clone heterozygous at two color loci: R/r and V_{S3}/v_s, in which R is red; r, purple; V_{S3}, solid color; and v_s, speckled white. This provides mutable (V) and stable (R) genes for simultaneous study of the bud-cluster response to irradiation. Purple and speckled sectors are scored for the mature flowers. At low acute doses, the V locus is more sensitive than the R locus. For example, at 15 R the V mutational yield per cell per roentgen is 3.5×10^{-5}, but at the stable locus the yield is only 0.087×10^{-5}. Furthermore, at low dose rates the somatic response of the V system is 10-fold greater than that of the R system, although in the germ line responses are similar.

The low dose response argues against deletion aberrations. Cell killing is ruled out by an experimental design which allows recovery of mutations from the mutable and stable loci from the same cell population. Sector formation is independent of tumor induction. These considerations and others suggest hypotheses involving either chromosome structure or cellular physiology.

Root Experiments

In the majority of field or forest studies, plant roots are shielded from radiation by the soil in which they are anchored. In addition to serving as plant anchors, roots have important functions in the absorption of water and mineral nutrients. Also, in perennials, they serve as a storage reservoir. The irradiation of artificially exposed roots has revealed one clear principle. A single, small radiation exposure to the meristematic region of the root tip causes growth inhibition (Davidson, 1960). The total damage to chromosomes is evident only in the course of a week or more.

Although the meristem is the source of new cells, increase in root length also depends on an elongation of cells situated behind the proliferative population. More than 10 kR are required to interfere with elongation. That is, the zone of growth completion is relatively insensitive because the destruction of extant auxin molecules such as indoleacetic acid (IAA) is accomplished only by massive doses. No evidence has been found for necrocytotic substances moving from irradiated to shielded parts of the root.

Absorbed Radioisotopes

Special consideration is due radiation sources which become part of an organism's physiology. Radioisotopes accumulate in particular tissues and regions as a result of growth, development, and metabolism.

We are about to discuss plants. Later chapters will consider internal isotopes in animals and in ecological situations. Much of the damage is due to emitted radiations, but some damage results when an incorporated element transmutates into another which may be inappropriate or even toxic. The nuclear reaction called radioactive decay can occur to atoms built into biologically important molecules.

Controlled Experiments. ^{32}P has been used widely, possibly because of its low cost and strong beta rays, but especially because of an indispensable association with the genetically important nucleic acids and the energy-storage-transfer mechanisms. Investigators had good reason to expect radiophosphorus to become associated with important cellular sites. With tomato plants, for example, they demonstrated that ^{32}P accumulated in young leaves and stem tips. Furthermore, more phosphorus accumulated in young fruit than in older fruit. The element is not permanently fixed in place, however. With low availability of phosphorus, retransport of ^{32}P from leaves to fruit can occur.

The damaging effects of absorbed radioisotopes were revealed when seeds and seedlings were subjected to radioactive nutrient solutions. The growth of shoot and root lengths was considerably curtailed (Figure 9.6). As little as 5 μCi applied to barley and wheat seed induced chromosome disturbances in more than half the subsequent cell divisions, a situation lethal to the seedlings. Compared with x-ray experiments, damage was equivalent to 25,000 R or more. Damage from internal radiation has also been demonstrated in trees and woody plants. Meristematic accumulation of ^{32}P followed radioisotope injections of peas, cherry and apple trees, and rose bushes. Leaf deformation and shoot bifurcation resulted. Autoradiography, a technique in which

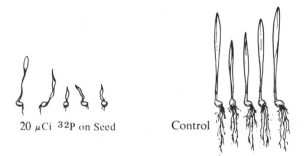

20 μCi ^{32}P on Seed   Control

Figure 9.6. Barley seedlings germinated in radioactive solutions, compared with controls. (Based on Ehrenberg *et al.*, 1949; with permission.)

radioactive areas reveal their activity in contact with photographic emulsions, demonstrated that ^{32}P concentrated quickly in the meristematic zones characterized by mitotic activity. Conspicuous clublike swellings often resulted from disruption of normal cell division.

Other radioisotopes have other patterns of distribution depending upon their chemical affinities. Space prohibits our considering all the essential and nonessential elements which are necessary for, or interfere with, mineral nutrition in plants. A number of sizable monographs and symposia have been published on these matters. However, we shall consider a few radioisotopes which have demonstrated patterns of damage.

^{35}S, which can become a constituent of many important proteins, typically has a general distribution and persistence. Experiments with plants showed it present not only in meristematic zones, but also abundant in stretching zones. ^{22}Na proved to be easily absorbed and easily eliminated, but not before reaching seed parts from which it transfers to the coleoptile and the first leaf.

Radiostrontium is a fallout element which has drawn much public attention. Jacobson and Overstreet (1948) demonstrated that tracer levels of Sr and other fission products including Y, Ce, Zr, and Cb caused severe injury to peas in a three-month period. However, a Canadian team (Spinks et al., 1948) discovered that plants can eliminate strontium chloride by concentrating it in their first two leaves, which wither and drop off. Practically all of a dose of ^{90}Sr given to wheat, barley, or sunflower seeds became localized in the first two leaves. These become expendable presumably after a lethal concentration of isotope is reached. Aarkrog (1969) confirmed that ^{85}Sr sprayed on the foliage of rye, barley, wheat, or oats was not translocated. In contrast ^{134}Cs and ^{54}Mn moved around and tended to concentrate in the grains. Other foliar absorption tests using common corrosion products from nuclear reactors (Aarkrog and Lippert, 1971) showed that 40% of either ^{65}Zn or ^{58}Co concentrated in the grains. ^{59}Fe translocated into the grain to far less extent (10%), while little ^{51}Cr reached the grains. When isotopes were incorporated via the roots, ^{137}Cs was more mobile than ^{85}Sr in bean, tomato and corn plants. Almost all ^{106}Ru was retained by the roots (Handley and Babcock, 1972).

Radioactivation of atmospheric nitrogen leads to the formation of ^{14}C by nuclear explosions. Incorporated into DNA it can be mutagenic, or when used as a tag for compounds containing carbon, reactor-produced ^{14}C can cause cell damage. In a study of medicinal plants used in the biosynthesis of radioactive drugs, Beal (1949) found that although routine dosages were not lethal, the pattern of tissue differentiation was altered. Leaf sections showed distorted epidermis, poorly defined palisade, and spongy parenchymal cells. There were numerous groups of dead or dying cells and practically no intercellular spaces.

For a study of chromosome aberrations broad bean shoots were exposed to ^{14}C as $^{14}CO_2$. The percentage of cells showing chromosome aberrations was 9 to 25 times as high as those receiving radiation from the exterior. Since ^{14}C was uniformly distributed, the aberrations cannot be explained by localized β radiation, and the results were interpreted as a transmutation effect. Onion root tips with incorporated [methyl-^{14}C] thymidine produced twice as many chromosome aberrations as [2-^{14}C] thymidine, which provides an additional example of transmutation. An increase in cell death from atomic decay is a reasonable inference. However, not all experiments are consistent. The snapdragon somatic mutation rate from incorporated ^{14}C was not significantly above that induced by comparable external irradiation (Krisch and Zelle, 1969).

In tissue culture, the long half-life of ^{14}C makes possible the study of retention during subsequent transfers and growth on a nonradioactive medium. Ball (1953) demonstrated that there was persistence through 10 months of growth and five transfers of a culture of *Sequoia*, with some movement of ^{14}C from old into new tissue. Morphologically, the isotope caused thickening of callus tissue by hypertrophy of internal parenchymal cells and more new cells forming at right angles to the flat surface. However, histological damage from incorporated radioisotopes was much more pronounced with other beta emitters, ^{32}P and ^{35}S. With ^{32}P, division ceased and cells hypertrophied. Groups of marginal meristem cells died. ^{35}S caused disintegration of internal parenchyma, hypertrophy of marginal meristems, and cessation of new cell formation. Progressive blackening of the whole culture was observed after ^{35}S incorporation, while patchy dark necrotic areas resulted from the action of incorporated ^{32}P. These reflections of the extent of damage may be correlated with the greater tissue absorption of energy from the softer β rays of ^{35}S, but there is also the toxic ^{35}Cl decay product of ^{35}S. It is difficult to determine the transmutation component of cell lethality.

Entry of Isotope from the Biosphere. When man is not imposing something as artificial as injection or tissue culture, the ultimate criterion of availability of an element, whether useful or damaging, is its uptake by the plant. Entry is either through root or foliage. The former, as the more orthodox route, is largely dependent on the composition of the soil solution and the metabolism of the plant. Until recently, land plants usually have not had access to mineral nutrients via the leaves, and research on foliar entry is a feature of concern about the consequences of fallout. Although absorptive surfaces of the leaves differ from those of the roots and there is no continuous liquid phase through which ions may travel from the environment, plant foliage can take in radioactive materials.

Whether substances falling onto the leaves of plants get into the cells depends first upon whether or not they are soluble. If insoluble, they may persist merely on the surface. If soluble, they may penetrate the cell wall; but if the ion is so unusual that there is no carrier at the plasmalemma which recognizes it, no transport into the cellular interior may occur. Many of the fission products in the Bikini test debris persisted for years in the leaf axils without contributing significant radioactivity to the interior of the plant (Biddulph, 1960). A periodic table of elements can be consulted in order to decide whether the isotope of interest bears similarity to any common element for which transport mechanisms may exist.

Concluding Remarks

In this chapter we have considered a range in expression of plant anomalies and of radiosensitivity which is bewildering at first encounter. Neither the size of the plant, nor its growth habits, nor its prevalence, nor its evolutionary niche furnish good clues. Even when studied by experts, little or no correlation exists between any of these factors and the radiation response of the plant. Instead, cellular characteristics have had to be studied to reveal the role played by the nucleus and its contents.

Now we are going to turn to studies with animal materials. Here, too, the most significant radiation damage has a nuclear basis, although as yet no comprehensive study of radiosensitivity has been made at the DNA level. Comparisons on the diploid basis may provide an explanation of relative radiosensitivity during development, but polysomaty may complicate studies of differentiated tissues. Another matter to consider is the fact that chronic exposure of a plant in a gamma installation is not really an irradiation of the whole organism. Roots are shielded by the soil around them. When root tips are exposed, root tips are the structures examined; the plant itself is not under consideration. With animals, whole-organism exposure is routine rather than exceptional.

References

Aarkrog, A. (1969). On the direct contamination of rye, barley, wheat and oats with Sr, Cs, Mn, and Ce. *Radiat. Bot.* **9**, 357–366.

Aarkrog, A., and Lippert, J. (1971). Direct contamination of barley with Cr, Fe, Co, Zn, Hg, and Pb. *Radiat. Bot.* **11**, 463–472.

Ball, E. (1953). Histological effect of absorbed radioisotopes upon the callus of *Sequoia sempervirens*. *Bot. Gaz. (Chicago)* **114**, 353–363.

Beal, J. M. (1949). Some histological effects of Carbon 14 on the leaves of certain medicinal plants. *Bot. Gaz. (Chicago)* **110**, 600–604.

Biddulph, O. (1960). "Radioisotopes in Plants: Foliar Entry and Distribution," pp. 73–85. University of Minnesota, Minneapolis.

Davidson, D. (1960). Mechanisms in seeds and roots. *In* Radiation Protection and Recovery" (A. Hollaender, ed.), pp. 175–211. Pergamon, Oxford.

Duggar, B. M., ed. (1936). "Biological Effects of Radiations," Vols. I and II. McGraw-Hill, New York.

Ehrenberg, L., and Granhall, I. (1952). Effects of beta-radiating isotopes in fruit trees. *Hereditas* **38**, 385–419.

Ehrenberg, L., Gustafsson, A., Levan, A., and von Wettstein, U. (1949). Radiophosphorus, seedling lethality and chromosome disturbances. *Hereditas* **35**, 469–489.

Gager, C. S. (1936). The effects of radium rays on plants. *In* "Biological Effects of Radiations" (B. M. Duggar, ed.), Vol. II, pp. 987–1014. McGraw-Hill, New York.

Gordon, S. A. (1957). The effects of ionizing radiation on plants. Biochemical and physiological aspects. *Quart. Rev. Biol.* **32**, 3–14.

Gunckel, J. E., and Sparrow, A. H. (1954). Aberrant growth in plants induced by ionizing radiation. *Brookhaven Symp. Biol.* **6**, 252–279.

Handley, R., and Babcock, K. L. (1972). Translocation of Sr, Cs, and Ru in crop plants. *Radiat. Bot.* **12**, 113–119.

Johnson, E. L. (1936). Effects of x rays upon green plants. *In* "Biological Effects of Radiations" (B. M. Duggar, ed.), Vol. II, pp. 961–986. McGraw-Hill, New York.

Jacobson, L., and Overstreet, R. (1948). The uptake by plants of plutonium and some products of nuclear fission absorbed on soil colloids. *Soil Sci.* **65**, 129–134.

Krisch, R. E., and Zelle, M. R. (1969). Biological effects of radioactive decay: The role of the transmutation effect. *Adv. Radiat. Biol.* **3**, 177–213.

Mericle, L. W., and Mericle, R. P. (1961). Radiosensitivity of the developing plant embryo. *Brookhaven Symp. Biol.* **14**, 262–283.

Sand, S. A., and Smith, H. H. (1973). Somatic mutational transients. III. Response by two genes in a clone of *Nicotiana* to 24 R of gamma radiation applied at various intensities. *Genetics* **75**, 93–111.

Smith, H. H. (1972). Plant genetic tumors. *Prog. Exp. Tumor Res.* **15**, 138–164.

Sparrow, A. H. (1962). The role of the cell nucleus in determining radiosensitivity. *Brookhaven Natl. Lab. Lect. Ser.* No. 17, BNL 766.

Sparrow, A. H. (1966). Research uses of the gamma field and related radiation facilities at Brookhaven National Laboratory. *Radiat. Bot.* **6**, 377–405.

Sparrow, A. H., and Christensen, E. (1953). Tolerance of certain higher plants to chronic exposure to gamma radiation from cobalt-60. *Science* **118**, 697–698.

Sparrow, A. H., and Singleton, W. R. (1953). The use of radiocobalt as a source of gamma rays and some effects of chronic irradiation on growing plants. *Am. Nat.* **87**, 29–48.

Sparrow, A. H., Underbrink, A. G., and Sparrow, R. C. (1967). Chromosomes and cellular radiosensitivity. I. *Radiat. Res.* **32,** 915–945.

Spinks, J. W. T., Cumming, E., Irwin, R. L. B., and Arnason, T. J. (1948). Lethal effect of absorbed radioisotopes on plants. *Can. J. Res., Sect. C* **26,** 249–262.

Underbrink, A. G., Sparrow, A. H., and Pond, V. (1968). Chromosomes and cellular radiosensitivity. II. Use of interrelationships among chromosome volume, nucleotide content and D_0 of 120 diverse organisms in predicting radiosensitivity. *Radiat. Bot.* **8,** 205–237.

CHAPTER 10   Animal Embryology

An embryo is not simply a miniature of the adult organism but an epigenetic system, or as Rugh (1960) puts it, a dynamic "changing mosaic of metamorphosing parts all integrated into an overall pattern by 'organismic' forces." These forces are influenced when the number of intact building blocks is altered by ionizing radiation. Cells which happen to be in the most vulnerable stage at the time of exposure are destroyed. The embryo constantly has an abundance of vulnerable cells provided by different organ systems at different times.

The embryo is a mosaic of developing centers, many of which are necessary for survival of the organism. Thus it is as radiosensitive as its most sensitive vital organ system at any particular period of development. At the same time, the embryo possesses great powers of repair and reconstitution. In the vertebrate, phagocytes are present to remove such debris as necrotic cells damaged by radiation. When these are gone, undifferentiated, undamaged cells attempt to fill in the deficiencies. Deficiency is tolerated to the extent that residual cells can take over the role of those destroyed. On occasion, reduction of cell mass in a topographically normal embryo results in stunted organisms and in smaller organs. Microophthalmia and microcephalia are striking examples.

Relative Radiosensitivity and Development

The most striking contrasts in radiosensitivity of developmental stages occur in insects. Packard's (1945) work is often cited. He found 190 R to be the mean lethal dose for early *Drosophila* embryos, whereas 100,000 R was required for adults. Also, whereas 165 R will kill all diploids and nearly all haploid early embryos, doses in excess of 100,000 R must be used to kill adult *Habrobracon*. Figure 10.1 shows the progressive loss of radiosensitivity in selected holometabolous insects.

Even in vertebrates, which are relatively sensitive as adults due to the vulnerability of important proliferative tissues, there is an early stage when the organism is more radiosensitive than at any other time. Trout

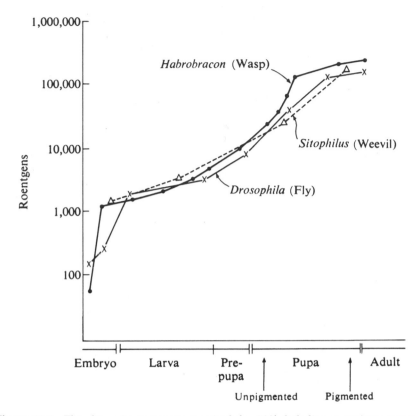

Figure 10.1 The doses in roentgens required for 50% lethality at various stages of development of holometabolous insects from three important orders.

embryos have an LD_{50} of little more than 50 R at the one cell stage; later, embryos from the same group tolerate up to 900 R. Similarly, in the fish *Fundulus* only a fraction of the dose later tolerated may be delivered safely during cleavage. Also, frog embryos tolerate only a fraction of the radiation dose used for larval and adult stages, and the LD_{50} for birds is lowest during the first few days of incubation. Dead mouse embryos result from only 50 R given before implantation, but the incidence of neonatal death is not increased by 300 R. For adults, the $LD_{50/30}$ may be as high as 700 rads.

In addition to death, still another aspect demonstrates that the embryo is more sensitive to ionizing radiation than at any subsequent stage. Deficiencies and abnormalities are produced by exposing the developing organism to relatively low levels of radiation. No matter what the level of radiation used, similar results cannot be obtained by exposing the adult.

Insect Development Abnormalities

Some malformations occur as a result of irradiating insect embryos, but a significantly higher frequency of noninherited adult abnormalities follow irradiation of larvae and pupae (Figure 10.2). It is in this extended period of development that proliferation of cells in the buds of adult structures occurs. In beetles, flies, moths, and wasps, deformities of head structures, appendages, and body segments are obtained which are serious enough to interfere with normal behavior. In addition to

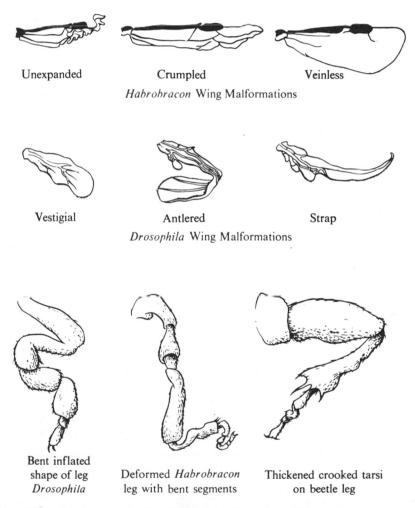

Unexpanded   Crumpled   Veinless

Habrobracon Wing Malformations

Vestigial   Antlered   Strap

Drosophila Wing Malformations

Bent inflated
shape of leg   Deformed *Habrobracon*   Thickened crooked tarsi
Drosophila   leg with bent segments   on beetle leg

Figure 10.2. Developmental abnormalities produced by irradiating larval and pupal insects. Some of them mimic known mutational changes but are not inherited.

these freaks, there is the phenocopy pattern of effect in which adults mimic known mutant types. Malformations in wing venation and structure have been most thoroughly investigated. During a critical stage in development, alternate pathways of growth and differentiation exist. An environmental influence such as radiation, rather than gene control, may determine which path is followed. Type of phenocopy depends on genotype and time at which radiation is delivered; the number obtained is related to the intensity and extent of exposure (Grosch, 1974).

Early Embryo

In Chapter 3 we considered radiation-induced cleavage delay. In this chapter our concern is mainly with the induced abnormalities, deficiencies, and teratologies. In all animals, cleavage and gastrulation are critical periods in development. The latter especially is a developmental crisis in which extensive cell movement and differentiation occur in a delicately balanced situation. The right kinds of cells must be present in the right place, in the right quantity, at the right time. In extensive work with amphibian embryos, imperfect gastrulation was the most commonly observed developmental abnormality in embryos surviving cleavage (Butler, 1936).

In some cases, interference with the mechanics of gastrulation reduced or destroyed potential structures yet the rest of the organism proceeded to develop for a while. A set of experiments in the fish *Fundulus* demonstrated development proceeding in the absence of a head. There were pulsating hearts connected to blood vessels and functional body and tail muscles, in evidence of a cephalic gradient of radiosensitivity. Suppression of the anterior development can result from exposure prior to visible differentiation. Thus production of the anomaly results not only from damage to neuroblasts but also from interference with cells destined for morphogenetic movement (Rugh and Grupp, 1959).

Mammals have not provided the most suitable material for investigating the effects of irradiation on development since the embryo cannot be exposed without also irradiating some maternal tissues. Nevertheless much is known concerning radiation effects on all embryonic stages, especially in rodents.

During the preimplantation stage, irradiation causes a high rate of prenatal mortality. In the mouse 200 R may kill up to 79% of the embryos. The whole litter may die and pregnancy terminate prior to implantation, or individuals may die before or after implantation (Rugh, 1960). This could mean a sorting out or a selection effect. At any rate, survivors are typically normal (Figure 10.3). The dose required and the stage at which lethality is expressed depends upon the stage irradiated. Included are stages nearly equivalent to the gastrulae of lower organisms.

There is no parallel to failure at implantation or loss through preimplantation deaths in egg-laying vertebrates. Major malformations can be recovered from eggs irradiated as early as cleavage. To some degree this reflects damage to chromosome and gene functions required later in development, rather than destruction of cells active in morphogenesis.

Later Stages, Period of Major Organogenesis

When the embryo has achieved the period of major organogenesis, death tends to be delayed until birth. Radiation-induced abnormalities recovered at that time can be very dramatic, and many cases of mis-

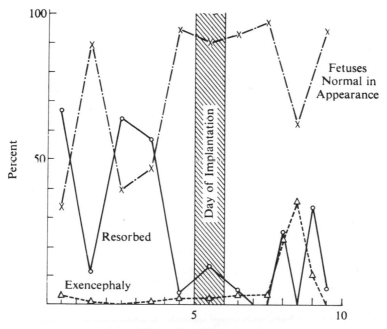

Figure 10.3. Some effects of 200 R of x radiation delivered to mouse embryos at different embryonic ages. Note the reciprocal relationship between resorption and normal fetuses during preimplantation. After implantation, fetuses with visible aberrations tend to persist. (Data by courtesy of R. Rugh.)

shapen heads, distended abdomens, and dorsally flexed tails were reported for amphibians in the early literature.

In birds, vascular disorders due to irradiation are very common: understandable on the basis of extensive extraembryonic pattern, high rate of development, and the far-reaching result of a small initial arrest in formation. An increase in radiosensitivity which obscures the responses of the intraembryonic structures is correlated with the development of the extraembryonic vascular bed, where blood vessels may be caused to break down even before they contain blood. Lead shielding as well as transplantation experiments point up this peculiarity of the material. In the chick embryo, anlagen exposed to doses that cause embryonic death develop normally when transplanted to normal chorioallantoic membranes.

In spite of the complications involved when part of the circulatory system is outside the embryo, patterns of developmental sensitivity can be demonstrated, yet again vascular damage is prominent. Internal hemorrhage is a main cause of death in 4-day chicks. Six-day chicks given 800–43,000 R responded with three independent sets of injury mechanisms. A pooling of blood in large veins was associated with death within 24 hr. Localized accumulations of fluid were characteristic of deaths within 2–5 days. In later deaths, hepatic lesions and hematopoietic failure predominated (Stearner et al., 1960). Damage to the developing beak which occurs before the seventh day is a serious structural defect usually fatal in birds, where it is used to break out of the shell (Moreng and Hollister, 1963).

Although Goff (1962) studied a graded series of chick embryos, the classic analysis was made on rodents by Russell (1950). Sensitive periods for the induction of almost all abnormalities are short. With the threshold dose of 200 R, many periods are restricted to a particular day. When the sensitive period extends over several days, one day stands out as the especially critical time. Figure 10.4 presents this principle in a few of the more than 100 morphological features examined in mice. A pattern of sensitive periods has also been shown for rat embryos. For example, when they are given 300–400 R at 8 days, the embryos which survive seem free of malformations, but only a day later (the ninth), brain deficiencies and facial deformities are frequent after exposure to only 150 R. The pattern of malformation depends upon when the exposure is made. Damage seen later in development occurs in organ anlagen and appendage buds that contain cells in sensitive stages at the time of irradiation. Figure 10.5 presents faithful representations of a selected assortment of radiation-induced malformations. Not all the possible teratisms appeared in the U.S. experiments. A paper by

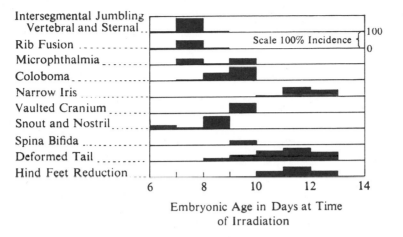

Figure 10.4. Critical periods for mouse abnormalities shown by doses of 200 R of x rays. Of all these and other features studied, only tail deformities span more than 3 days. (Data by courtesy of L. B. Russell.)

Kriegel *et al.* (1962) reported many additional mouse abnormalities, including protruding abdominal organs. Among the larger mammals, deformities have been induced in calves, lambs, pigs, and puppies.

The consequences of acute doses above 100 R are well established, but relatively little is known about the effects of small doses. Jacobsen (1970) addressed himself to the question using large samples of mice exposed *in utero* to 5, 25, and 100 R on the eighth day of pregnancy. Despite controlled temperature and humidity, the differences between summer and winter results in Denmark were so large the dosage responses would have been submerged if statistical analysis had not been by seasons. Particular attention was given to skeletal deviations from normal. As an example of rising incidence with increased dose, consider the ratios of defects per fetus for cervical vertebrae in summer data: control = 0.29, 5 R = 0.34, 25 R = 0.53, and 100 R = 1.02. A valid demonstration of a threshold seems an unlikely prospect from doses lower than 5 R. The 95% confidence limits for the means of control and 5 R data overlap in each of more than a score of morphological features assessed. Theoretically, a threshold for teratogenesis could exist when the critical number of associated cells in a particular organ has been damaged.

The developing gonads have received more specific attention than the visceral organs. An early period of radiosensitivity, identified in both sexes, is associated with a high mitotic activity of primordial germ cells. Nash (1969) demonstrated a peak in radiosensitivity at 10½ days when

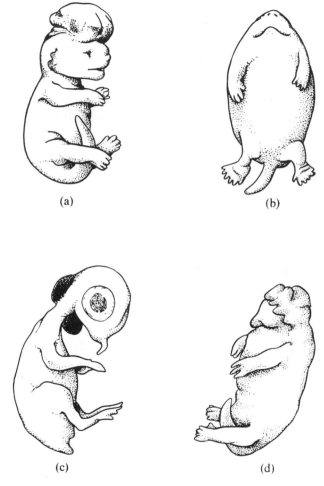

(a)

(b)

(c)

(d)

Figure 10.5. Vertebrate examples of induced developmental abnormalities of the more drastic type (teratologies). (a) Exencephaly of mouse fetus with areas of hemorrhage on extruded brain. 200 R at 3½ days (after Rugh, 1960). (b) Newborn mouse with many abnormalities. Note the short tail, thickset neckless trunk, paddle-shaped six-toed hind feet. 300 R at 10½ days (after Russell, 1950). (c) Chick embryo with vesicles containing bloody fluid, deformed beak, and retarded development of toes. ^{60}Co gamma rays delivered to the egg (after Stearner *et al.*, 1960). (d) Anencephaly and loss of all facial features in a mouse which received only 50 R of x rays at the 4–8 cell stage (after Rugh, 1960).

the mouse gonads are still histologically indistinguishable. During the final stages of embryonic development, oogonia provide the cellular basis of radiation damage in both birds and mammals. Later during fetal life, all oocytes enter meiotic prophase.

The question of whether low doses of x rays during the human embryonic period can lead to significant increases in childhood cancer has been examined retrospectively by a number of groups. Stewart and Kneale (1970) found a significant increase in childhood cancer for those irradiated *in utero*, particularly during the first trimester. The cancer risk was found to be proportional to the number of radiological films. The doubling dose was estimated to be approximately 2 rads. This figure is considerably lower than the figure of 20 rads for adult exposure. However, other retrospective studies have not indicated an increase for such doses. Possibly other factors make the embryo more or less susceptible to carcinogenesis.

Fetal Period

After the organs are formed and the body shape is essentially complete, the term fetus is applied to the developing vertebrate. The majority of the structures increase in size by division of stem cells. During this period, morphologically smaller organs and decrease in overall body size result from adequate irradiation. Those who have sought it usually found a depression in birthweight directly proportional to dose, although the main interest of investigators has been drawn to the preceding period of development when so many areas of the embryo are sensitive.

Because of quick compensation for cell loss, the hematopoietic system is an exception. Exposure of mouse fetuses to 100 R caused only transient leukocytosis and anemia (Rugh and Somogyi, 1968). Both these deviations from normality were rectified quickly, so that shortly after birth, blood counts from those x-rayed *in utero* and from parallel controls were indistinguishable.

Finally only the nervous system is particularly radiosensitive. In fetal rats and mice, as little as 40 R given to the whole body of the mother produces nerve cell necrosis which is visible within 4 hr. Neurectoderm can be totally destroyed by 600–800 R. In contrast, newborn or adult rat neurons can tolerate at least 1500 R with no visible damage, and in some cases neurons persisted after 25,000 R (Van Cleave, 1963). Obviously, the fetal sensitivity to destruction of nerve cells is an outstanding difference from adult conditions. *Differentiating* cells of the nervous system are among those most easily destroyed by ionizing radiation.

Hicks and D'Amato (1966) have contributed to a great deal of information on the radiosensitivity of all parts of the developing rat's nervous system. With special attention to the retina, they demonstrated a range of induced malformations from eyelessness to all types of histological abnormalities. The kinds of cells killed or spared in the retina paralleled the responses in the brain and spinal cord until about the thirtieth day, when the retina diverged toward transient radiotolerance.

As evidence of a pattern of radiosensitivity accumulated, it became apparent that ionizing radiations could be used to locate regions of active differentiation in the nervous system and brain. The rat cerebellum, one of the last portions to differentiate, is not radiosensitive until just before birth. Correlated with the presence of cerebellar neuroblasts, the sensitivity persists for several weeks after birth.

Psychological Research

Although it is evident that prenatal irradiation has long-lasting sequellae, much remains to be done in psychological research, even though long ago Pavlov's laboratory used x-ray injury to the nervous system as a tool in psychological analysis. Most of the literature concerns doses above 90 R, but recently a few experiments have been performed at lower doses. Even 25 R may alter motor performance somewhat and increase the susceptibility to audiogenic seizure. Evaluations of activity and emotionality by inclined plane and open field tests, and by maze learning, revealed differences between rats irradiated in the earlier and in the latter half of gestation. Maze scores indicate that the learning ability of fetally irradiated rats is decreased in proportion to the amount of radiation given. Also such rats are more nervous than controls and engage in what would be termed antisocial behavior in humans. For postnatal irradiation, the greatest differences in learning ability occurs in rats irradiated before they were four days old. The persistence of infantile motor patterns revealed in vertical-rod climb and rope-descent tests is another consequence of neonatal radiation.

Species differences occur. Mice have not always given the same response as rats. Comprehensive tests have not yet been made on birds irradiated before hatching from the egg. However, posthatching approach behavior and color preference were unchanged for duck and chick embryos given doses ranging from 200–1000 R, which suggests a less sensitive system than that of mammals (Oppenheim *et al.*, 1970).

Human Abnormalities

Recorded examples of malformations in human babies after the irradiation of pregnant women fortunately have been few since 1950, but earlier more than 60 cases of radiogenic microcephaly had been reported in medical journals. Other malformations were mentioned less frequently.

By 1910 it was realized that irradiation in the first days of pregnancy usually results in abortion, and repeated attempts were made to utilize this response therapeutically. In recent decades attitudes have changed (Dalrymple and Barnhard, 1973). The most serious aspect of human exposure is that the majority of deaths and abnormalities from radiation occur during the first six weeks in women not aware of their pregnant condition. Therefore the use of diagnostic radiation procedures should be delayed when possible if pregnancy cannot be ruled out. Many hospitals have instituted a form that includes a checklist of factors which may eliminate the potential of pregnancy: birth control, menopause, tubal ligation, menstrual period less than 14 days previous.

If an irradiated human embryo or fetus is not aborted, the baby could be abnormal. Figure 10.6 shows a case of severe developmental damage. Direct fetal injuries, imbecility, mongolism, as well as hydro-, hemi-, and ancephaly have been reported along with damage to the sensory organs, especially the eyes. These latter abnormalities typically follow

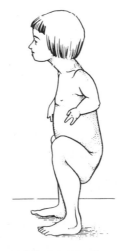

Figure 10.6. Severe developmental damage in the case of a child irradiated *in utero*. Note the unusual stance, the short arms, and the missing fingers. (After Cutler and Buschke, 1938; courtesy of M. Cutler.)

irradiation during the later months of pregnancy, and the papers report-
ing them appeared long before Hiroshima.

Dr. Plummer of the Atomic Bomb Casualty Commission examined
over 200 Japanese children who had been exposed *in utero* to the
Hiroshima detonation (Plummer, 1952). Thirteen percent of them
showed malformations. This may be contrasted with records from
Tokyo which indicate congenital malformations of less than one percent
for a 20-year period. Nearly half of the abnormal Hiroshima children
had heads significantly smaller than normal. Correlated with this was
mental retardation. Children 4½–5 years old had a mental age below
that of the average 1-year-old child. Such results are disturbingly
similar to experimental findings with rodents.

Profound mental retardation was not seen for doses below 50 rads,
but decreases in head circumference were detectable after doses of
10–19 rads in Hiroshima. In Nagasaki, no effects on mental or physical
retardation were seen for doses less than 150 rads. The difference in the
two cities is attributed to the neutron component of Hiroshima.

Internal Radioisotopes

X-ray experiments have shown that the sensitivity of an embryo
changes during the period of development with respect both to lethality
and to the production of malformations. Conceivably a similar pattern
of response may follow injection or ingestion of radioisotopes. However, interpretation of the response may be more complicated due to
persistence of an emitter long after the initial exposure. Also uptake by
maternal tissue becomes involved. Factors of indecisiveness may have
discouraged investigations. Whatever the reason, few isotopes have
been used in investigations with embryos.

For rats, the lethal dose of injected ^{32}P increases between the sixth and
tenth days of gestation. Malformations were evident in those for which
exposure began on the eighth, ninth, or tenth day (Sikov and Noonan,
1957). Also, birth weights decreased. A dose-related pattern of mal-
development of teeth was obtained from ^{32}P given as phosphate a few
days before birth. Most sensitive were the odontoblasts and amelo-
blasts toward the roots, where cells had recently differentiated.

The same isotope injected into chicken eggs has given rise not only to
stunting but also to a variety of defects. Consistent with the generalization based upon x-ray research, the least sensitive organs were those
undergoing the least developmental activity at the time of injection.
Thus structures like the heart, notochord, and lens could be undamaged

while branchial arches, neural tube, and optic cup showed considerable alteration.

Developmental delay along with developmental abnormalities became apparent also when immature insects were fed moderate doses of ^{32}P. Appendage abnormalities are most common because their buds are full of proliferating cells during larval and pupal development. Also, the insect is able to complete metamorphosis even though an appendage is malformed. Equivalent damage to internal organs may not be borne so easily. In wasps, diploid types were found to be more resistant than the haploid males, both in their ability to complete metamorphosis and also to do so without suffering structural aberration from a burden of ^{32}P.

Other isotopes can damage immature arthropods and have been proved transmissable from mother to embryo in laboratory mammals. Researchers concerned with the problems of an Atomic Age have studied selected examples of the transuranium elements and uranium fission products. Plutonium and radiostrontium have been chosen typically as interesting and troublesome specimens from the two categories. ^{89}Sr is a β emitter, ^{85}Sr provides γ rays, and ^{239}Pu is an α emitter. Observed sequellae include an increased proportion of stillbirth, retarded growth, anemia, bone malformation, and osteogenic sarcoma.

Radioiodine, a fission product, has been featured as much as any isotope in vertebrate studies. The concentration of ^{131}I in the developing thyroid corresponds with the first appearance of follicles and concomitant secretion of thyroglobin from which thyroxine is derived. Reports are available for rodents, domestic animals, birds, and humans. However, an enthusiasm to demonstrate onset of function must be tempered by the realization that ^{131}I localization can lead to damage. Fibrotic thyroids, compensatory hyperplasia, adenoma, and colloid goiters are direct evidence. Retarded growth and reduced female reproductive activity of fetally exposed rodents are additional aspects of concern. Although the administration of radioiodine to pregnant humans has been discouraged, a few cases of congenital hypothyroidism have been traced to such treatment.

Iron also has a special place in mammalian biology. In the fetus, liver is the critical organ, accumulating ^{59}Fe during the period when it is the major site of hematopoiesis. Later the bone marrow and spleen become more important. Comprehensive experiments have been performed in rats and verification obtained with a small series of human fetuses.

The cross-placental transfer and fetal organ-accretion rates are discussed at length for many other isotopes in hundreds of papers. Useful guides to the literature are (1) the International Symposia on Trace Element Metabolism in Animals, 2nd (1974), and (2) the U.S. Atomic

Energy Commission Symposium No. 17 (Sikov and Mahlum, eds., 1969). Most of the investigations used isotopes as tracers for studies of metabolism in which organ damage is undesirable. However, special efforts were made to demonstrate tritium damage to rat fetuses.

Rats maintained throughout pregnancy at equilibrium body–water levels of tritium up to 100 μCi/ml had small litters of underweight offspring with dwarfed internal organs. Also, there was a dose-related decrease in head and brain size. In order to provide whole-body irradiation in which cell nuclei would receive a higher dose than the cytoplasm, tritiated thymidine was administered by infusion pump via the catheterized tail vein of the mother, continuously from day 9 of pregnancy. At doses above 3.2 μCi/g/day, the frequency of stillbirth increased along with marked bone-marrow depression. After infusion of 8.0 μCi/g/day, all fetuses were malformed and dead at term. Some lacked vital organs such as the heart or brain.

In general, the radiation dosage from internal radioisotopes differs for mother and offspring. In a sense, pregnancy is protective because the embryo competes with the mother's system for the isotope (Finkel, 1947). Accordingly, the mother's tissues accumulate less of it and experience less damage. Selective accumulation and retention by a relatively small mass of tissue results in the newborn experiencing radiation doses up to 20 times that sustained by an adult from the same quantity of radionuclide. Furthermore, on a per weight basis an infant's air and water uptake is much greater than an adult's, and a contaminated environment is proportionately more hazardous.

Mechanism

Although massive radiation doses to the mother may indirectly affect the viability of a mammalian embryo, there is little doubt that embryonic abnormalities are due to the action of radiation directly on the embryo. A few investigators have gone so far as to expose embryos in surgically exteriorized uteri, and obtained results similar to those from whole body exposures.

At 30 rads or above, the selective destruction of certain classes of embryonic cells can be seen at various sites. The consequences are analogous to those of the extirpation or cautery experiments performed in bird and amphibian embryos. Differentially distributed cell damage explains the relatively specific changes in certain characters when irradiation is delivered at a particular time. Since cell death must be explained, a hypothesis which appeals to us is that of chromosomal damage (see Chapter 13). Uniformly distributed ionizations may be expected to cause chromosomal aberrations sufficient to interrupt or impede mitosis in cells vulnerable because of their nuclear condition. Damaged but surviving cells might influence development through their descendants. Dead cells and the failure of regulatory potency of the remaining cells would contribute to abnormality. The degree of abnormality may be related to the number of cells irrevocably damaged or seriously insulted by the radiation exposure. Hypoxia markedly protects against radiation-induced developmental abnormality, a fact not inconsistent with a chromosomal hypothesis.

Concluding Remarks

From this chapter we have obtained some appreciation of the vulnerability of animal tissues and organs which depend upon division and movement of radiosensitive cells for their development. Indeed, vulnerability is intimately associated with processes requiring normal chromosome structure and function. Nothing presented in this chapter is inconsistent with the evidence in other chapters that chromosome aberrations are intimately involved in radiation-induced cell death.

References

Butler, E. G. (1936). The effects of radium and x rays on embryonic development. In "Biological Effects of Radiation" (B. M. Duggar, ed.), pp. 389–410. McGraw-Hill, New York.

Cutler, M., and Buschke, F. (1938). "Cancer: Its Diagnosis and Treatment." Saunders, Philadelphia, Pennsylvania.

Dalrymple, G., and Barnhard, H. (1973). Protection of potentially pregnant women. In "Medical Radiation Biology," p. 301. Saunders, Philadelphia, Pennsylvania.

Finkel, M. P. (1947). The transmission of radiostrontium and plutonium from mother to offspring in laboratory animals. Physiol. Zool. 20, 405–421.

Goff, R. A. (1962). The relation of developmental status of limb formation to x-radiation sensitivity in the chick embryo. I. Gross study. J. Exp. Zool. 151, 177–200.

Grosch, D. S. (1974). Environmental aspects: Radiation. In "The Physiology of Insecta" (M. Rockstein, ed.), 2nd ed., Vol. 2, Chapter 3. Academic Press, New York.

Hicks, S. P., and D'Amato, C. J. (1966). Effects of ionizing radiations on mammalian development. Adv. Teratol. 1, 196–250.

International Symposia on Trace Element Metabolism in Animals (1974). 2nd Symp. Univ. Park Press, Baltimore, Maryland.

Jacobsen, L. (1970). Radiation-induced fetal damage. Adv. Teratol. 4, 95–124.

Kriegel, H., Langendorff, H., and Kunick, I. (1962). Die Einwirkung von Röntgenstrahlen auf die Embryonalentwicklung der Maus. *Embryologia* **6,** 291–318.

Moreng, R. E., and Hollister, K. W. (1963). Morphology and hatching power of the developing chick embryo following x-irradiation. *Proc. Soc. Exp. Biol. Med.* **114,** 99–103.

Nash, D. J. (1969). Lifetime reproductive performance of mice exposed as embryos to x-irradiation. *Biol. Bull. (Woods Hole, Mass.)* **137,** 189–201.

Oppenheim, R. W., Jones, J. R., and Gottlieb, G. (1970). Embryonic motility and post-hatching perception in birds after prenatal gamma irradiation. *J. Comp. Physiol. Psychol.* **71,** 6–21.

Packard, C. (1945). Roentgen radiations in biological research. *Radiology* **45,** 522–533.

Plummer, G. (1952). Anomalies occurring in children exposed *in utero* to the atomic bomb in Hiroshima. *Pediatrics* **10,** 687–692.

Rugh, R. (1960). Gametes, the developing embryo, and cellular differentiation. *In* "Mechanisms in Radiobiology" (M. Errera and A. Forssberg, eds.), pp. 1–94. Academic Press, New York.

Rugh, R., and Grupp, E. (1959). Ionizing radiations and congenital anomalies in vertebrate embryos. *Acta Embryol. Morphol. Exp.* **2,** 257–268.

Rugh, R., and Somogyi, C. (1968). Hematological recovery of mouse following fetal x-radiation. *Biol. Bull. (Woods Hole, Mass.)* **134,** 320–324.

Russell, L. B. (1950). X-ray induced developmental abnormalities in the mouse and their use in the analysis of embryological pattern. I. External and gross visceral changes. *J. Exp. Zool.* **114,** 545–602.

Sikov, M. R., and Mahlum, D. D., eds. (1969). "Radiation Biology and the Fetal and Juvenile Mammal," Symp. No. 17. U.S. At. Energy Comm., Div. Tech. Inf., Oak Ridge, Tennessee.

Sikov, M. R., and Noonan, T. R. (1957). The effects of irradiation with ^{32}P on the viability and growth of rat embryos. *Radiat. Res.* **7,** 541–550.

Stearner, S. P., Sanderson, M. H., Christian, E. J., and Tyler, S. A. (1960). Modes of radiation death in the chick embryo. *Radiat. Res.* **12,** 286–300 and 301–316.

Steward, A., and Kneale, G. W. (1970). Radiation dose effects in relation to obstetrics, x-ray and childhood cancer. *Lancet,* **1,** 1185–1187.

Van Cleave, C. D. (1963). "Irradiation and the Nervous System," Chapter 5. Rowman & Littlefield, Inc., New York.

CHAPTER 11   Somatic Histopathology

The literature presenting the effects of radiations on tissues and organs is enormous. As early as 1936, Warren could cite 18 reviews, mainly on the damage from external sources. A definitive compendium which included information on internal sources was the volume of the National Nuclear Energy Series edited by Bloom in 1948. Subsequently, the techniques of microscopy have provided data for thousands of reports. Here we can give only the major patterns of damage.

Very early (1906), Bergonié and Tribondeau recognized that there were differences in the radiosensitivity of various types of cells. X-ray damage tended to be greater where there was cell reproduction and for cells less fixed in morphology and function. In other words, mitotically active, undifferentiated tissue proved sensitive. The so-called law is historically important since it focused attention on the tissues containing dividing cells. Actually, it reflects how soon and to what extent radiation damage will lead to evident consequences in a cell population.

In general, progenitive tissue is most susceptible to ionizing radiations. Among such tissues, whose primary function is to proliferate cells, are the blood-forming components, the alimentary tract mucosa, the skin and associated structures, and the lens of the eye. Germinal epithelium, to be considered in the next chapter, should also be recognized in this category. In some organisms, notably certain adult insects, the only proliferative tissue present may be in the gonads.

Vertebrates are vulnerable to radiation because of their dependence upon proliferative tissues for lines both of defense and of supply. Their cells unable to survive the crisis of mitosis are lost. This is reflected in a depletion of mature cells as the need for replacement continues. Debility results when there are not enough mature cells to maintain the vital function of the tissue. Restoration may result from proliferative repopulation of the tissue based upon relatively insensitive interphase cells. Conversely, death from acellularity and toxicity might occur.

The responses of progenitive tissue have three things in common: (1) Each such tissue has a stem cell component, damage to which is a central feature of irradiation sequellae; (2) progenitive tissues involve processes of renewal and maturation of cells; and (3) they elaborate a

191

product of some kind, such as erythrocytes, squama, crystalline fibers, gametes, and so on, by cellular transformation.

Human skin is an excellent example of a progenitive tissue. Indeed, early investigators organized the relative sensitivity of tissues by taking that of the skin as unity (Table 11.1). Another way of organizing relative radiosensitivity is shown in Table 11.2. Although exact placement differs, in either case progenitive tissues are shown to be more sensitive than connective tissue, muscle, bone, and nerves. However, we must remember that this is from the viewpoint of the pathologist, who classified on the basis of morphological changes visible under the microscope. When function has been studied, nervous tissue has not proved highly radioresistant.

Skin

Before more physical types of measurement were developed, a biological basis of dosage widely employed was reddening of human skin. This, the skin erythema dose (SED), depends on a number of

TABLE 11.1

Relative Sensitivity of Normal Tissues to X Radiation[a]

Leukocytes	Dermal structures	Viscera
2.5 Lymphocytes	1.4 Hair Papillae	0.8 Intestine
2.4 Polymorphs	1.3 Sweat Glands	0.7 Liver, Pancreas
	1.2 Sebaceous Glands	0.6 Uterus, Kidney
Germinal cells	1.1 Mucous Membrane	
2.3 Ovarian	1.0 Skin[b]	Connective tissue
2.2 Testicular	0.9 Serous Membrane	0.5 Fibrous
		0.4 Muscle
Blood forming		0.4 Fibrocartilage
2.1 Spleen		0.3 Bone
2.0 Lymphatic		
1.9 Bone Marrow		Nervous tissue
		0.2 Nerve
Endocrine		
1.8 Thymus		Storage
1.7 Thyroid		0.1 Fat
1.6 Adrenal		
Blood vessel		
1.5 Endothelium		

[a] From Clark (1955; copyright McGraw-Hill Book Co.; used by permission).
[b] Skin taken as unity.

TABLE 11.2

Tissues Listed in the Order of Their Decreasing Radiosensitivity

1. Lymph tissue, especially lymphocytes[a]
2. White blood cells and immature red cells of the bone marrow
3. Cells lining the gastrointestinal tract
4. Gonadic cells
5. Skin, especially the proliferating layer
6. Blood vessels and body cavity lining
7. Tissues of glands and the liver
8. Connective tissues
9. Muscle
10. Nerves

[a] The prime example of a radiosensitive differentiated cell vulnerable due to sensitive membrane systems.

factors including time, wavelength, and size of the field. More radiation is tolerated if the intensity is low, the rays more penetrating ("harder"), and the field small. Also, regional differences occur, decreasing in the order of neck, chest, abdomen, thigh, back, and face. For a more detailed discussion see Ellinger's 1941 book. The general form which skin reactions take after administration of an SED is shown on Figure 11.1.

As shown, a transient reaction develops within hours. Then a latent stage lasting a few days precedes the main reaction. The main erythema gradually subsides while pigmentation appears. In the absence of the pigment migration typical of sun tan, the coloration may persist for years.

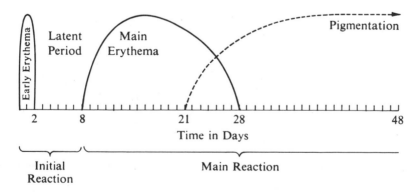
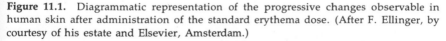

Figure 11.1. Diagrammatic representation of the progressive changes observable in human skin after administration of the standard erythema dose. (After F. Ellinger, by courtesy of his estate and Elsevier, Amsterdam.)

Erythema is explained by the liberation of histamine or other capillary dilators when cells are damaged. The course of events may depend upon differences in cell sensitivity and upon whether division occurs promptly or at a deferred time. A portion of cells killed immediately results in the transient early response; delayed necrosis of other cells could contribute to the main reaction. However, a circulatory compensation for arteriole occlusion or venule collapse can also give rise to capillary dilation.

In addition to reversible reactions, serious irreversible reactions of the skin may be produced. Melanization is a common response of the skin to injury of any kind, but its appearance during exposures to ionizing radiation is a warning that the accumulated dose is approaching that for degenerative changes such as dermatitis, ulcer, and carcinoma (Figure 11.2). Acute lesions have resulted from overexposure and faulty technique, while chronic lesions have been associated with repeated exposures—often a professional hazard in the early days of medical radiology.

Upon overexposure, the skin turns dark red or purple and small blisters form which eventually coalesce into large vesicles. These result from cell destruction followed by a collection of fluid between the cell layers. Considerable tension may develop. Then the blisters rupture, exposing the basal layer or even the raw surface of the dermis. After a very heavy dose, cells of both epidermis and dermis are killed and a deep ulcer results. Blood vessels are very important structures of the epidermis, and we shall give them special attention below. For the present let us consider healed or healing areas.

Contracting scars are less vascular, deficient in elastic tissue, and

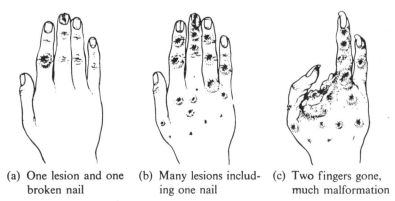

(a) One lesion and one   (b) Many lesions includ-   (c) Two fingers gone,
    broken nail   ing one nail   much malformation

Figure 11.2. Drawings of hands of early radiologists showing increasing degrees of tissue damage.

more fibrous than normal dermis. Pressure on sensory nerve endings from contracting fibrous tissue may be uncomfortable. Also, the destruction of a protective thickness of skin results in hypersensitive areas. Exaggerated perception in the finger tips was a danger signal to the radiologists in the early days.

Structures Associated with the Skin

Hair, nails, claws, and glands are subject to reversible and irreversible damage. Temporary or permanent loss of hair, depression of sebaceous and sudiferous gland function, and cracked, brittle nails are well-known examples of these effects. Indeed a response to x irradiation by the hair was one of the earliest observed biological effects. Only a year after the announcement of Roentgen's discovery, a case of scalp epilation was reported following fluoroscopy. In this phenomenon the degree of damage depends upon the amount of injury to the hair follicle. Often a regrowth of unpigmented hair occurs as a reflection of damage to the melanocytes which deliver pigment to the developing hair cells. In most mammals, because of the profuse hairy covering, hair changes are more commonly studied than skin erythema. The statistically significant increase in white and gray hairs in mice flown at high altitudes is one of the most clear effects of cosmic radiation. Chase and associates (1963) have stressed the importance of studying the response of individual hairs. The backs of cattle exposed to the fallout from nuclear weapons testing showed areas of gray hair and keratinized scars for years afterward. Paradoxically, graying of the hair and hyperpigmentation of the extremities can occur in the same animal. The melanin is produced by melanocyte activation in the basal layer of the epidermis (Quevedo and Grahn, 1958).

The sebaceous glands of mammals and man are radiosensitive. Therefore attempts have been made to employ radiation for acne therapy. However, recent knowledge of the associated hazards led to discontinuing this practice.

In birds, feathering changes have been studied.

Hematology

A change in the blood, the prompt decrease in lymphocyte count after irradiation, is one of the most sensitive indicators of radiation exposure of a mammal. Other changes also occur in the peripheral blood, but these are revealed later, the life span of each type of cell being involved. Normally there is a balance between the rate of utilization and the rate of the production of cells. After an exposure, the cellucidal action of radiations seriously interferes with cell production. Also, indirectly, whole-body irradiation may increase the rate of cell utilization. Again we meet a situation in which the formed elements are relatively radioresistant, while formative cells are damaged. An exception to this is the great radiosensitivity of formed lymphocytes, explained by the paucity of cytoplasmic organelles (Goldfeder, 1963). Observed changes can be traced back to damage of the hematopoietic centers. These include the spleen, the thymus, lymph nodes, and the bone marrow.

In the mouse, McCulloch and Till (1960) demonstrated the 37% dose to be in the neighborhood of 100 rads. A dose of 215 rads reduced the erythropoietic cells of mouse bone marrow to 8.5% surviving, while 400 rads destroyed all but 1%. Complete depletion of hematopoietic cells occurred within a week after 800 rads. Bone marrow was reduced to fat cells, collapsed sinuses, and intracellular jelly (see Bloom, 1948). A lack of reliable morphological criteria for distinguishing the various cell types in the early stages makes it impossible to prepare a tabulation of radiosensitivities such as that presented for spermatogenesis in the next chapter.

Figure 11.3 shows the rates of change in various types of blood cells

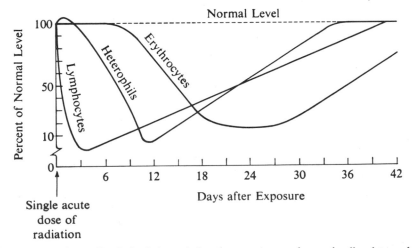

Figure 11.3. Generalized depiction of the changes in numbers of cells observed in peripheral blood subsequent to a dose of several hundred roentgens to a mammal. The scale is different for each type of cell and for each type of animal. Also, a family of curves differing in the slopes of decline and recovery result from a series of doses.

after an exposure of the organism. The rate of change reflects the typical life span, which for lymphocytes is a few hours; for granulocytes and platelets, a few days; and for erythrocytes, months. Note when the lowest value for cells per unit volume is reached. For lymphocytes it occurs within hours; for granulocytes, days; and for erythrocytes, weeks. At higher doses, recovery takes longer. If the dose is high enough, months may elapse before the peripheral blood returns to preirradiation levels in all aspects. At doses high enough to stop cell production completely, the rate of disappearance of cell types from the blood approaches the utilization rate.

The people exposed to atomic bombs and industrial accidents (Chapter 14), and the crew of a vessel that strayed into the Bikini test area (Table 11.3), experienced impressive decreases in both circulating cells and precursors in the bone marrow (Lapp, 1958).

The restoration of the leukocyte count after moderate irradiation is achieved partly by discharge of cells from storage spaces and partly by release of cells at an earlier stage of development than that at which they are normally released. In polymorphonuclear types, the younger cells can be recognized because they have fewer lobes in the nucleus. For lymphocytes, an abortive early peak often seen may be a mobilization phenomenon. Visible morphological changes for damaged lymphocytes found in circulating blood include pyknotic, fragmented, and "owl-eyed" nuclei. Cytoplasmic inclusions which take nuclear stains are demonstrable after as little as 100 R (Rugh, 1964). To the abnormal picture may be added vacuolated granulocytes, nucleated red blood cells, and phagocytized nuclear masses and red blood cells, especially after high doses.

TABLE 11.3

Quantitative Changes in the Cellular Complement of the 23 Fishermen of the *Fukuryu Maru (Lucky Dragon)*

Cell types	Normal (per mm^3)	4 to 6 weeks after voyage (per mm^3)
Leukocytes	5000–9000	5 below 2000
		1 below 1000
		1 below 800
Erythrocytes	5,400,000	Below 4,000,000
Platelets	200,000–900,000	10,000–20,000
Bone marrow	150,000	10,000
Sperm	120,000	0–1

Blood Vessels

Arteries and veins have complex walls, with inner linings of flattened cells known as the endothelium. Damaged cells are replaced by the division of reserve cells. The radiosensitivity of endothelial cells is difficult to determine because the cells undergo sporadic division. Their sensitivity, measured in systems where they are induced to divide, appears to be somewhere between the rapidly dividing stem cells and the nondividing differentiated cells.

Layers of muscle and of elastic connective tissue complete the walls of the tubes and give them resilience, and it is such structure which confers relative radioresistance to the large blood vessels. However, radiation inhibits replacement of worn-out endothelium, so there is a vulnerable aspect. Vulnerability is most evident in smaller tubes, especially in the capillaries which are formed from a single layer of endothelium. A multitude of tiny hemorrhages have been discovered in and on large organs upon autopsy of irradiated animals (Behrens, 1953). Even permeability changes of the capillary endothelium and its intercellular cement can contribute to early circulatory failure after an acute lethal exposure. Lower doses may destroy only a few cells but these may serve as a site for clot formation.

Reparative processes involve either cells which were beyond the field of intense exposure or cells which were in an insensitive state that enabled survival. Alternate routes for the blood may be established and collateral circulation may check damage to other tissues. Possibly damaged linings may be restored. In some cases overgrowth and narrowing of the lumen may occur. However, it is possible that thickened endothelium may be an optical illusion resulting when loss of collagen and muscle leave the endothelium most prominent. Histochemical changes to the collagen are more evident than any other damage observed at lethal doses and higher in laboratory animals.

An impaired vascular system contributes to the changes in other tissues. Of particular importance is the damage which may develop in normal tissue over several years after radiation-induced alteration of the blood supply.

Spleen and Lymph Nodes

Space will not permit us to consider all the details of the histological changes in organs containing lymphatic tissue. Let us take the spleen as a dramatic example of what can happen after irradiation.

The mammalian spleen, much like a lymph node, has a collagenous framework within which is suspended a reticular framework. The former consists of a capsule from which branching trabeculae penetrate the organ to serve as supports. Collagenous fibers continue directly into the reticular fibers of the red pulp. The space in and around the connective tissue is taken up by white pulp, red pulp, blood vessels, and venous sinuses. The white pulp, concentrated around the arteries, is characterized by lymphocytes. All types of blood cells are found in the red pulp and many types are formed there.

Soon after severe radiation exposures, mitosis ceases and careful microscopic examination discloses clumped nuclear chromatin in lymphocytes and hemocytoblasts. Debris in both white and red pulp is removed by phagocytosis and catabolic processes, accompanied by shrinkage of the organ. As a result, the amount of connective tissue per unit volume increases. The sometimes-misinterpreted increased density of fibers appears to be due entirely to depletion of other tissues (Figure 11.4).

The effects of a damaging total-body radiation dose can be divided into four phases: (1) destruction, during which nearly all lymphocytes are destroyed; (2) elimination of debris, when the spleen shrinks and reticular cells become prominent; (3) a period of inactivity, with some consolidation of reticular cells and some attempted regeneration by

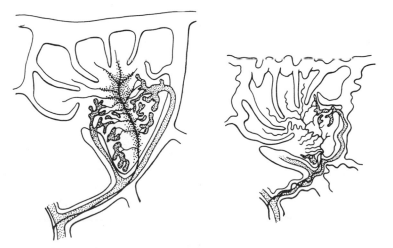

Figure 11.4. A spleen lobule, normal and after loss of white pulp and depletion of red pulp. A view of a limited area of the lobule would give the impression of an increase in the amount of connective tissue. The stippling represents white pulp.

reticular cell transitions; and (4) reconstitution, which involves active mitotic proliferation.

Depending upon dosage, the first two phases are accomplished in hours, the third in days, and the fourth in weeks. The lower the dose, the shorter is the inactive period and the more rapid is regeneration. In terms of x-ray dose, below 175 R there is little apparent disruption of spleen tissue.

Destructive, eliminative, and reconstitutive phases are also seen for the lymphatic bodies stationed like guards at appendage-trunk junctions and along vessels which might become potential routes of invasion. These lymph nodes can be severely depleted of lymphocytes. The degree of destruction is correlated with the amount and intensity of irradiation. A nodule-free period is typical of doses which approach the lethal level for the organism. Histological changes produced in other lymphoid and lymphatic tissues follow a similar pattern and exhibit a similar correlation between histopathological changes and amount of irradiation.

Digestive Tract

The digestive tract has a lining which is simply a continuation of the outer surface of the body; however, unlike the skin, it is composed of only a single layer of epithelial cells for most of its length. These cells are radiosensitive.

Ulceration and erosion of the lining of the mouth is the most obvious consequence of exposing the upper tract. The pharynx and esophagus are relatively radiotolerant. Cells of the stomach's glandular epithelium degenerate after moderate doses of radiation, and ulcers appear several weeks after irradiation. The large intestine is comparably radiosensitive. The small intestine is more sensitive than other sections, and the duodenum has proved highly vulnerable in a variety of vertebrates. Microscopic examination subsequent to irradiation reveals crypt epithelium more damaged than villus epithelium (Williams et al., 1958). The numerous folds can become so cluttered with degenerating and fragmented crypt cells that function is curtailed. The extent and duration of mitotic depression and decrease in tissue weight are dose-dependent. After doses higher than 2000 rads, uncompensated loss of cells from the extrusion zone of the villi results in a striking histological change. Within a day the villi shrink from long projections to stubby knobs. The remaining epithelium changes from columnar through cuboidal to a squamous arrangement.

Recovery is rapid after doses of 200 to 600 rads. As in other organs, its onset is marked by resumption of mitosis, occurring earlier at lower doses. In rats, new cells cover the villi in less than a week. When cell regeneration is insufficient, denudation leads to ulceration, hemorrhage, and gangrenous inflammation. When gastrointestinal (GI) injury is the principal cause of death, the symptoms show up in the number of days postirradiation required for the stem cells to divide, mature, and differentiate into the types comprising the cellular surface of the villi.

Some of the functional changes, such as decreased absorption, are coincident with damage to the epithelial layer. Others, such as the amplitude of churning action and the rate of propulsion of intestinal contents, involve the parasympathetic nerves and the muscle layers. Still others, including diarrhea and attendant loss of fluids and electrolytes, are conditioned by changes in the microflora.

Nervous Tissue

The usual criterion of cell damage, loss of reproductive integrity, is not applicable to the nerve cells of adult mammals, and the evaluation of any type of cell loss is most difficult in the unique cellular architecture of nervous tissue. The absence of lysosomal enzymes and nucleic acids confers extreme radiotolerance on the nerve fibers, but their metabolic dependence on glial cells renders them sensitive to delayed radionecrosis (Zeman, 1961). In addition to altering the population of interstitial neuroglia, radiation impairs capillary circulation and causes permeability changes. Glial cells disappear rapidly after doses of 10,000 rads or more, and their loss may contribute as much to the central nervous system (CNS) syndrome as does damage to the neurons. However, species differences in sensitivity to irradiation of the head may depend upon circulatory differences. Vascular changes explain the death of burros with CNS symptoms after only moderate doses (Brown *et al.*, 1962). Congestion with concomitant increase in the size of perineuronal, periglial, and other spaces was characteristically prominent. Extravasation of plasmatic fluid and perivascular cuffing with neutrophils was common.

The Eye

In the eye, the part most easily injured by radiation is the lens. X-ray doses above 15 rads increase the incidence of opacities in mice, while the threshold in man is considerably higher. The effect, related to the dose rate, is often delayed to old age. Neutrons are more effective than x or γ rays by at least a factor of 10. Many hundreds of rads are required to cause completely opaque lenses, and at least 20 krads must be delivered to produce permanent damage in other parts of the eye.

Damage to individual cells of the lens epithelium is recognized by the decrease in mitotic activity and abortive attempts to differentiate normal lens fibers. Abnormal cells and debris accumulate at the lens poles (Evans *et al.*, 1960). The mammalian lens cannot rid itself of this material, but the bird lens profits from a rapid lysis and removal system.

Neurophysiologists employ different criteria in their investigations of response to environmental agents. The recording of action potentials during and following irradiation indicated a high radiosensitivity of retinal rods, but indicated radiotolerance when alteration of the conductivity of the nerve fiber was considered.

Bone

In our consideration of the skeletal system, it is necessary to distinguish between bone which is still growing and bone which has completed its growth. Furthermore, for the present we are concerned only with the supportive and morphological aspect of this tissue and not with the marrow of hematopoietic function.

We have seen that bone is traditionally classed among the more radioresistant tissues, but actually this holds true only for the bony substance and not for the interior contents. Cell death is inconspicuous in the former, but of massive proportions in the latter. However, although bone may appear histologically normal, after heavy irradiation fractures become common, and healing processes proceed more slowly than normal. This sort of experiment, in which thousands of roentgens may be delivered, requires local irradiation since laboratory animals die too quickly following whole body irradiation in excess of a few hundred roentgens. A month or more must elapse before the bone breaks occur. Presumably, modification of the material is involved. Histologically, bone cells are more sensitive than the interstitial substance of the bone cartilage.

When growing bones are exposed, radiation damage is more obvious. The stunting of bone growth known from the years of early application of x rays has been a consistent caution to radiologists, even when histological indications of damage would be indecisive. Growth in length results from continued multiplication of the epiphyseal cartilage cells, calcification of the stroma between them, and concomitant invasion of the calcified zone by vascular connective tissue from the bone marrow. With so much cellular activity, it is reasonable to expect radiosensitivity such as in fact does exist for the epiphyses in immature mammals. Most significant is cessation of multiplication of cartilage cells.

Experiments in which either shafts or ends of bones were shielded are instructive. For example, in one series of experiments with rabbits, shafts were unaffected by 1500 R, yet 400 R delivered to the entire leg stunted growth. A dose of 200 R was enough to alter disk thickness and produce irregular cell arrangements in epiphyses. There seems to be good reason for shielding epiphyses in children who must undergo radiation therapy. Figure 11.5 concerns a classic case in which epiphyses were not protected (Bisgard and Hunt, 1936).

Bone Marrow

The active marrow of the mammal consists of a loose framework of reticular fibers and cells, plus blood sinusoids lined with phagocytes. Groups of stem cells and the precursors of several types of blood cells occur within the reticulum. In humans, myelocytes are found in all cavities of all bones during the first few years but their distribution diminishes with age, so by age 21 they are demonstrable only in the rib cage, shoulder girdle, and ends of long bones of appendages. The

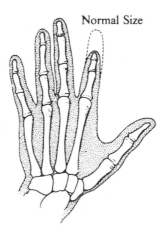

Normal Size

Figure 11.5.   Interference with bone growth by irradiation of the index finger at an early age. (Based on a roentgenogram by courtesy of J. D. Bisgard.)

radiosensitivity of this tissue is reflected in two ways: (1) dilation of sinuses with fatty or gelatinous replacement of hematopoietic cells, and (2) decrease in the cells found in peripheral circulation when degeneration of blood-forming sites alters the output which formerly was in equilibrium with utilization.

Opinions have differed concerning the relative sensitivity of various cell lineages, but in general, younger cells are more sensitive than older forms of the same cell type. Within a few days after a whole-body exposure near the lethal level, the bone marrow becomes almost completely devoid of immature red and white cells. Recovery from this state requires several weeks. During the process, the dilated venous sinuses regain normal size and successful proliferation of stem cells must occur. These are derived from mitosis of a few resistant undifferentiated cells or by transformation from reticular cells. Marrow at the ends has proved more sensitive than that in the shaft both in the development of damage and in the timing of regeneration. Unfortunately, this corresponds with the localization of bone-seeking radioisotopes which accumulate at the growing ends. After severe or prolonged exposure to radiation, regardless of its source, abnormal fibrous bone tends to replace gelatinous marrow, and tumors may result.

Bone-Seeking Isotopes

Essentially the same type of tissue injury is produced by ionizing radiation regardless of whether the source is external or internal. However, localization of the emitter can be important when its rays have a limited penetration.

Most of the agents which are likely to become internal hazards in vertebrates are bone-seekers causing disproportionately great damage to bone and bone marrow. Involved are the divalent, trivalent, and quadrivalent cations. In lower animals, shellfish, of course, lay down calcareous material, but the great range and variety of invertebrates lack shell or skeleton to serve as a site for such deposits. Exoskeletons not of the same constitution are disposed of by molting.

Radium is most notorious in man as a bone-seeker, and because of long years of study we know much about its effects. In 1925 Hoffman's statistical survey of deaths and disability among girls employed in painting numerals on watch dials was followed closely by an autopsy of a fatal case of anemia by Martland and associates (1925). Their report also included the first demonstration of gamma emission from a living human burdened with radioactive material. The work of this group was an important factor in removal by the AMA of internal administration of radium from the list of nonofficial remedies, but not before several hundred patients received injections.

Case histories for individuals who ingested radium or to whom it had been administered twenty to thirty years ago have become available. Hematologically, findings were neither striking nor diagnostic, but the osseous lesions were clearly correlated with the body burden of radium. A list of abnormalities includes destruction of the heads and streaked imperfections of the shafts of long bones, punched out areas of the skull, necrosis of vertebral bodies, and sarcomas (Looney et al., 1955). The deposition of radium was not homogeneous and the energy of the α rays was absorbed close to the site of deposit. The "clinical triad" summarized the responses as (1) anemia from bone marrow destruction, (2) osteitis followed by osteonecrosis, and (3) osteosarcoma. With few exceptions, no increase in chromosome aberrations has been demonstrated by culturing peripheral leukocytes. In two individuals with the highest body burdens of 3.55 and 8.6 μCi, dicentrics and ring chromosomes were discovered. In addition to bone associated damage, some of the dial painters developed tumors of the central nervous system.

A somewhat related health problem is that of patients who received injections of Thorotrast, a colloidal sol containing $^{232}ThO_2$. Despite its alpha emission and decay to radioactive daughters, Thorotrast was once used extensively in medical radiology because of its radiopacity. Bone marrow is an important site of deposit. In addition to damaging hematopoiesis, the induction of lung and liver cancers can occur. Nineteen out of a sample of 20 patients who received Thorotrast 19 to 27 years previously showed chromosome aberrations in peripheral blood cultures (Hoegerman, 1976).

Concern about fallout hazards drew attention to the strontium isotopes which are incorporated into bone in somewhat the same way as the more common alkaline earth, calcium. Their effects are similar to radium, differing chiefly in the amount of material required to produce a particular change. Degeneration and necrosis is accompanied by reactive formation of new bone which may be atypical, possibly leading to malignancy.

In experimental mice injected with ^{89}Sr, one of the first signs of injury to the femurs was a depletion of hematopoietic cells in the metaphysis. At high enough dosage, these cells completely disappear, and the space once occupied contains dilated sinuses, gelatinous and fibrous marrow, and fat. In immature animals, a premature aging, a sealing off of the zone of growth from the metaphysis, is an additional result that warns us that both increase in bone as well as replacement of blood cells can be disturbed by bone seekers.

Miscellaneous Internal Emitters

We cannot spare the space to consider all the groups of elements in detail. Some of them such as tritium and the alkali metals of group 1 have an essentially uniform distribution throughout the body. With others, ^{65}Zn for example, the highly penetrating gamma rays make distribution in the body of secondary significance (Durbin, 1960).

Because of its function as a filtration device featuring phagocytic cells, the liver has sometimes been placed in vulnerable circumstances by experimental procedures. Radiogold disappears from the peripheral blood within minutes when injected in colloidal form. Ninety percent of a dose is deposited in the liver, the other 10% in bone marrow and lymphatic sites. Hepatic cell giantism as well as necrosis and distortion of the lobular pattern follows. Subsequently, hepatic dysfunction becomes evident, with liver failure the major cause of death (Koletsky and Gustafson, 1952). The colloidal form must be used because in tolerated form at physiological pH gold is insoluble.

The best illustration of damage by an isotope localizing in a specific tissue is provided by the ^{131}I affinity for the thyroid gland where it is incorporated into thyroglobulin and thyroxine. In rats, single doses above 250 μCi destroy the entire gland within a week following the prompt appearance of collapsed or ruptured follicles and necrotic lining cells. The gland is replaced by hyalinized fibrous scar tissue. Accordingly, pathological conditions, ordinarily associated with surgical thyroidectomy, appear in the organism. Most notable are vascular calcification and cardiac enlargement. In animals as large as sheep, 5 μCi of ^{131}I per day result in reduced size of the gland and an increase in its connective tissue (Bustad et al., 1957). Tissue in close proximity to the thyroid may show damage due to radiations emanating from it. Constriction of the trachea is a resultant common aberration.

Most of the anions, including the halogens, oxygenated and halogenated oxidation states of the fourth, fifth, and sixth groups, and platinum metals, are eliminated rapidly, chiefly by the kidney; although ^{14}C and ^{32}P enter the skeleton as carbonates and phosphates. When isotopes become part of organic molecules, their distribution and retention are influenced by the compound which contains the radioisotope. Adequate pursuit of this theme would require a coverage of the entire field of biochemistry, something far too ambitious and not entirely pertinent. We have already mentioned phosphorus as part of the genetically important nucleic acids in discussing plants. In addition, it is a constituent of many organic energy-storing and -transferring systems and is essential to life as we know it. Sulfur is almost as important, and brief reference to it is in order since its distribution depends upon whether the molecule containing it is inorganic or organic. ^{35}S has been employed to show that sulfate tends to become incorporated into the mucopolysaccharides associated with connective tissue. On the other hand methionine, an essential amino acid important in protein synthesis, localizes in active proliferating epithelia and in glands (Nunez and Mancini, 1956).

Routes of Entry

In our daily life we do not have to contend with injected radioisotopes. Our concern is with normal routes of entry. The two most important routes into terrestrial animals are ingestion and inhalation. This section concerns vertebrates. Other forms differ structurally, the most notable difference being the direct tracheal supply of air to every tissue in insects.

The amount of radioactive material absorbed from the contents of the gastrointestinal tract depends upon the specific element, its chemical form, and the makeup of the diet. Transportable radionuclides identical to or congeners of the mineral nutrients are mainly absorbed from the small intestine. If transfer into the portal vein is efficient, damage may be negligible.

Food residue spends more time in the large intestine than in any other compartment of the GI tract. Therefore, poorly absorbed radioisotopes tend to induce damage in the lower tract. Gold, silver, lanthanide, and actinide isotopes are included in this category (Eve, 1966). In experiments with small beads, only 70% of those fed were recovered in the stool within 72 hours. More than a week was required for total recovery of the beads.

In upper parts of the respiratory tract, ciliary movement of mucus-trapped material clears out the inhaled particles, but in the distal portions of the lung, removal is slow, involving phagocytosis and lymphatic drainage (Holtzman and Ilcewicz, 1966). Plutonium oxides are retained in the lungs for months while the more soluble radioactive materials are translocated within a week. Most of the insoluble plutonium compounds are trapped in the tracheobrancheal lymph nodes after leaving the lungs (Bair and Thompson, 1974). Solubilized material is translocated to the liver and skeleton. In dogs, $^{239}PuO_2$ entering by way of the lungs was demonstrable up to 10 years after inhalation. Deaths later than three years were due to pulmonary neoplasia induced by an accumulated 5300 rads from 1.2 μCi of initial lung burden. At higher doses, beagles died in less than a year from pneumonitis and pulmonary fibrosis. In both lungs and intestines, all the energy of alpha particles is absorbed locally by the epithelial cell lining.

In addition to the occupationally exposed humans, wild animals of the Nevada Test Site carry transuranium elements in their bodies. Also, ^{239}Pu has been demonstrated in respirable dust offsite downwind from a Colorado Nuclear Weapons Plant. A more mundane matter is the elevated amounts of ^{210}Pb and ^{210}Po in the lung alveoli of smokers. Presumably these elements come from the phosphate fertilizers used on tobacco fields.

Concluding Remarks

This chapter demonstrates that tissue-oriented research evolved into a concern for cells and cell potentialities. The key to understanding the problem appears to lie in chromosome behavior associated with the normal tendency of cells to divide. Chapter 5 provides necessary background for deliberation. In addition, we needed to explore the deleterious consequences of blocking proliferation. In establishing the vulnerability of tissues with mitotically capable cells, we have not considered it necessary to treat all types of tissue in great detail, but we will devote the entire next chapter to a discussion of gonad histopathology. Isotopes have been given some attention because of their propensity for localization rather than because of any characteristic radiation effect. Vertebrate studies seem to have been preemptory for somatic tissues, but in the next chapter we shall have something to say about insect gonads.

References

Bair, W. J., and Thompson, R. C. (1974). Plutonium: Biomedical research. *Science* **183**, 715–722.
Behrens, C. F. (1953). "Atomic Medicine." Williams & Wilkins, Baltimore, Maryland.
Bergonié, J., and Tribondeau, L. (1906). Interprétation de quelques résultats de la radiothérapie et essai de fixation d'une technique rationnelle. *C. R. Hebd. Seances Acad. Sci.* **143**, 983–985.

Bisgard, J. D., and Hunt, H. B. (1936). Influence of roentgen rays and radium on epiphyseal growth of long bones. *Radiology* **26**, 56–64.

Bloom, W., ed. (1948). "Histopathology of Irradiation from External and Internal Sources," Natl. Nucl. Energy Ser., Div. IV. v. 22 I. McGraw-Hill, New York.

Brown, D. G., Bassmore, D. P., and Jones, L. P. (1962). Acute central nervous system syndrome of burros. *In* "Response of the Nervous System to Ionizing Radiation" (T. J. Haley and E. S. Snyder, eds.), pp. 503–511. Academic Press, New York.

Bustad, L. K., George, L. A., Jr., Marks, S., Warner, D. E., Barnes, C. M., Herde, K. E., and Kornberg, H. A. (1957). Biological effects of I^{131} continuously administered to sheep. *Radiat. Res.* **6**, 380–413.

Chase, H. B., Straile, W. E., and Arsénault, C. (1963). Evidence for indirect effects of radiations of heavy ions and electrons on hair depigmentation. *Ann. N. Y. Acad. Sci.* **100**, 390–398.

Clark, G. L. (1955). "Applied X-rays," 4th ed. McGraw-Hill, New York.

Durbin, P. W. (1960). Metabolic characteristics within a chemical family. *Health Phys.* **2**, 225–238.

Ellinger, F. (1941). "The Biological Fundamentals of Radiation Therapy." Am. Elsevier, New York.

Evans, T. C., Richards, R. D., and Riley, E. F. (1960). Histologic studies of neutron- and x-irradiated mouse lenses. *Radiat. Res.* **13**, 737–750.

Eve, I. S. (1966). A review of the physiology of the gastrointestinal tract in relation to radiation doses from radioactive materials. *Health Phys.* **12**, 131–161.

Goldfeder, A. (1963). Cell structure and radiosensitivity. *Trans. N. Y. Acad. Sci.* [2] **26**, 215–241.

Hoegerman, S. F. (1976). The cytogenetic effects of internal alpha emitters on human lymphocytes: A review. *In* "The Health Effects of Plutonium and Radium" (W. S. S. Jee, ed.), pp. 779–791. J. W. Press, Salt Lake City, Utah.

Holtzman, R. B., and Ilcewicz, F. H. (1966). Lead-210 and polonium-210 in tissues of cigarette smokers. *Science* **153**, 1259–1260.

Koletsky, S., and Gustafson, G. (1952). Liver damage in rats from radioactive colloidal gold. *Lab Invest.* **1**, 312–323.

Lapp, R. E. (1958). "The Voyage of the Lucky Dragon." Harper, New York.

Looney, W. B., Hasterlick, R. J., Brues, A. M., and Skirmont, E. (1955). A clinical investigation of the chronic effects of radium salts administered therapeutically. *Am. J. Roentgenol., Radium Ther. Nucl. Med.* [N.S.] **73**, 1006–1037.

McCulloch, E. A., and Till, J. E. (1960). The radiation sensitivity of normal mouse bone marrow cells determined by quantitative transplantation into irradiated mice. *Radiat. Res.* **13**, 115–125.

Martland, H. S., Conlon, P., and Knef, J. P. (1925). Some unrecognized dangers in the use and handling of radioactive substances. *J. Am. Med. Assoc.* **85**, 1769–1776.

Nunez, C., and Mancini, R. E. (1956). Comparative study of incorporation of S^{35} by tissues of adult rats both as sodium sulfate and as DL methionine. *Proc. Int. Conf. Peaceful Uses At. Energy, 1st 1955* Vol. 12, pp. 461–465.

Quevedo, W. C., and Grahn, D. (1958). Effect of daily gamma-irradiation on the pigmentation of mice. *Radiat. Res.* **8**, 254–264.

Rugh, R. (1964). An anomalous lymphocyte: Possibly diagnostic for exposure to ionizing radiations or radiomimetic agents. *Am. J. Roentgenol., Radium Ther. Nucl. Med.* [N.S.] **91**, 192–201.

Warren, S. L. (1936). The physiological effects of radiation upon organ and body systems. *In* "Biological Effects of Radiation" (B. M. Duggar, ed.), Chapter 14. McGraw-Hill, New York.

Williams, R. B., Toal, J. N., White, J., and Carpenter, H. M. (1958). Effects of total body x-radiation from near threshold to tissue lethal doses on small bowel epithelium of the rat. *J. Natl. Cancer Inst.* **21,** 17–48.

Zeman, W. (1961). Radiosensitivities of nervous tissues. *Brookhaven Symp. Biol.* **14,** 176–199.

CHAPTER 12   Gonad Histopathology

This chapter concerns the response of the gonads to radiation, but even an entire chapter does not provide enough space for an exhaustive treatment of a subject which has received much special attention. Here the emphasis will be upon induced cell destruction and tissue changes. Genetic implications are covered in other chapters.

Much of the volume of a gonad is made up of cells which share many aspects of the progenitive type of tissue, including radiosensitivity. Such tissue features primitive stem cells which give rise to units exhibiting processes of renewal, maturation, and cellular transformation. Acellularity for certain types of gametogenic cells is a typical result of irradiation. Development of the condition relates to the length of time required for normal maturation and the duration period of mature cells.

However, in all males and in the females of many species the mature cell produced is a gamete dispensed or deposited outside the organism. Since the cellular products have no function in the organism, gonad destruction has negligible influence on the survival of the individual, although hormonal dysfunction is a consequence in vertebrates where the gonad has a double function, endocrine in addition to gamete production. In birds, the female may possess a rudimentary testis which may enlarge and produce male hormones if the functional ovary is destroyed.

Testes

Weight Loss. A change in testicle weight is the basis of a simple quantitative method of measuring radiation injury to mammals. Qualitatively, the dramatic changes following irradiation were noted by the earliest investigators shortly after the turn of the century. However, extensive quantitative studies did not occur until 40 years later in Lorenz' laboratory at the United States National Cancer Institute (see Kohn and Kallman, 1955).

211

Testicular weight loss depends only upon the dose delivered to the testes and appears to be an exponential function of that dose (Grahn, 1954). Primarily, the loss is of germinal epithelium and correlates well with the histological changes revealed by microscopic examination. In mice, about four weeks are required for the testes to reach a minimum weight after 1000 R or more. The exact time and dose required to accomplish the same for rats, rabbits, hamsters, and other experimental animals differs somewhat, but the pattern is similar for sizable acute doses.

When the rate at which a dose is delivered is varied, results may be quite different (Kohn and Kallman, 1965). Testes supplied one of the earliest demonstrations that fractionation can enhance x-ray damage. Apparently the secondary doses can be spaced to catch the cells surviving the initial dose as they progress into a more sensitive phase. On the other hand, with long interfraction periods or extremely protracted chronic exposures the rate of injury is reduced below the rate of recovery, and testicular weight may be unchanged.

Histological Examination. The vertebrate testis is comprised of a number of greatly convoluted tubules with supportive tissue between. Figure 12.1 diagrams cross-sections of normal and irradiated seminiferous tubules as seen through a microscope. Such examinations reveal that the weight loss of irradiated testes results from degeneration and resorption of the germinal components (Nebel, 1958). Sertoli cells and

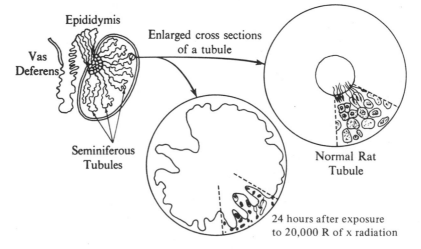

Figure 12.1. Diagram of a testicle showing cross-sections of normal and irradiated seminiferous tubules.

interstitial tissue remain relatively unchanged, short of the massive doses which destroy the most resistant tissue components.

Both the testis as a whole and the individual tubules shrink markedly in size as the degeneration of damaged cells is completed. Also, some decrease in volume can be traced to spermatocytes and spermatids which complete development and are discharged from their tubules as mature sperm. Intermediate spermatogonia are the most radiosensitive cells (see Table 12.1). Their depletion results in ultimate depletion of spermatozoa. The order of disappearance follows the order of the sequence in the developmental series (Oakberg, 1975).

The remaining tissue components are crowded into a reduced volume as the tubules shrink both in length and diameter. Therefore, uncorrected counts per cross section of tubule are subject to large error. To this complication are added disagreements concerning cell classification and specific steps of normal spermatogenesis.

In 1903, Albers-Schönberg's demonstration of aspermy without disappearance of sexual instincts was hailed as the first report of a profound effect on an organ by a specific external agent. Since that time, a voluminous literature has accumulated from experiments on laboratory

TABLE 12.1

Development Times and Radiation Sensitivity for Successive Spermatogenic Stages in the Mouse[a]

Germ cell type	Days taken to reach ejaculate	LD_{50} (R)
Type A spermatogonia		
A_s (stem cell)	Over 42	33–200
A_1		
A_2		23
A_3		
A_4		
Intermediate spermatogonia	35–37	21
Type B spermatogonia	34–36	
Primary spermatocytes		
Resting (preleptotene)	33–35	205
Leptotene	32–33	492
Zygotene	30–32	520
Pachytene	23–30	
Diplotene	22–23	564
Diakinesis—metaphase I	21–22	837
Secondary spermatocytes	21–22	1000
Spermatids	7–21	1500
Spermatozoa	0–7	60,000

[a] Based upon Oakberg (1969), and Searle (1974).

animals including primates. Also, there are a few reported cases of
human testicular injury, one being a response to only 15 R of localized
radiation. Generally, the minimum acute dose required to induce a
temporary infertile period is 100–300 R depending on the species and
genetic strain. In men exposed in criticality accidents, the time required
for the sperm count to return to normal has varied from a year after 100
rem to over three years after near-lethal exposure. The permanently
sterilizing dose for male mammals exceeds the acute lethal dose applied
to the whole body.

Degeneration of cells coincides with multiplicative periods. However, mitotic changes of degenerate cells can be identified only in early
necrosis. Rapid liquefaction results in such loss of nuclear detail that
most of the cells in advanced necrosis are classed as interphase. Certainly abnormal nuclei implicate the nuclear mechanism as vulnerable,
but there is evidence that the first meiotic division may be blocked and
that the unreduced cells migrate to the basement membrane. Despite
technical difficulties, Casarett and Casarett (1957) obtained consistent
counts of the terminal spermatogonia still at the basement membrane in
tubule cross sections. In rats, 325 R of acute x rays reduced these
prespermatocytes to a low near zero, reached at 25 days posttreatment.
For substantial persistent depression from daily exposures, 2–3 R/day is
required for mice, rats, guinea pigs, and rabbits, while 0.5 R/day suffices
for dogs. After cessation of chronic irradiation, the recovery phase takes
at least 50 days. Mouse testes exposed to 2560 R contained cells so
seriously damaged that they degenerated before entering mitosis
(Bryan and Gowen, 1958).

Regardless of the time element or differences in dosage, one pattern is
consistent for all species. After a sublethal dose of whole body irradiation, males continue to void sperm derived from surviving spermatocytes and spermatids. Finally, after the epididymis has emptied, maturation depletion results in temporary sterility. Subsequent recovery of
fertility is determined by the species-specific dynamics of spermatogenesis which provide for spermatogonial repopulation.

Surprisingly few studies of radiation damage to invertebrate testes
have been made, in view of the tremendous number of genetics experiments in which male insects are irradiated. However, in lower animals, testes are not located superficially nor are ejaculate samples easily
obtained. Furthermore, at eclosion, insect testes principally show transforming spermatids and maturing spermatozoa. The spermatogonia
and spermatocytes found in the apical portion of the testes have not
attracted investigators. When studied by Welshons and Russell (1957),
the cytological reaction of Drosophila testes was found quite similar to

that observed by Oakberg (1955) in mice. The radiosensitivity of secondary spermatogonia and young spermatocytes and the resultant temporary period of aspermy following moderate radiation doses was revealed. Studies in pest control add the observations that a decrease in testes size can be induced by irradiating insects during metamorphosis.

Semen Analysis

Not much is known about the number of sperm produced by insects where collection is infeasible. Some data has been obtained from dissecting seminal vesicles and pressing out their contents (Nilakhe and Earle, 1976). A total dose of 6250 rads from ^{60}Co delivered in five daily fractions to adult weevils decreased the sperm count by 33%. A similar regime for pupae caused a 96% decrease.

Because sacrifice of mammals is unnecessary, and quantitative data can be obtained before, during, and after experimental treatments, changes in sperm counts have been demonstrated for the larger farm animals as well as the smaller laboratory types. Initially, the most extensive information came from a long-term experiment with beagle hounds to supplement information from male exposures at Hiroshima (Murakani, 1959), Rongelap, and the associated *Fukuryu Maru* incident (see Table 11.1).

For years, Casarett's group (see Casarett and Hursh, 1958) studied the various histological responses of beagles receiving daily exposures totaling 0.3, 0.6, and 3.0 R per 5-day week. The lowest dose was chosen to correspond with the maximum permissible chronic dose in industry. Only the highest protracted dose caused marked changes in spermatogenesis. The progressive decline in absolute sperm count began after 20–30 weeks of exposure. Lowest values were reached in less than a year when the accumulated exposure exceeded 150 R.

A Colorado State University team investigated the effects on semen of x-ray doses ranging from 50 to 800 R delivered to bull testicles. The legs, perineal region, and lower abdomen were shielded with 3 mm of lead. Changes in ejaculate samples were evident within a month but the nadir point in the family of dose-related curves occurred at about 14 weeks posttreatment. Recovery approaching the control level was observed between 30 and 40 weeks. The fructose production by accessory sex organs, the seminal amino acids, and ascorbic acid levels remained relatively unchanged (Gillette *et al.*, 1964). Other investigations on boars, rams, and monkeys complete a spectrum of animal types which include smaller forms common to the laboratory.

Malfunction or morphological aberration of spermatozoa seems to be due to early damage. Once the sperm is formed, no effects on viability, motility, or appearance have been observed with a variety of mammals and birds, up to dose levels above which breeding experiments become impractical. With invertebrates, exposures of sperm samples have withstood impressive doses. For example, spermatozoa of the clam *Spisula* were unaffected by 264,000 R when motility and fertilizing power was scored (Rugh, 1953). However, because of chromosomal and genic damage, ability of a sperm to reach and penetrate an egg is no guarantee that a normal embryo or a healthy adult will result.

Abscopal Effect

The changes in a testis produced by small to moderate doses of radiation occur when energy absorbed in its cells cause their destruction. The situation may be more complicated when the dose approaches a lethal level for the organism. In guinea pigs, sperm output was depressed below a million cells per ejaculate for 12 weeks after 300 R whole-body irradiation, for 6–7 weeks after testes exposure (head and body shielded), and for 1 week after head and body exposure (testes shielded). Freund and Borelli (1965) recognize that the testes received 15 rads (5% of the 300 rads) from scatter, but consider the severity and time course of the effect to indicate abscopal action. However there was no effect on sperm production from irradiating the head alone, which ruled out hypothalamic–hypophyseal influences. A generalized body reaction or stress syndrome is speculative. This and other results in other species pose unanswered questions.

Ovaries

There is a basic similarity in the ultimate pattern of response by reproductive systems of female animals. However, because of the variety of structural detail, we need to consider the experimental results separately. The ovaries of some animals, including mammals, are solid masses; in others like the frog they are saclike; and in insects they are composed of tubular units. Furthermore, there are differences of physiological significance. The most highly developed corpora lutea appear to be associated with viviparity in mammals, and aside from the mammals there is no clear evidence that they are essential for the maintenance of pregnancy. Figure 12.2 diagrams the histologically visible sequence of events.

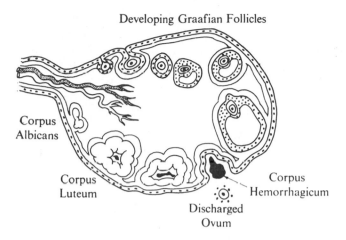

Developing Graafian Follicles

Corpus Albicans

Corpus Luteum

Corpus Hemorrhagicum

Discharged Ovum

Figure 12.2. Conventionalized diagram of the sequence of events in a transected mammalian ovary. The order is not regular as shown, and all space is packed with connective tissue, interstitial cells, and potential ova.

Mammals. Severe x-ray injury accompanied by a decrease in the size of ovaries was first demonstrated about the same time as testes damage, but the classic study was performed about half a dozen years later. This was in 1913 when Lacassagne made thousands of slides of rabbit ovaries following delivery of 3500 R (see Lacassagne and Gricouroft, 1941). To his surprise, sterilization was not complete; a few primitive ova began to develop after some months had elapsed. In succeeding years mice, rats, and other laboratory animals, including monkeys, have provided additional evidence that developing follicles are radiosensitive. Mature follicles are somewhat more resistant, and primary follicles most radiotolerant. The corpora and interstitial tissues are relatively insensitive. The oogenetic sequence is more radiosensitive in most mammals than in rabbits, but with the exception of small rodents, the quantity of radiation necessary to cause dissolution of the majority of primary follicles is in excess of that which kills the animal. In cattle, massive cell destruction requires 900 R, yet 300–400 R whole-body irradiation is lethal. In both man and monkeys, pregnancies are on record after 2000 R delivered to the ovaries!

The primary follicles of mice are especially sensitive to radiation (Rugh and Wolff, 1956). Normally the ovary of a sexually mature mouse contains three to eight corpora lutea and about the same number of developing follicles. A few months after a 50 R exposure, examination discloses no maturing follicles and only rare primary follicles and peripheral groups of presumptive follicles. If 150 R is delivered, not even presumptive follicles will remain. It is difficult to determine any details in the compact mass of connective tissue stroma. With higher doses the body of the ovary is reduced in volume so that the tunic layer appears relatively thick and is thrown into folds.

Higher doses cause the histological changes to develop more quickly. After 1500 R, atresia develops within 2 to 4 hours. Thus with acute doses we see that the rapidity with which damage is revealed depends upon the amount of radiation delivered. On the other hand, at levels as low as 1–5 R/day it may take as long as a year of continued whole-body irradiation before growing follicles disappear. However, an ovarian concentration of radioisotope can cause serious damage. As little as 25 μCi of ^{32}P injected into mice reduced the ovarian size. A diminished number of follicles and an absence of corpora lutea was accompanied by marked condensation of the stroma.

Species differences in the structure of oocyte nuclei provide a clue to differences in radiosensitivity. In the mouse, the dictyate stage of the nucleus is diffuse, while a lampbrush structure is present in the oocyte nuclei of rabbits, cows, humans, and monkeys. Nuclear changes such as pyknosis and karyolysis precede cell death. Mitochondrial and other cytoplasmic responses are transient (Parsons, 1962).

The pathologic changes described in oocytes and follicles following irradiation resemble the necrobiotic changes associated with ovulatory failure in hormone insufficiency. However, endocrine gland changes in function occur too slowly to account for the ovarian response at doses adequate to alter hormone output. Nevertheless, rats given high doses of x radiation retained germ cells in the ovary that were capable of responding to subcutaneous injection of gonadotropin (Spalding *et al.*, 1957). On the other hand, x irradiation of the pituitary glands of monkeys resulted in no obvious changes in their ovaries (Vermande-Van Eck, 1959). Hyperemia was the main physiological result when both ovaries and pituitaries were in the radiation field. Perhaps the period of hyperemia evokes growth of new follicles after damaged units have been cleared away. In spite of destruction and because of temporarily increased nourishment, small follicles will start to grow. These should be able to mature provided they lack gross nuclear damage. The load of recessive mutations induced in potential eggs is something to be revealed only in future generations, perhaps many generations hence (see Chapter 8).

Birds. Although the obvious qualitative experiments have been performed with domestic birds, it is surprising that a great deal of quantitative data on egg production has not been obtained. As we shall see with insects, egg laying lends itself to a study of oviposition per unit time. Wild birds have been neglected except by Weatherbee (1966).

Irregularity in the laying records of x-rayed adult hens may take the course of a gradual decrease to total cessation, or there may be exaggerated periods of oviposition separated by prolonged rest periods. Analytical attention has been directed more to histological studies than to egg production. In the mature ovary, doses of 1200 R and up are necessary to produce atrophy in which only connective tissue remains. A single dose of 400 R reduces some areas of the germinal epithelium to a single layer, but in other regions epithelium several cells thick persists (Essenberg and Karrasch, 1940). There, both mitosis and primary follicles are evident. From this standpoint, the gonads of birds appear somewhat more resistant than those of mammals, but during development only 80 R destroys the rudimentary ovary (Essenberg and Zikmund, 1938).

A normal anatomical feature confers a propensity to sex reversal in hens. Only one ovary is differentiated; the other is rudimentary. If the functional ovary is destroyed by disease or irradiation, the rudimentary organ develops into a testis. When this secretes hormones, the male comb, tail feathers, and sex instincts develop.

Egg laying involves more than release of the ovum from the ovary. At that time there is only nucleus and yolk. The bird must provide additional material in making what we call an "egg." Passage down a bird's oviduct results in secretion of albumen, shell membranes, and shell. Irradiation can influence this course of events. In one study, surgically exposed oviducts were irradiated with graded doses of x rays (Smith *et al.*, 1956). Lead plates were used to shield the rest of the bird. Afterwards, the laparotomy was repaired. Above 1000 R, albumen formation showed a logarithmic inhibition with increase of radiation dose. A related aspect was the decreased quality of broken-out eggs scored by the U.S. Department of Agriculture system. Above 4000 R, eggs lacked thick albumen. At higher doses, shell defects were common and egg shape sometimes bizarre with tail-like appendages and other irregularities. However, at autopsy there was no significant reduction in oviduct weight. Because of the doses employed, the oviduct is considered to be relatively radioresistant.

Insects. The insect ovary has supplied some of the most convincing evidence that the pattern of radiosensitivity varies with the cytological state of the oocyte or the oogonial stem cell. The tubular nature of the ovaries provides especially suitable material for such studies.

Within a single tube, known as an ovariole, differences occur depending upon the species. Two principal types of ovarioles are known. These are distinguished by the presence or absence of specialized nutritive cells (Figure 12.3). A further subdivision is made according to the position of these nurse cells or trophocytes in the egg tube. Species also differ in the number of ovarioles per ovary, and in their ability to store matured oocytes. Flies and wasps, the insects most used for irradiation experiments, have tubes of the polytrophic type in which a group of nurse cells accompanies each oocyte in its progress down the ovariole.

Typically, a threshold is demonstrable above which lifetime egg production decreases with increasing radiation dose. In contrast to the situation in mammals, this threshold requires the delivery of thousands rather than hundreds of roentgens. No comparative studies have been made on the basis of absorbed dose.

The wasp *Habrobracon* (*Bracon hebetor* Say) has proven to be especially suitable for studying the radiation sensitivities of cells. We have already referred to this fact in Chapter 5. Usually there are only four ovarioles, the contents of which are in synchrony. Each contains a single seriation of developing units ranging from oocytes in first meiotic metaphase to interphase oogonia (Figure 12.4). At the time of exposure, differentiated, transitional, and primitive cells are present. Eggs are dispensed in order and each deposited egg can be accounted for. Therefore, gametes obtained at any designated time may be traced back to their cytological condition at the time of exposure, and quantitative modifications in numbers of eggs or hatchability may be correlated with the cellular state during a critical period.

Eggs deposited during the first three to five days were already differentiated into oocytes and accompanied by trophocytes at the time of exposure. Although physiological states such as dehydration and star-

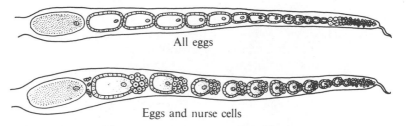

All eggs

Eggs and nurse cells

Figure 12.3. The two main types of insect ovarioles. The number of such tubes depends on and is typical of the species. Also, the number of nurse cells has taxonomic significance.

vation are effective in altering the output of the first few days, irradiation is relatively ineffective, short of massive doses which may damage the female's nervous system. In contrast, the cells from which oocytes are derived are vulnerable because several mitotic divisions are required to change an oogonium into an oocyte and its nest of nurse cells. Irradiation modifies egg production to give a family of curves characterized by a valley reflecting the vulnerability of cells in or near mitosis when exposed (Figure 12.4). The valley deepens and broadens as more radiation is delivered. When it reaches the base line we observe a period of infecundity. At higher doses, adequate to destroy all oogonia, permanent infecundity occurs. This impressive destruction of all the stem cells giving rise to oocytes occurs after deliver of 4–5 kR of hard x rays delivered as an acute dose; but permanent infecundity does not necessarily follow considerably higher doses if the radiation is spread out in time by chronic exposure or fractional delivery. Furthermore, temperature is important. Below 15°C, little recovery occurs between successive fractions of a divided dose experiment, presumably because

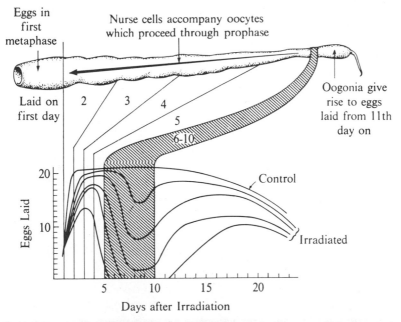

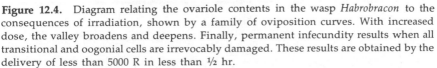

Figure 12.4. Diagram relating the ovariole contents in the wasp *Habrobracon* to the consequences of irradiation, shown by a family of oviposition curves. With increased dose, the valley broadens and deepens. Finally, permanent infecundity results when all transitional and oogonial cells are irrevocably damaged. These results are obtained by the delivery of less than 5000 R in less than ½ hr.

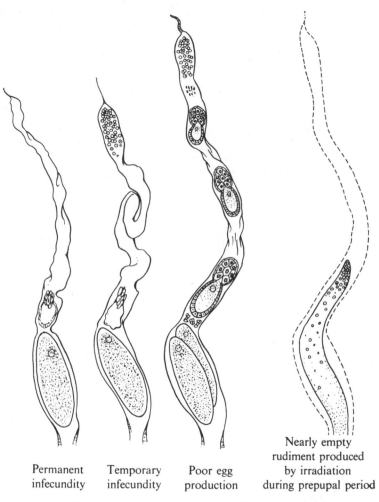

Permanent   Temporary   Poor egg   Nearly empty
infecundity   infecundity   production   rudiment produced
                                                    by irradiation
                                                    during prepupal period

Figure 12.5.   Ovarioles from irradiated *Habrobracon* females.

enzyme-mediated steps are inoperative. Chemical inhibitors also interfere with the oogonial recovery phase, but they also change the pattern
of response by decreasing oocyte vitellogenesis.

Pyknotic degeneration of oogonia and resorption of oocytes occurs
both in wasp and fly ovarioles (Mandl, 1964; Theunissen, 1977). King
(1957) reported radiation induced ovarian tumors in *Drosophila*.

Insect ovaries are more radiosensitive during their development than
in their adult differentiated form. Doses which selectively influence
only certain cell types in adult oogonia destroy ovarian anlagen. There

are periods in embryonic and larval development when radiation castration is possible. That is, the aggregation of cells destined to become ovaries can be completely eliminated so that no evidence remains in the adult. Finally, when the ovariole sheath is well-developed, it proves more radioresistant than its contents. For example, delivery of 3000–4000 R of x rays to last instar braconid larvae produces the empty sheath in adult wasps shown in Figure 12.5.

Concluding Remarks

The last two chapters, concerned with tissue response to irradiation, have emphasized that death at the cellular level is the significant feature reflected in the observations made, or in the data accumulated. In turn, tissue health is decisive for the continued life of organisms, somatic tissue for survival of the present generation, and gonadic tissue to provide future generations. This theme will still be present in the following chapters of the next section.

References

Albers-Shönberg, H. E. (1903). Uber eine bisher unbekannte Wirkung der Roentgenstrahlen auf den Organismus. *Muench. Med. Wochenschr.* **50,** 1859.

Bryan, J. H. D., and Gowen, J. W. (1958). The effects of 2560 r of x rays on spermatogenesis in the mouse. *Biol. Bull.* **114,** 271–283.

Casarett, A. P., and Casarett, G. W. (1957). Histological investigations of x ray effects on spermatogenesis in the rat. U.S. At. Energy Comm. Documents UR-496 and UR 497. Washington, D.C.

Casarett, G. W., and Hursh, J. B. (1958). Effects of daily low doses of x rays on spermatogenesis in dogs. *In* "Nuclear Radiation in Food and Agriculture" (W. R. Singleton, ed.), Chapter 17. Van Nostrand-Reinhold, Princeton, New Jersey.

Essenberg, J. M., and Karrasch, R. J. (1940). An experimental study of the effects of roentgen rays on the gonads of the sexually mature domestic fowl. *Radiology* **34,** 358–365.

Essenberg, J. M., and Zikmund, A. (1938). An experimental study of the effects of roentgen rays on the gonads of the developing chick. *Radiology* **31,** 94–103.

Freund, M., and Borelli, F. J. (1965). Semen production after x-irradiation of the testis, of the body, or of the head (guinea pig). *Radiat. Res.* **24,** 67–80.

Gillette, E. L., Hopwood, M. L., Carlson, W. D., and Gassner, F. X. (1964). The effect of x-irradiation of bovine testicles on semen. *Radiat. Res.* **22,** 264–275.

Grahn, D. (1954). Genetic variation in the response of mice to total body x irradiation. II. Organ weight response of 6 inbred strains. *J. Exp. Zool.* **125,** 63–83.

King, R. C. (1957). The cytology of the irradiated ovary of *Drosophila melanogaster.* *Exp. Cell Res.* **13,** 545–552.

Kohn, H. I., and Kallman, R. F. (1955). The effect of fractionated x-ray dosage upon the mouse testis. *J. Natl. Cancer Inst.* **15**, 891–899.

Lacassagne, A., and Gricouroff, G. (1941). "Actions des radiations sur les tissues." Masson, Paris.

Mandl, A. M. (1964). The radiosensitivity of germ cells. *Biol. Rev. Cambridge Philos. Soc.* **39**, 288–371.

Murakani, N. (1959). Disturbance of spermatogenesis due to radiation by atomic bomb explosion and fallout in Hiroshima and Bikini. *Geka No Ryoiki* **7**, 1070–1083 (see Nuclear Science Abstract 22024, Sept. 1961).

Nebel, B. R. (1958). Fine structure of chromosomes in man and other metazoa and testicular recovery from x rays in mammals. *Proc. U. N. Int. Conf. Peaceful Uses At. Energy, 2nd, 1958* Vol. 22, pp. 308–318.

Nilakhe, S. S., and Earle, N. W. (1976). Sperm production in normal vs. sterile boll weevils. *J. Econ. Entomol.* **69**, 609–613.

Oakberg, E. F. (1955). Sensitivity and time of degeneration of spermatogenic cells. *Radiat. Res.* **2**, 369–391.

Oakberg, E. F. (1969). Radiation response of the testis. *Prog. Endocrinol., Proc. Int. Congr. Endocrinol. 3rd, 1968* pp. 1070–1076.

Oakberg, E. F. (1975). Effects of radiation on the testis. *In* "Male Reproductive System" (D. W. Hamilton and R. O. Greep, eds.), pp. 233–243. Williams & Wilkins, Baltimore, Maryland.

Parsons, D. F. (1962). An electron microscope study of radiation damage in the mouse oocyte. *J. Cell Biol.* **14**, 31–48.

Rugh, R. (1953). The x irradiation of marine gametes. A study of the effects of x irradiation at different levels on the germ cells of the clam *Spisula. Biol. Bull. (Woods Hole, Mass.)* **104**, 197–209.

Rugh, R., and Wolff, J. (1956). X irradiation sterilization of the female mouse. *Fert. Steril.* **7**, 546–560.

Searle, A. G. (1974). Mutation induction in mice. *Adv. Radiat. Biol.* **4**, 131–209.

Smith, A. H., Hage, T. J., Julian, L. M., and Redmond, D. M. (1956). The effect of x irradiation of the oviduct on egg production and egg quality in the fowl. *Poul. Sci.* **35**, 539–545.

Spaulding, J. F., Wellnitz, J. M., and Schweitzer, W. H. (1957). The effects of high-dosage x ray on the maturation of the rat ovum and their modification by gonadotropins. *Fert. Steril.* **8**, 80–88.

Theunissen, J. A. B. M. (1977). "Aspects of Gametogenesis and Radiation Pathology in the Onion Fly, *Hylemya antiqua.* II. Radiation Pathology," Monogr. Meded. Landbouwhogesch., Wageningen, Netherlands.

Vermande-van Eck, G. J. (1959). Effect of low-dosage x irradiation upon pituitary glands and ovaries of the rhesus monkey. *Fertil. Steril.* **10**, 190–201.

Welshons, W. J., and Russell, W. L. (1957). The effect of x rays on the *Drosophila* testis and a method for obtaining spermatogonial mutation rates. *Proc. Natl. Acad. Sci. U.S.A.* **43**, 608–613.

Wetherbee, D. K. (1966). Gamma irradiation of birds eggs and the radiosensitivity of birds. *Mass., Agric. Exp. Stn. Bull.* **561**.

PART IV THE ORGANISM

We now turn our attention from specific alterations in the diversified structures of organisms to more general matters, leading finally to consideration of the entire individual. Although the activities of life are carried out by cells, tissues, and organs differing in structure and separate in function, the parts are mutually dependent. Specialization has resulted in such interdependence that malfunction or injury to one part may result in the death of the whole. However, loss of health or loss of life may be scored without concern for cause, or at least without investigations designed to reveal the ultimate basis.

The following two chapters concern investigations of survival and death of the individual. Although disruption of architecture often is involved, emphasis in this work has been directed to organic processes, typically in a collective sense.

CHAPTER 13   Modifiable and Nonmodifiable Damage, Protective Measures, and Regeneration Processes

Restoration Processes

This chapter concerns recovery of the organism or its parts from radiation. The word restoration can be used only in the sense of its application to a deteriorated historical building. No steps that are taken can bring back the original structure. Instead it is a case of taking steps to minimize damage, repairing that which is reparable, or substituting new structure for that which was impaired. Neutralization of the primary effects produced by the direct action of radiation at the molecular level does not seem feasible. This is not only a matter of ignorance; intervention is difficult when damaged molecules rapidly undergo further change within 10^{-5} sec. The protective measures which will be discussed later in the chapter must be employed, rather than restorative action. This means that the substance or condition must be present at the time of irradiation rather than be provided subsequently.

The course of events appears to be more amenable at the cell and tissue level. Intracellular recovery is obtained by the resynthesis of destroyed or inactivated molecules, and promoted by the neutralization of secondary effects. The recovery of tissues and organs, expressed as their ability to carry out vital functions, involves accommodation or adaptation. The process may occur within the individual cell (or structural unit), or it may involve cell populations. In the adult mammal we find tissues with cells which never divide (nerve), which divide only when called upon for regeneration (liver), and which continually divide (hematopoietic and epithelial tissue). At one end of the scale there are irreplaceable cells in which no division occurs to precipitate death, while at the other end of the scale both damage and replacement are promoted by a propensity for division. A prominent feature in the latter case is the replacement of dead cells by cells derived from the active division of stem cells. For survival of the organism, the question may resolve itself into damage or repair of the weakest histological link, and the outcome may depend upon whether scar tissue forms or cell replacement occurs. If replacement occurs, we say that a capacity for regeneration exists.

In earlier chapters, cell replacement was featured in tissue recovery. Now again at the organism level we must invoke the classic cell doctrine: All higher animals (metazoa) and plants (metaphyta) are made up entirely of cells and the products of cells. All the normal activities of the organism both constructive and destructive are the result of the activities of cells.

Death Defined

Death is usually defined as the irreversible stoppage of vital activity. It may occur as the ultimate conclusion of the process of senescence (see Chapter 14), or it may occur earlier due to an environmental agent. Induced death is regarded either as a response to any one type of insult exceeding its tolerance limit, or the result of a sum of varied kinds of injury exceeding a critical threshold, depending upon whether the investigator tends toward a multiple or unitary viewpoint. In either case, a series of biochemical events is triggered which causes death of the organism. The intricacy of the scheme of events increases in proportion to the complexity of the organism, but this can be resolved by identifying the most important cell types.

At the single cell level, death is usually specified in terms of reproductive ability. Defunct bacteria are those which fail to divide. In higher forms, the individual is considered dead when activities have ceased in the cells which are essential for coordination of the organism. Certain tissues or even separate cells may remain functional for hours or days after the organism is considered dead. When death is an individual occurrence which takes place cell by cell, the question arises whether a particular dose of radiation kills a critical number of all cells or a decisive proportion of special cells. The classification by leading organ of early deaths in irradiated mammals supports the special cell approach. In order of increasing dose, these are hematopoietic tissue, intestinal syndrome, and central nervous system modes of death. The tissues of the first two classes depend on cell proliferation for functional maintenance. Furthermore, a relationship exists between the death of stem cells or their daughters, the transit time of these cells, and the death of the organism. After medium doses, the time when a mammal dies coincides with either cytopenia of the blood or with denudation of the small intestine's epithelium.

There have been no adequate investigations of lethal syndromes in invertebrates except insects. Only some species have a radiosensitive midgut in which cell death occurs at division (Ducoff, 1972). Little attention has been given to radiation effects on the blood cells of adult insects. On the other hand, CNS damage occurs after massive doses to all types of insects. This implies ionizations sufficient to disrupt interphase cells.

An adequately high dose of radiation given to any cell in any stage can cause prompt death. However, massive doses which influence practically all organic substances are not as important in everyday life as are moderate doses which nevertheless may have lethal consequences. Exposure to a few hundred roentgens produces little chemical change in the cell as a whole, but in Chapters 3–8 we have learned about the vulnerability to such doses of the genetically important nuclear material. At modest doses, instead of instant dissolution, the end of cell life must be viewed as progress through several periods. There is a period during which deterioration is reversible, followed sequentially by irreversible intracellular damage, loss of cellular organization, and finally necrosis.

Cytological Vulnerability

Since we are now confining our discussion to the irradiated generation, recessive point mutations are important only in those organisms which have a well-developed haploid phase of the life cycle. Thus Lea (Chapter 2) could use them to interpret the killing of bacteria and viruses. In normally diploid organisms, recessive lethal mutations would not be effective due to the presence of a normal allele at the same locus on the homologous chromosome. In exception to this are the sex-linked loci in organisms possessing a sex simplex for the X-type chromosome.

In diploid organisms, changes in chromosomal material have been suggested as the main cause of lethality at the cellular level. This may be extended to organism mortality by graphic manipulation of vital statistics and of induced chromosomal aberrations. Relations can be adduced which correspond in all but the scale units. Similarities in response are found in the dependence on dose, exposure time, and radiation quality.

Bridges and chromosome fragments at division, and genetic imbalance afterward are phenomena which can explain death precipitated by division. Respectively, cells are hindered from completing division, or they lack coordination in physiological mechanisms after division. However, the picture is complicated by the delay in division which is induced by a radiation exposure as well as chromosome and gene changes. Few investigations have been concerned simultaneously with both types of phenomena. One study by Conger already cited in the introduction to Part III revealed that delayed cell division did not account for the dose-related decrease in ascites cell populations. Cell counts were made five days after a measured number of cells had been inoculated into mice. At even the largest dose, 600 R, division was inhibited only 12 hr more than in the control. At the most, such a delay does not account for more than one-third of the observed decrease, which approaches 25% of control values.

In organized complex tissues, further complications are introduced by the alternatives presumably open to a cell. In addition to division with or without degeneration, a cell might elect the alternatives of differentiation and/or migration. Under such circumstances, an absolute quantitation of radiosensitivity could not be based on a fall in mitosis or upon an increase of degenerating units in the zone of proliferation. Nevertheless, in suitable material, cell degeneration is regional in distribution and typically restricted to areas where cell division normally occurs. Furthermore, as shown in Figure 13.1, return of mitotic activity coincides with the appearance of degenerating cells (Spear, 1953). Characteristically the peak of mitosis precedes the peak of cell degeneration.

Evidence from Cultured Cells

When Puck and Marcus (1956) first measured the ability of a single cell to undergo proliferation after irradiation, they noticed that a number of cells were able to divide several times but did not continue dividing long enough to form a colony. The lethal effect was genetic but not due to simple gene inactivation.

More recent time-lapse cinemicrographic studies have revealed additional information about the death process. The majority of cell lines studied retain the ability to undergo at least one division, even for doses of 500–1000 rads where over 90% of the irradiated cells will not

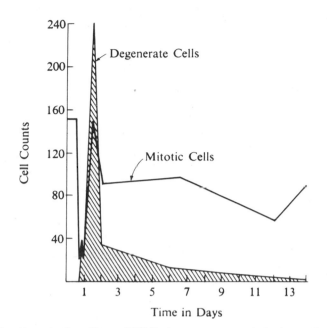

Figure 13.1.   Quantitative effects of 268 R of gamma rays on tadpole eye tissue. (Spear, 1953; by permission of Wiley, New York, and Strangeways Research Lab.)

survive to form a colony. Then in subsequent generations the probability of division decreases gradually with each generation to less than 0.5, until after five generations or more (depending on the dose). It increases again when the few survivors take over the population. The generation times are lengthened in these postirradiation generations but are usually not as long as the generation time of the irradiated generation. Hurwitz and Tolmach (1969) found a strong correlation between the generation time and impending cell death; i.e., the generation time for a parent cell was significantly longer if the daughter cell died.

The patterns of cell death seem to show some variability among cell lines. HeLa cells undergo a high incidence of death in mitosis. The cells reach mitosis and remain in the rounded state with a metaphase plate evident for periods of 3 to 24 hr. Then they die a sudden death by blebbing or disintegration. The incidence of death in mitosis of L cells is much less; instead, some morphologically intact cells persist for many days. The lymphoid cell L51787 appears to disintegrate in the G_1 phase.

Before the cell actually disintegrates, other abnormalities are evident. The irradiated cell may give rise to two daughters which fuse together after several hours. When this cell reaches mitosis, a multipolar mitosis may produce four cells, which may fuse all together or one at a time.

Eventually, this abnormal behavior leads to cell death. For low doses, several divisions are required; these may allow for the dilution of essential components present before irradiation or for the segregation of the damaged gene(s).

This overall pattern of cell death provides some insight into the mechanisms of how the initial damage to a cell leads to its final demise. The prolonged aspect suggests damage to the nuclear material. In contrast, cells die immediately after very high doses (> 20 krads), possibly due to membrane or other cytoplasmic damage. Then no time is available for remedial steps.

Carrano (1973) demonstrated a significant correlation between chromosome aberrations and cell death. By determining transmission and survival parameters for specific aberrations, he found it possible to predict the fraction of the cell population surviving at any time subsequent to irradiation. The presence of chromosome bridges may explain both the earlier death and the cell fusion, while acentric fragments may account for the cell death that occurs over several generations. A loss of all copies of homologous material do not seem necessary to cause cell death. The loss of substantial regions of the genome suffice. However, one or more cell generations may be required for depletion of the accumulated intracellular substances manufactured under the direction of the genetic information in the lost fragment. Thus even though a class of cells may not die during a division stage, their death is the consequence of cell proliferation.

Interdependence of Organelle and Organism

A mass of direct and inferential evidence indicates that radiation damage to the contents of the cell nucleus is a major cause of cell death. Only a portion of the ionized-induced changes seems to be modifiable. The repair systems of Chapter 4 and the chromosomal rejoining of Chapter 5 are involved, but their interrelations are not yet understood. An additional complication is that they are not autonomous. Synthetic processes even in the nucleus depend upon energy-generating series of reactions in cytosomal structures.

Mitochondria play a major role in cell respiration. By isolating mitochondria from rat livers at successive times postirradiation, and using a variety of substrates, Hall *et al.* (1963) demonstrated impaired efficiency of phosphorylation, decrease in the rate of adenosine triphosphate (ATP) synthesis, and a drop in mitochondrial protein. Tremendous doses of radiation did not cause comparable damage to mitochondria *isolated* from liver, spleen, or thymus glands. Routinely after total-body irradiation there is a depression of oxidative phosphorylation in rodent spleen and thymus glands, but the reproducibility of the *in situ* liver response was debated. Finally Yost *et al.* (1967) discovered variability of the liver response to depend on the condition of individual rats. Furthermore, there was a seasonal effect on all rats in their colony. In liver tests, the uncoupling of oxidative phosphorylation was not demonstrable during the summer. Such dependence on intrinsic differences between organisms suggests an abscopal effect.

The function of mitochondria and other organelles is intimately associated with a characteristic structural organization. Reduction in structural complexity results in a loss of ability. Thus the capacity for implementing the complete citric acid cycle is lost when the sac-within-a-sac arrangement is disrupted, while electron transport persists as long as there are fragments of single membranes. Ultimately reductional techniques provide structural proteins. At this point, the cellular environment rather than organismal influences becomes the more important conditioner of the response to radiation.

Isolated structural proteins are relatively radioresistant (Errera, 1954). This earlier conclusion has been borne out in more recent studies with hemoglobin. Even in an aqueous system, massive doses of 4–5 Mrad were required to alter sedimentation constants, limiting viscosity value, and electrophoretic behavior. Furthermore, the sulfhydryl enzymes shown to be sensitive *in vitro* are not inactivated *in vivo* by radiation doses that kill cells. In the cell, such compounds are associated with glutathione and other types of protective agents. Among the cell constituents are vitamins E and C, which are antioxidizing agents for lipids and aqueous systems (Table 13.1) respectively. Gunckel and Sparrow (1961) reported the *in vivo* inactivation doses "fairly high" for a long list of plant enzymes.

The situation in plants is more readily interpretable. Vertebrates, by contrast, are not ideal for a demonstration of specific biochemical or physiological lesions. In a higher animal, the mechanisms for retaining physiological balance complicate matters. Compensatory or buffering processes are evoked in response to any significant stress.

Respiration Studies

Plant studies of respiration have the advantage of avoiding the effect of thyroid hormones on the mitochondria. Irradiated bulbs, roots, and seedlings have been used for such investigations. Mikaelsen's (1953)

TABLE 13.1

Ascorbic Acid Content (mg/100 g fresh wt) and Relative Radioresistance of Green Plants[a]

| | Relative Resistance to Irradiation | | |
Species	Resistant	Moderately resistant	Low resistance
Cabbage	200–300		
Gladiolus	300–400		
Soybean		120–150	
Snapdragon		100–120	
Cosmos			90–100
Nicotiana			50–60
Xanthium			70–100
Hyoscyamus			30–40

[a] Cooke (1953).

x-ray experiments on barley are instructive (Figure 13.2). A Warburg constant-volume respirometer was adapted to the measurement of seed respiration.

Barley seeds irradiated dry and germinated immediately showed no adverse respiratory effect until after four or five days. Even then the effect was merely a failure of the oxygen consumption to increase at the control rate, for doses above 5000 R, Respiration was unaffected by 2500 R.

The histology and cytology of the seedling offer an interpretation. The growth of embryonic tissue at first is by cell elongation. When mitosis begins, nuclear disturbances become apparent. However, neither these nor induced mitotic delays interfere with completion of the first mitotic division, but further growth is initiated by a period of lively cell multiplication with which damaged nuclei cannot efficiently cope. The growth rate and associated metabolism is related directly to the number of cells capable of mitosis.

Consistent with this explanation are the findings in other plants that in the depression of respiration the apical region is most sensitive while the coleoptile is least sensitive. Leaves and primary roots are intermediate.

Some confusion has resulted from reports of respiratory increases after the irradiation of such diverse materials as frog skin, fowl erythrocytes, grasshopper eggs, and rat tissues. These can be explained by an uncoupling effect in which the phosphorylation of adenosine diphosphate (ADP) is inhibited but oxidation continues, often at an

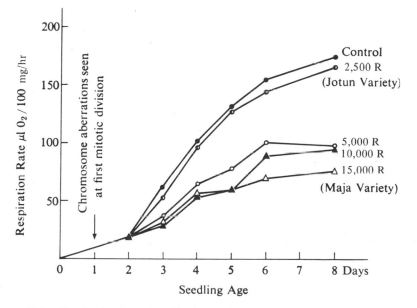

Figure 13.2.   Respiration intensity of barley seeds during the first 8 days of germination. Dry dormant seeds were irradiated. No influence is noted during emergence of primary root and coleoptile. Differences develop during the period of lively cell multiplication. (Based on Mikaelsen and Halvorsen, 1953; with permission of the Scandinavian Soc. for Plant Physiology.)

increased rate. Investigations on potato tubers which exhibit clear cases of the phenomenon indicate that the enzyme systems of respiration are more resistant than the capacity for growth.

Protective Conditions

The discovery of the oxygen effect and an appreciation of the importance of the indirect action of ionizing radiations encouraged exploratory attempts to protect vertebrates. Lowering the oxygen tension can reduce the quantity of free radicals produced from irradiation of water. Consistent with this view is the reduced injury from radiation in mammals where breathing is restricted or circulation is impaired (Dowdy *et al.*, 1950). Experimental techniques included the strapping of chests, the tying of blood vessels, tourniqueting, and bleeding to produce severe anemia. However there was the criticism that other essential metabolites may fail to reach the cell in adequate quantity and that wastes would not be removed.

Gas chamber experiments became popular. To avoid secondary reactions, extreme anoxia was obtained for the brief duration of irradiation. For rats x-rayed in 5% oxygen/95% nitrogen, the LD_{50} was pushed from 600 R to above 1200 R.

Frigid temperatures can reduce radiation mortality by lowering oxygen tension. For infant mice, the survival of refrigerated (about 5°C) litter mates is twice that at room temperature, almost as if they had been irradiated in a nitrogen atmosphere. To round out the picture, anoxia combined with refrigeration does not enhance the radiation protection and the benefit derived from chilling is less if animals are placed in pure oxygen.

Reduced body temperature during exposure also affords protection to adult mice. Adults have been irradiated when all heart and respiratory movements have stopped and the colonic temperature has neared 0°C. Under such conditions, the 30-day LD_{50} dose is more than four times that required at normal body temperature. However, although low temperature may influence mammals in this way, different results occur in lower animals. Because of the greater solubility of oxygen, diminished oxygen tension is not expected for simple organisms in a refrigerated aqueous medium exposed to air. Even chilled frogs are probably not anoxic, since oxygen passes easily through moist amphibian skin.

Hypoxia explains the protective action of carbon monoxide in mammalian whole-body irradiation, and brings forward the question of protective compounds. In fact, CO may be given either in an exposure chamber or by injection.

Protective Substances

A variety of compounds in one way or another associated with the production of anoxia have been used to protect mammals. Some, like p-aminopropiophenone, operate through the formation of methemaglobin; others such as epinephrine, influence the parasympathetic nervous system. However, alterations by such means are indirect and somewhat removed from the cellular sites of radiation damage.

Respiratory Inhibitors. As a result of the research interest in the oxygen effect (see Chapter 5), equivalent attention to cellular respiratory inhibitors was inevitable.

Herve and Bacq (1949) showed that cyanide near the lethal dose protects 80% of injected mice against the minimum x-ray dose lethal for controls. Confirmation of the protective effect is available in experiments on a variety of forms including peas, barley, insects, bacteria, and ciliates. In organisms suitable for cytological or genetic study, significant decreases in chromosomal abnormalities or mutations are noted.

On the other hand, there are reports in which cyanide is claimed to increase the effect of radiations, typically on tumors. A reasonable explanation is that with oxygen consumption inhibited, the oxygen tension of the tissue may be increased. Thus the protective action might be offset by an increased radiosensitivity due to an oxygen effect.

Agents other than cyanide which inhibit cytochrome oxidase and metal enzymes have been tested. Sodium azide, for example, may protect mice and bacteria from lethality. However, the relationship between inactivation and mutagenic action has not proved simple in the microorganism experiments. In some bacteria, azide may increase the mutation rate while decreasing lethality.

Dangerously toxic compounds like cyanide, carbon monoxide, and other enzyme inhibitors are not substances which lend themselves to medical practice or employment by disaster fighters, but there are substances being developed which may.

Aminothiol Compounds. The group led by Patt (Patt *et al.*, 1949) is given credit for the "breakthrough" in this field. They discovered that cysteine injected into rats and mice before x irradiation increased the proportion of the total which survived. Injection of cysteine immediately after the exposure was ineffectual. This is the essence of protection. A substance protective against radiation damage is one which must be present at the time of irradiation (Patt, 1953).

In their experiments, control and injected rodents received 800 R of x radiation in a brief single exposure. The amount of cysteine and the pH of the injection were varied. Nevertheless, in a critical experiment, if all rats receiving cysteine before irradiation were considered as a single group, 92 of 126 cysteine-treated animals survived as compared with only 18 from 134 irradiated untreated. In other words, 73% survived instead of only 13%, a highly significant difference statistically. As is customary, this score was taken at the end of 30 days.

Subsequently, the term "protection" has been used in various ways, depending upon the type of experiment performed. With experimental mammals it is employed when a larger proportion of animals survives a given dose of radiation or when they have tolerated a larger dose than usual. This does not mean that animals surviving an appreciable dose of radiation are normal. A histological examination of protected rats will demonstrate most of the tissue abnormalities discussed in Chapter 11, but somewhat decreased quantitatively. Furthermore, despite protection, fertility is altered and mutation rate is increased.

Immediately following irradiation, the protected mammals show the same responses as an uprotected group receiving the same radiation dose. The initial damage to the thymus, intestine, and hemopoiesis occurs in both groups. The important difference is that the recovery phase, especially in hemopoiesis, occurs earlier and is more intense.

Hundreds of compounds were screened for their protective effect on mortality and weight loss in laboratory mammals. Clearly the SH group alone did not confer protective properties upon a molecule. The molecular structure that is particularly effective includes an amino group separated from a sulfhydryl or disulfide group by not more than three carbon atoms. That is, the most effective compounds are aminothiols. Some, like glutathione, are effective only if injected (Patt *et al.*, 1950). Others, like cysteamine, may be used orally.

Despite 20 years of research, none of the aminothiols was proven clinically useful, mainly because humans do not tolerate the doses required for protection. Finally the U.S. Army Medical Research and Development command synthesized a class of drugs known as phosphorothioates. These are phosphorylated derivatives of cysteamine in which a phosphate covers the sulfhydryl group. In the mammal, these are enzymatically dephosphorylated to the protective free SH form, but in tissue cultures on standard media where the conversion does not take place, no protection is conferred. WR-2721, perhaps the most effective phosphorothioate, protects mice against all modes of radiation damage except CNS death (Yuhas *et al.*, 1973, 1977).

Theories of Action. There are several possible mechanisms whereby the effects of ionizing radiation may be decreased, since SH-type protectors are hydrogen- or energy-transfer agents and radical scavengers. A widely accepted premise has been that such compounds act as absorbing material for oxidants formed in intracellular water after irradiation. Another possibility is that effective compounds might compete for oxygen itself, which promotes production of HO_2 radicals. These concepts emphasize indirect action (Adams, 1972).

An idea which explains resistance against both direct and indirect action involves the formation of mixed disulfides. Important compounds modified by reaction with the radiation protector should become resistant if sensitive S—S bonds are involved in the reaction. However cystine which easily forms mixed disulfides does not act protectively. Also, although DNA lacks sulfur, it is protected by cysteamine.

A more general mechanism, envisaged by Bacq and Alexander (1961) concerns peroxidized targets. By reacting with a protector, an organic radical might be saved from a highly unstable peroxyl condition, the decomposition of which would mean its inactivation. Although they favored this interpretation for protection in mammals, these authors were careful to point out that SH protectors are so reactive that they could be functioning simultaneously in a variety of ways within the same system. The restoration of induced free radicals to an inactive state by the donation of H atoms from a protector is still another explanation of recent popularity.

Since protection has been confirmed for isolated cells, the phenomenon is not confined to vertebrate organ system physiology. As a means of simplifying the work of screening chemical compounds and as an aid in understanding some aspects of the action, chemists have employed synthetic systems such as aqueous polymethacrylic acid. However, studies of polymers fail to give information on metabolizing systems which may alter radiosensitivity. Furthermore, the action of protective compounds in a complex organism is influenced by variations in penetration, distribution, and detoxification.

Unrestricted Utility. Cultures of bacteria have been favored for living cell research. Here, as with mammals, survival has been the standard criterion of protection, but there are several advantages of conducting experiments with microorganisms. They can be handled in large numbers; results become available in a short time; measured quantities of chemicals can be applied directly to cells in suspension; and biochemical functions can be investigated directly.

Results with one of the more successful compounds are shown in Figure 13.3 Hollaender and Stapleton, 1956), where there is increasing protection with increasing concentration until a plateau is reached. Careful technique must be used to demonstrate the clearest expression of protection. Preirradiation growth conditions are often as important as added factors on survival of cells after irradiation.

In certain strains it is possible to protect against the production of mutations of the nutritional reversion type, provided there is a minimum of population pressure. Population pressure can obscure the protective phenomenon. Synchronization of division to produce a

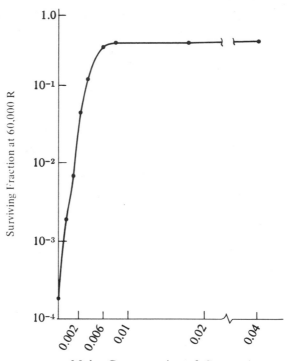

Figure 13.3. Effect of cysteamine on the survival of *Escherichia coli* B/r during exposure to 60 kR of 250-kV x rays. (From Hollaender and Stapleton, 1956; used with permission from Churchill, London)

homogeneous population is difficult. Also, the controversial state of bacterial cytology is disadvantageous.

Some investigators have managed to set up ingenious *in vitro* experiments with vertebrate cells and tissues. The Patt group studied cells from minced thymus glands after washing and suspending them in serum-buffered Ringer solution (Patt *et al.*, 1952). Damaged thymocytes could be detected by their eosin stainability. Undamaged cells do not take up the stain. Radiation damage appeared at 50 R, a dosage similar to the threshold for lymphopenia (see Chapter 11). Figure 13.4 demonstrates how cysteine displaces the radiation dose–response curve by a constant percentage over a wide dosage range. The Bacq group demonstrated that reticulocyte maturation can be protected. However, massive doses were necessary in this study. (Bacq and Alexander, 1961).

If the right amount of a substance like cystamine-HCl is supplied to chick-heart fibroblasts before irradiation, tissue cultures are more likely

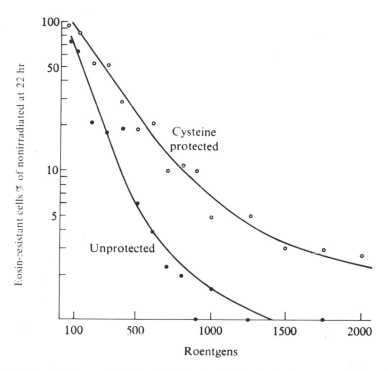

Figure 13.4. Cysteine, added 15 min before irradiation to obtain a concentration of 19.2 mM, displaces the radiation dose–response curve for thymocytes by a constant amount over a wide dosage range. (Based on Patt *et al.*, 1952; with permission of the Society for Experimental Biology and Medicine.)

to survive the critical phase which occurs several transfers after exposure. The influence is not in mitotic inhibition, but probably upon the continuity of hereditary material itself.

With insects, results were disappointing until Grosch (1960) studied the fate of dividing and differentiating cell types of the ovariole sequence. Evidently static mature sperm and differentiated adult tissues are not optimum for demonstrating aminothiol protection.

Direct investigation of a protective effect on the nuclear contents has been pursued chiefly with plant chromosomes. Root tips can be irradiated in nutrient solution containing various concentrations of substances anticipated to be protective. After exposure, slides may be prepared using an acetocarmine or other "squash" technique. Table 13.2 shows results from a *Tradescantia* experiment in which glutathione conferred protection. Other compounds like cysteine and dimercaptopropanol (BAL) have proved effective, and several different plants have

TABLE 13.2

Effect of Different Concentrations of Glutathione on Frequencies of Chromosome Fragments and Bridges after Chronic γ Irradiation of *Tradescantia* Root Tips[a]

Conc. added (M)	Total no. anaphases	No. fragments	Fragments per 100 cells	No. bridges	Bridges per 100 cells
None	661	115	17.40	20	3.03
1×10^{-5}	250	42	15.20	2	0.63
1×10^{-4}	235	29	11.17	2	0.67
3×10^{-4}	474	40	8.63	5	1.03
1.5×10^{-3}	298	25	8.13	5	1.74

[a] Mikaelsen, 1952.

proved useful in this work. Onion roots have been particularly popular. The depression in growth has been correlated with the cytological picture. One of the main problems is whether the chromosomal disturbances constitute the main cause of death for the cells and the organism, and whether the protective effect of SH substances is due to alleviation of chromosome breakage.

Chelating Agents. Chelating agents are a type of compound which first caught the attention of radiobiologists, because of the need for therapeutic agents to aid in the removal of radioisotopes from the living organism. They also have been considered for their protective possibilities. However, only a few of the sequestering agents of industrial chemistry can be used safely in mammals (Bacq and Alexander, 1961). Furthermore, despite success with mice, the results were negative with bacteria, yeast, plants, and insects. Table 13.3 demonstrates that a combination of x radiation and EDTA lowers life span significantly at a radiation dose which in itself had no effect on wasps. Most of the commercially available agents have been assessed using life span and females' fecundity. None have shown protective promise in insects.

In theory, a stable chelate of copper or any other important cation would be invulnerable to oxidation, an indirect effect of radiation. Even aminothiol protectors are believed to have this ability.

Miscellaneous Substances. Practically every class of chemical compounds at one time or other has been considered for protective ability (Ellinger, 1956; Rugh and Grupp, 1960). The test organism has usually been a bacterium or a rodent. Agents which cause hypoxia were men-

TABLE 13.3

Effect of Ingested Disodium Versenate and X-Irradiation on Survival of *Habrobracon* Females[a]

Conditions	Mean life span (days)	Standard error of mean
Control	22.8	2.7
2500 R	22.9	1.0
0.075 M EDTA	16.5	2.3
Both[b]	12.4	2.4
0.09 M EDTA	16.3	2.7
Both[b]	9.1	2.8
0.025 M EDTA	18.1	1.5

[a] Courtesy of L. E. La Chance.
[b] Both indicates combined EDTA + x-ray treatment.

tioned earlier. In addition, anesthetics, sedatives and tranquilizers are effective for related reasons, but they are not as potent as aminothiols.

The effectiveness of radioprotective chemicals can be expressed as a dose reduction factor (DRF) obtained from the ratio of the radiation dose required to give the same effect in protected and unprotected individuals. Aminothiol DRFs for the mouse LD_{50} are about 1.7. The best pharmaceutical drugs give DRFs less than 1.5.

Chemical Radiosensitization

The converse of radioprotection is radiosensitization, which means that an agent increases a cell's response to irradiation by altering the cell's internal environment. This can be particularly useful in cancer therapy for promoting destruction of the anoxic parts of a tumor.

Prompted by the knowledge that N-ethylmaleimide (NEM) was an industrially useful SH poison, Bridges (1960) demonstrated a sensitizing effect in bacteria. Later it became evident that SH suppression was not as important as originally believed. Two other modes of action are indicated by mammalian cell-culture investigations (Sinclair, 1973). NEM inhibits the repair process either by competing with, or binding with, intracellular compounds involved in the reconstruction of damaged molecules. An SH-containing enzyme may be the most critical cell component.

More recently, Diamide [diazenedicarboxylic acid bis(N,N-dimethylamide)] has been identified as a radiosensitizer of anoxic cells, which oxidizes endogenous reduced glutathione (GSH). Previously no reagents were known which would perform this feat without also reacting extensively with protein-bound sulfhydryl groups (Harris and Power, 1973).

Other classes of radiosensitizers under investigation include a range of electron-affinic compounds. Indirect action via electron transport from hydrated atoms was the original hypothesis, but now a direct action mechanism is favored. This postulates that the sensitizer increases the probability of electron trapping and promotes migration to increase the number of free radicals at ionization sites. In most cases, the maximum degree of sensitization does not exceed the sensitizing effect of oxygen (Adams, 1972).

Somewhat different is the halogenated pyrimidine analogue effect. If a bromine, chlorine, or iodine atom is substituted for the methyl group in thymine, the molecular and cellular effects or irradiation (visible light, ultraviolet, and xrays) are enhanced. The halogen atom acts as a trap for electrons liberated along the length of the DNA strand. The strand is more susceptible to single-strand breaks and to chromosome aberrations produced by irradiation. Cells *in vitro* and *in vivo* are sensitized to x rays by a factor of approximately 1.5. Since the sensitization effect is dependent upon the analogue being incorporated into DNA, maximal sensitization occurs when the cells have replicated their DNA for several generations in the presence of the analogue. Attempts to use bromodeoxyuridine to sensitize tumor cells have been unsuccessful as a result of dehalogenation before the agent reaches the tumor, although more recent studies have attempted to use intraarterial infusion directly into the tumor.

Regeneration

In the broad sense, protected organisms retained superior regenerative ability. Here "regeneration" is used in the strict sense: Destruction of an organ or appendage can reawaken morphogenetic processes at an advanced stage of development of the organism. Earlier in Chapter 11 we considered reconstitution of tissues damaged by radiation. There is another type of experiment in which part of an organ or appendage is surgically removed and its ability to regenerate determined after irradiation. In mammals, the liver and kidney have conditional ability to renew cells. That is, once fully developed, these organs show little cell proliferation unless they must compensate for a loss of functional organ mass. In rats, irradiation interferes with the regeneration of surgically removed liver lobes (Fabricant, 1968), and with the burst of mitotic activity in the kidney remaining after one kidney is removed. Depending on dose, irradiation prior to partial hepatectomy may delay or eliminate the regenerative ability. A lag in the mitotic response is evident even if surgical removal is delayed for some days.

Animals from the more primitive phyla exhibit impressive ability to regenerate entire body parts. Coelenterata, the lowest animals with definite tissues, are relatively radiotolerant for this among other reasons. Much of the cytological research on regeneration has been performed on worms, chiefly planarians. If the posterior is shielded by lead, flatworms can even regenerate a head region necrotized by x rays. The partial regeneration of segments amputated immediately after whole-worm irradiation can occur, despite suppression of all mitosis, if the cell types which provide necessary RNA are still well stocked.

A majority of the radiation investigations on vertebrates has been done with amphibians, which possess a greater ability to regenerate lost parts than any other member of the group. The tail, whole limbs, and even parts of the head may be restored after injury or amputation. Ionizing radiation not only prevents regeneration in amphibian appendages (Figure 13.5), but it also proves universally preclusive in all organisms tested. Demolition processes are unchecked. However, subsequently a regeneration bud fails to develop because the required undifferentiated cells are incapable of reproduction.

The doses used in typical experiments are not adequate to cause loss of a limb. Instead, the member is amputated to enable study of its rate of reconstruction. Often an irradiated leg differs from normal only in one aspect—it lacks the capacity to regenerate. Treated animals may be kept for the rest of their lives without developing structural or functional differences. Even histological techniques fail to demonstrate a change from normal. Nevertheless, if an irradiated limb is amputated, a permanent stump results instead of a regenerated appendage. The passage of months or years between irradiation and amputation makes no difference. Apparently, regional autonomy is so pronounced that cells do not migrate from unexposed regions to compensate for the nondividing local tissue cells. Brunst (1961a,b) refers to the situation as an induced stable state which can persist for the remainder of the life span. In some of his experiments, irradiated individuals remained alive for such a long period that death resulted presumably from other causes.

Experiments have also been performed on limbs in the process of regeneration. Radiation may either retard or stop limb regeneration, depending upon dose and dose-rate. Acute x-ray doses between 5000

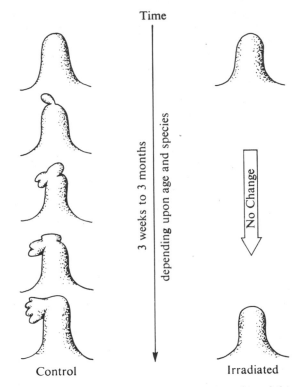

Figure 13.5. Ionizing radiation can prevent regeneration of amphibian appendages.

and 7000 R have completely halted regeneration in newts. Instead of developing skeleton and muscle, the limb bud may fill with connective tissue, followed by partial or complete resorption. At lower doses, a stunted appendage may result if differentiation occurs, but the number of cells is too small to form a structure of normal size.

Shielding experiments reinforce the evidence that local cellular elements are responsible for regeneration. If the distal end of the appendage is shielded but a portion nearer the body is irradiated, the distal end can regenerate despite its being connected to the body by an irradiated section. However, the amputation must leave some shielded tissue distal to the stump.

Regeneration of the irradiated end of an extremity may occur if normal epidermis is grafted upon it. This makes possible renewed contact between nerves and epidermis, a condition Rose (1970) considers important for restoring the "polarized message-transport systems."

Concluding Remarks

Because of their common foundation in the cellular basis of organism survival, restoration processes (other than DNA repair) and protective measures have been combined in this chapter. An extension of the classic doctrine identifies the cell as the important structural unit for death as well as for life of an organism. Depending on their nature, lethal alterations may express themselves either at cell division or during interphase. At face value this suggests nuclear and nonnuclear causes. However, caution is advised against conclusions drawn from tissue investigations limited to a single cellular aspect. A cytosomal change may be an effect attendant to a moribund condition rather than its cause.

The replacement of cells is important in the repair and regeneration of organs and appendages. Protective conditions and protective substances can enhance the likelihood of replacement by altering stem-cell environment during irradiation. Discovery of the oxygen effect stimulated many of the early investigations, while in recent years methods were sought for inactivation of free radicals. The converse of protection, radiosensitization, has also been demonstrated.

These cell-based matters are of general significance to all organisms. Of more restricted occurrence but great theoretical interest is the complete regeneration of organs and appendages found in more primitive animal phyla. In higher organisms, conditional regeneration occurs only in certain tissues. The next chapter on somatic mortality extends consideration to events in which regeneration is inadequate, or deterioration occurs instead of restoration.

References

Adams, G. E. (1972). Radiation chemical mechanisms in radiation biology. *Adv. Radiat. Chem.* **3**, 126–208.

Bacq, Z. M., and Alexander, P. (1961). "Fundamentals of Radiobiology." 2nd ed., Chapter 19. Pergamon Press, New York.

Bridges, B. A. (1960). Sensitization of *E. coli* to gamma-radiation by N-ethylmaleimide. *Nature (London)* **188**, 415.

Brunst, V. V. (1961a). Some problems of regeneration *Q. Rev. Biol.* **36**, 178–206.

Brunst, V. V. (1961b). Roentgen regression in the axolotl. *Am. J. Roentgenol., Radium Ther. Nucl. Med.* [N.S.] **85**, 158–178.

Carrano, A. V. (1973). Chromosome aberrations and radiation-induced cell death. *Mutat. Res.* **17**, 341–343 and 355–366.

Cooke, A. R. (1953) Effect of gamma irradiation on the ascorbic acid content of green plants. *Science* **117**, 588–589.

Dowdy, A. H., Bennett, L. R., and Chastain, S. M. (1950). Protective action of anoxic anoxia against total body roentgen irradiation of mammals. *Radiology* **55**, 879–885.

Ducoff, H. S. (1972). "Causes of death in irradiated adult insects. *Biol. Rev. Cambridge Philos. Soc.* **47**, 211–240.

Ellinger, F. (1956). Pharmacological studies on irradiated animals. Part V. The effects of postirradiation administration of vitamin K on x ray induced mortality. *U.S. Nav. Med. Res. Inst. Rep.* **14**, 55–64 (see *Proc. Soc. Exp. Biol. Med.* for other papers in this series).

Errera, M. (1954). Action of ionizing radiation on cell constituents. *In* "1954 Liège Radiobiol. Symp." (Z. M. Bacq and P. Alexander, eds.), pp. 93–103. Academic Press, New York.

Fabricant, J. I. (1967). Cell proliferation in the regenerating liver and the effect of prior continuous irradiation. *Radiat. Res.* **32**, 804–826.

Grosch, D. S. (1960). Protective effects on fecundity and fertility from feeding cysteine and glutathione to *Habrobracon* females before x irradiation. *Radiat. Res.* **12**, 146–154.

Gunckel, J. E., and Sparrow, A. H. (1961). Ionizing radiations: Biochemical, physiological and morphological aspects of their effects on plants. *In* "Handbuch der Pflanzenphysiologie" (W. Ruhland, ed.), Vol. 16, pp. 555–611. Springer-Verlag, Berlin and New York.

Hall, J. C., Goldstein, A. L., and Sonnenblick, B. P. (1963). Recovery of oxidative phosphorylation in rat liver mitochondria after whole body irradiation. *J. Biol. Chem.* **238**, 1137–39.

Harris, H. W., and Power, J. A. (1973). Diamide: A new radiosensitizer for anoxic cells. *Radiat. Res.* **56**, 97–109.

Hervé, A., and Bacq, Z. M. (1949). Cyanure et dose léthale de rayons X. *C. R. Seances Soc. Biol. Ses Fil.* **143**, 881–883.

Hollaender, A., and Stapleton, G. E. (1956). The influence of chemical pre and post treatments on radiosensitivity of bacteria, and their significance for higher organisms. *Ioniz. Radiat. Cell Metab., Ciba Found. Symp. 1956* pp. 120–135.

Hurwitz, C., and Tolmach, L. J. (1969). Time lapse cinemicrographic studies of x-irradiated HeLa S3 cells. *Biophys. J.* **9**, 607–633 and 1131–1143.

Mikaelsen, K. (1952). The protective effect of glutathione against radiation induced chromosome aberrations. *Science* **116**, 172–174.

Mikaelsen, K., and Halvorsen, H. (1953). Experiments on the respiration of x-irradiated barley seeds. *Physiol. Plant.* **6**, 873–879.

Patt, H. M. (1953). Protective mechanisms in ionizing radiation injury, *Physiol Rev.* **33**, 35–76.

Patt, H. M., Tyree, E. B., Straube, R. L., and Smith, D. E. (1949). Cysteine protection against x irradiation, *Science* **110**, 213–214.

Patt, H. M., Smith, D. E., Tyree, E. B., and Straube, R. L. (1950). Further studies on modification of sensitivity to x rays by cysteine. *Proc. Soc. Ex. Biol. Med.* **73**, 18–21.

Patt, H. M., Blackford, M. E., Straube, R. L. (1952). Effect of x rays on thymocytes and its modification by cysteine. *Proc. Soc. Exp. Biol. Med.* **80**, 92–97.

Puck, R. J., and Marcus, P. I. (1956). Action of x rays on mammalian cells. *J. Exp. Med.* **103**, 653–666.

Rose, S. M. (1970). "Regeneration." Appleton, New York.

Rugh, R., and Grupp, E. (1960). Protection of the embryo against the congenital and lethal effects of x irradiation. *Atompraxis* **6,** 143–148 and 209–217.

Sinclair, W. K. (1973). N-Ethylmaleimide and the cyclic response to x rays of synchronous chinese hamster cells. *Radiat. Res.* **55,** 41–57.

Spear, F. G. (1953). "Radiations and Living Cells," p. 72. Wiley, New York.

Yost, M. T., Robson, H. H., and Yost, H. T. (1967). Uncoupling of oxidative phosphorylation in rat liver and spleen mitochondria by exposure to total body irradiation. *Radiat. Res.* **32,** 187–199.

Yuhas, J. M., Proctor, J. O., and Smith, L. H. (1973). Some pharmacologic effects of WR-2721: Their importance in toxicity and radioprotection. *Radiat. Res.* **54,** 222–223.

Yuhas, J. M., Yurconic, M., Kligerman, M. M., West, G., and Peterson, D. F. (1977). Combined use of radioprotective and radiation sensitizing drugs in radiotherapy. *Radiat. Res.* **70,** 433–443.

CHAPTER 14   Somatic Mortality: Radiation Sickness, Aging, and Carcinogenesis

In this chapter we shall consider the response of the organism expressed as sickness and death. The consequences of exposure vary not only with dose but also with the kind, rate of administration, and penetrating ability of the rays. Animal size and structural detail also become important when comparative radiosensitivity is considered. Most of the research has been focused on mammals, and therefore, this will be our particular concern.

The characteristic pattern of mortality for mammals is shown in Figure 14.1 (Upton, 1957). Individuals which do not die immediately nevertheless have a decreased life expectancy. Between the periods of early and late deaths there is an interval of low mortality which varies inversely with dose. At doses lower than shown, the interval of low mortality is prolonged. At higher doses the interval is shortened, and finally disappears. Separate sections will deal with the early and delayed effects of irradiation.

Early Effects

Radiation Sickness. Table 14.1 summarizes our inferences about human symptoms. However, a nuclear explosion is accompanied by the emission of both neutrons and γ rays. In addition, radioactive decay of fission products contributes α, β, and more γ rays. This combination of rays complicates interpretations of dosage. Identifying the symptoms of radiation sickness was not always possible at Hiroshima and Nagasaki under stress situations for patients suffering from blast injuries and flash burns (Glasstone, 1962). Mass disasters provide a complex situation.

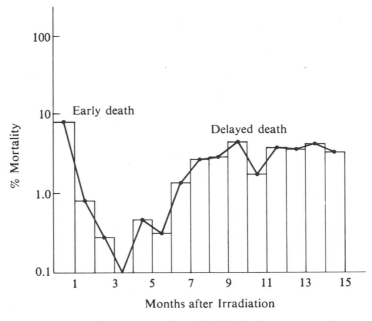

Figure 14.1. Mortality of mice exposed to 600–700 R of gamma rays from a nuclear explosion. (After A. C. Upton with his permission and also that of the *Journal of Gerontology*.)

More amenable to interpretation are the accidental exposures of people working in atomic establishments, but there, too, the dosage may be inferred from circumstantial evidence. Yet the clinical information is obtained in optimum hospital conditions. A useful check is provided by the experience accumulated from therapeutic irradiation of cancer patients. Depending on health at the time of exposure, and rest and medical attention after exposure, the lethal doses can be higher than shown, or with poor health and meager care lower doses may have an increased effectiveness. At lower doses, the hematopoietic tissues are the primary concern but the gastrointestinal tract provides the leading organs at the lethal threshold. For doses larger than those tabulated, the role of the central nervous system becomes more prominent and death occurs more promptly. In mice, the sequence of events goes through an ataxic, a lethargic, and a convulsive stage followed by death. Fortunately, such serious exposures are not common in human experience.

Radiation sickness follows a pattern of early reaction, latent period, and secondary stage (Cronkite and Bond, 1960). Two 1958 accidents,

TABLE 14.1

Symptoms of Radiation Sickness in Man in Relation to Time after Exposure.

Survival:	Probable	Possible	Improbable
Dose:	Moderate 100–300 R	Median lethal 400–700 R	Lethal 800 R
Weeks after exposure			
1		Nausea, vomiting	Nausea, vomiting
	Latent phase		Diarrhea
			Inflamed mouth
	No definite		and throat
	symptoms		Ulcers
			Fever
			Emaciation rapid
2		Epilation	Death
		Loss of appetite	
		Malaise?	
		Sore throat	
		Petechia	
3	Epilation	Diarrhea	
	Loss of appetite	Emaciation	
	Malaise	Death	
	Sore throat		
	Petechia		
4	Diarrhea		
	Emaciation		
	moderate		

one in Oak Ridge, Tennessee, the other in Vinca, Yugoslavia, have instructive value (Andrews, 1962). In the Oak Ridge incident, five men receiving 300 rads experienced nausea, and within 12 hr four of them vomited. These symptoms of nervous system origin persisted for two days. During this time the lymphocyte count fell, for all five cases, but hematological depression did not become prominent until the fourth week. The delay in depression resulted from the longer life spans of the other formed blood elements (see Chapter 11). Bleeding tendencies probably contributed to this situation. Subsequently, recovery occurred without recourse to transfusions or bone marrow transplants. Although they expressed feelings of weakness and dull aches in the legs, the men were discharged from the hospital on the forty-fourth day. Finally these symptoms disappeared and even the sperm counts returned to normal.

However, regaining blood cell counts within the normal range does not ensure complete normality. At the chromosomal level, persistent damage was demonstrable even $3\frac{1}{2}$ years after the 1958 incident (Bender and Gooch, 1962). Both gross and minor chromosomal damage were evident in cultured leukocytes (Bender and Gooch, 1962). In 1962, blood samples were obtained as early as 4 hr after the "Recuplex" criticality accident at Hanford. Subsequent samples were taken periodically for over two years. The frequencies of deletions, acentrics, and dicentric chromosomes peaked during the first 4 weeks, but some abberrations were found in samples taken 2 years later (Bender and Gooch, 1966).

Clinical evidences of injury were considerably more severe for the Yugoslavian group, and physical evaluation of the dose places it higher, in one case 1000–1200 rem. The most heavily irradiated man experienced diarrhea, insomnia, and headache; and, despite a marrow graft, he died after four weeks of gastrointestinal complications. Skin pigmentation and epilation was pronounced for the entire group. Menstrual irregularity resulted for the one female in the group.

The counteraction of radiation sickness by pharmacological means has been investigated with experimental mammals. The goal of therapeutic studies is to eliminate undesirable side effects of irradiation or to otherwise counteract radiation death. The postirradiation administration of vitamin K reduces mammalian mortality by alleviating hemorrhagic manifestations (Ellinger, 1955). Shifting the mortality curve by stimulating the reticuloendothelial system is another approach. Lipid therapy may benefit mammals in a third way.

In medical practice however, no specific agent is used on patients from a radiation accident unless there are clear-cut clinical indications that it is needed. More important in the management of radiation injury are proper rest, good nutrition, and the maintenance of fluid and electrolytic balance (Saenger, 1973). This provides the best opportunity for the organism's defences and restoratory processes to operate. Furthermore, minimizing the exposure to bacteria and other pathogens is one of the main benefits of hospital isolation.

Some symptoms cannot be assessed by histological techniques. When there are subtle changes in the nervous system, humans can describe how they feel, but there is no positive way of determining this for experimental animals except through observations of their behavior. Ingenious methods for demonstrating changes in nonintellectual behavior after irradiation include running wheel activities, pedometer manipulation, visual curiosity tests, taste aversion trials, and stress-avoidance of noxious stimuli. Although modifications in the performance of these feats follow whole body exposure to moderate doses, a mammal's capability for learning is not radically changed by massive doses of radiation (Van Cleave, 1963).

Reflex and Neuromuscular Experiments. Before World War II, relatively little had been published about radiation-induced disturbance in the nervous system, except in Russian. Opinions differ on the significance of this work because of the complicated systems considered where change may result from vascular, endocrine, or other disturbance. Dependent upon many interrelated systems are conditoned reflexes such as salivation in dogs. Also complex are such matters as the amplitude of cerebellar response to sciatic stimulus.

At the University of Georgia, a facility was constructed in the Animal Behavior Laboratory which permitted simultaneous recording of salivary secretion, leg flexions, electroencephalograms, heart rate, respiration rate, and general activity during Pavlovian conditioning. Changes in response to stimuli in the course of exposure to repeated low doses of whole-body radiation were evaluated by computer processing of the data. During 5 years of intense investigation, James and Peacock discovered that Russian findings could be duplicated only by selecting individual conditioning protocols to illustrate a particular point (see James *et al.*, 1966). Objective analysis failed. The variability within and between subjects was so great that statistical significance could not be established by experimental designs which pool subjects without regard for their constitution or prior experience. Unfortunately the contributing factors to the existence of two or more response categories are not yet identified. The occurrence of morphologically different types of nervous systems in dogs or other mammals is not generally accepted.

Subsequently, Peacock's interest shifted to radiation-induced taste aversions which provide clearcut results from less than 50 R spread over 4 hr (L. J. Peacock, personal communication, 1977). Within a few years a sizable literature on conditioned avoidance of food, water, and alcohol has accumulated (see the bibliography by Riley and Baril, 1976).

The most convincing evidence of low-dose alterations to the functional activity of the nervous system in intact animals has come from the susceptibility to audiogenic seizure in certain strains of mice (Miller, 1962). These sound-induced convulsions are remarkably radiosensitive, being influenced even by changes in the level of radioactive fallout in Chicago from 1957 through 1959. In experiments, a total dose of 0.14 rads received in the first 30 days increased the frequency and severity of seizures. A broad picture of the situation is provided by the Haley and Snider book (1962), and the IAEA Symposium (1962).

Simpler systems do not necessarily provide demonstrations of radiosensitivity. For example, consider the simple motor reflex provided by isolated nerve–muscle preparations. A decrease in amplitude and an increase in reflex time has been claimed after 1000 R. Indeed, even below 100 R, an increased scatter around the mean has been claimed. However frog preparations did not show changes in contractile irritability or refractory periods until they received more than 20,000 R (Rosen and Dawson, 1960). By a factor of 2 or 3, this is lower than the doses necessary to influence contractility of the muscle or to produce changes in the action potential or other measurable qualities of isolated nerves. Therefore it seems possible that neural synapses and neuromuscular junctions may be *relatively* radiosensitive. However, these dose levels are high compared to the lethal doses for vertebrates.

In weighing nervous system research, it is important to remember that nerve cells have a high capacity for protein regeneration, which may provide physiological as well as morphological tolerance (Zeman, 1961). Furthermore, Butler's (1956) comment about the general status of radiobiological research seems particularly appropriate to the nervous system. We are much like the man trying to comprehend a telephone exchange by observing some of the results of throwing bricks into it.

Stressor Agent Hypothesis. Although specific neuromuscular reactions have been given small consideration, nonspecific neuroendocrine reactions have had much attention. The idea is that every strongly harmful agent acting as a stress stimulates nerve centers which influence the anterior pituitary to secrete more adrenocorticotropic hormone (ACTH) while inhibiting its secretion of other hormones. Accordingly, the adrenal cortex becomes overactive and produces unusual amounts of steroid hormones including those of the cortisone type. In turn, lymphatic structures shrink and bleeding ulcers appear in the stomach and upper intestine. Thus three interdependent types of change comprise the stress syndrome: enlarged adrenal cortex, gastrointestinal ulcers, and thymolymphatic shrinkage (Selye, 1973).

Unfortunately the extreme sensitivity of lymphoid tissue to irradiation (see Chapter 11) complicates the use of a favorite criterion of the reaction to stress, lymphoid tissue atrophy. In whole-body irradiation, cytolysis from the radiation reaching the tissues is so intense that it obscures adrenal effects on lymphoid tissue. Also, removal of adrenals does not seem to influence weight changes of spleen and thymus when several hundred roentgens have been delivered to rodents.

On the other hand, remote effects on the thymus and spleen have been described when radiation has been delivered only to the anterior of the animal. Spleen–thymus atrophy has also been produced by localized irradiation of regions of the gut, although the syndrome seems to result only if exposure of a particular body region alters the total economy of the animal, thereby imposing a condition of stress. Under such circumstances, we can appreciate the fact that fatty liver and stomach ulcers may appear as part of the stress reaction. More subtle criteria have been sought for irradiation-stress studies. Among them is the fatigue curve of skeletal muscle, which has been featured in some of the Russian work.

Large localized doses of radiation delivered to the adrenal or pituitary result in neither stimulation nor interference with their function in producing the stress syndrome. Likewise, whether the adrenals are shielded or not seems insignificant for changes occurring to the cortical region. A notable prompt reaction to irradiation is a marked simultaneous decrease of ascorbic acid and cholesterol of the adrenals supposedly associated with cortic steroid synthesis. Consistent with this idea are reports of histological growth in the glomerular zone. This has been called the first phase. A second, later adrenal reaction occurs which is probably associated with the serious condition reached by animals preceding death.

Defenses against Infection. In mammals, a serious consequence of irradiation is disruption of the lines of defense against invaders. Not only do the mechanical barriers of skin and mucous membrane break down, but the secondary lines of defense involving leukocytes and lymphatic tissues are also damaged. In addition, a final line of defense, the ability to form antibodies, is decreased, because immunological incompetence results from the destruction of lymphoid tissue. A complete failure of antibody response can occur in a mammal sublethally but heavily irradiated. No antigen injected 24 hr later is able to elicit antibody production. Even the engulfing capacity of cultures of irradiated phagocytes is decreased, more by death of cells than by loss of cell function. Therefore infection is of grave concern since even an insignificant scratch may be serious for any animal not reared under highly artificial conditions. Incidentally the survival curve is shifted upward by a germ-free condition (Wilson, 1963).

If antibiotics are used therapeutically, it is the small lesion which is treated. The popular view of such agents as miracle drugs has not been shared by physicians who realize that antibiotics are antimetabolites which can depress tissue regeneration. Penicillin is a possible exception since its action on bacterial cells is not important in mammalian cells. However, only certain types of bacteria are sensitive to penicillin.

In the absence of skin wounds or burns, infection of intestinal origin can occur, as has been shown by blood culture of experimental animals. Furthermore, sublethal irradiation has increased the mortality from experimental infection with virulent *Salmonella*, and this was unaffected by a variety of antibiotics. Also, none of the available antibiotics hindered the spread of endogenous bacteria, nor prevented the death of noninoculated mice exposed to lethal doses of radiation in Korner's (1959) experiments. In contrast, penicillin enabled eradication of intraperitoneally introduced pneumococci and reduced mouse mortality. Many experiments have been carried out on other laboratory animals. An antibiotic such as aureomycin may control an aspect like diarrhea so that the death rate is modified, but an antibiotic can not save the life of an animal that has received too much radiation. Although one type of defect may be allayed, too many other aspects have been altered. Antibiotics function best when an organism's natural defenses are in good condition.

Although it is clearly established that whole-body irradiation approaching a lethal amount decreases immunity and lowers antibody formation, results from moderate and partial-body irradiation are difficult to interpret. The degree of inhibition varies for different criteria of antibody response and depends upon the temporal relation of the exposure and of the antigen injection. Reports that small amounts of x rays, often administered locally, may enhance antibody formation and immunity are unclarified. For an optimum response of the organism, the induction process requires an intact, nonirradiated mammal. Rabbits irradiated as long as a month prior to antigen injection fail to produce normal amounts of antibody. The secondary anamnestic response seems to be less radiosensitive.

Experiments on Shielding Part of the Body during Irradiation. For the ultraviolet wavelengths, pigmented cuticle, feathers, pelt, or clothing suffices as shielding, but for x rays, lead is the optimum material. During the first decade following the discovery of x rays, it became evident that shielding the abdomen conferred some kind of protection to a mammal. Finally, in 1949, Jacobson and his associates (1949a,b) demonstrated that if mouse spleens were exteriorized and enclosed in lead boxes (Figure 14.2), more than 1000 R were required to kill a strain of mice which ordinarily barely withstands 700 R. Lead-protected spleens compensate so rapidly and effectively for interruption of bone

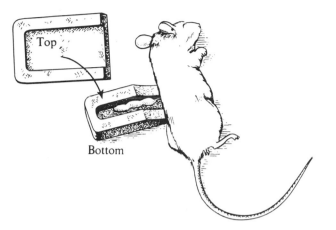

Figure 14.2. Mouse with surgically exteriorized spleen within bottom of lead box. When covered with the lead top, the spleen is well shielded from radiations. (Based upon a photograph by courtesy of L. O. Jacobson.)

marrow activity that anemia does not develop and the leukocyte decrease is slight. During compensation, the lymphatic tissue of shielded spleens may decrease due to stem-cell migrations between shielded and exposed organs.

Lead shields placed over other parts of the trunk offer some protection against whole body irradiation, but the regions of the liver, cecum, or lung do not have a capacity equivalent to the spleen for sparing an experimental animal from the lethal effects of exposure. Furthermore, unless the protected organ has been exteriorized—a very delicate operation—one is never positive that shielding regions of the skeleton may not contribute to the results. Actually, a lead screen over the thigh is as effective as shielding many visceral organs. Also small epicondylar lead cuffs enabled survival of dogs after doses up to three times the dose lethal to unprotected animals (Cole *et al.*, 1967).

In fish, when the head is shielded and the body exposed, survival after irradiation approaches control values. Osmoregulatory imbalance is the important factor in the death of unshielded fish. A head shield protects both the gills themselves and the site of neurohypophyseal hormone production involved in control of gill function.

Up to this point, the tests cited were made with shields which were small in comparison with the size of the animal. When large shields are used and more area is shielded than exposed, damage rather than protection is the aspect likely to be considered. Regional irradiation, particularly at doses exceeding those lethal when delivered to the entire body, gives rise to specific syndromes depending on the region exposed as shown below:

Region exposed	Syndrome[a]
Abdomen	Intestinal
Thorax	Acute pulmonary
	Esophageal (above 2250 R)
Head	Oropharyngeal
	Neurogenic (above 12,000 R)

[a] Details of these syndromes may be found in the report from Maisin's laboratory to the Second U.N. International Conference (Geneva, 1958).

Injections of Tissue Derivatives. A natural course of investigation following the success of spleen shielding was the grafting of spleens, and, even more satisfactory, the injection of spleen homogenates or suspensions. Survival of injected mice was impressive. Normally 950 R is lethal for 100% of the CBA strain. Even single survivors would have been significant. In actuality, a majority of spleen-injected mice not only survived for the conventional 30 days but for an appreciable time beyond this period. Bone marrow and fetal liver injections also promoted survival.

Two contrasting theories developed, the humoral and the cellular; and because heterospecific material from guinea pigs and rats could aid the recovery of mice, many authorities favored the humoral theory. However, this basis of objection finally provided evidence in favor of the cellular theory. Replacement of host bone marrow by injected donor cells occurs in heavily irradiated mice injected with rat bone marrow. A definite check is possible because the rat chromosome complement differs from that of the mouse. In one survey by Ford's laboratory, none of 1400 marrow cells examined could be identified as belonging to the mouse host (Ford et al., 1956). More evidence of an exacting cytological nature came from injections of mouse spleen cells which carried a reciprocal chromosome translocation. Cells characterized by the nuclear aberration showed up in bone marrow, spleen, thymus, and lymph nodes weeks after injection. These results substantiate immunological findings that implanted marrow gives rise to the antigenic tags of a majority (up to 80%) of the peripheral erythrocytes. Biochemical and biophysical methods are also being developed for the identification of cell origins.

A complete return of immune capacity must include cell-mediated immunity as well as the production of circulating antibodies. The dual nature of the immune system depends upon lymphocyte differentiation into two kind of cells: T cells, which combat fungi and viruses and reject tissues; and B cells, antecedents of those which manufacture immuno-globulin. "T" refers to the thymus-mediated differentiation.

Bone-marrow cells fail to return full immune capacity to neonatally thymectomized mice, or to older mice subjected to thymectomy plus near-lethal doses of radiation. Thymic cells must be used as a source of T-type stem cells. Alternatively for older mice, bone marrow plus thymic tissue in millipore chambers may suffice. Thus the simultaneous operation of a humoral factor is not completely excluded. If isolatable, a nonantigenic stimulatory agent would be advantageous to avoid the ultimate consequences of implanted foreign cells.

Incompatibility Reactions. Supralethal irradiation temporarily abolishes the mammal's natural immunological defenses, not only to invading organisms but also to injected cells or transplants of foreign origin. This is why rat cells can become established in a mouse. The mouse can temporarily tolerate rat cells. However, since immune mechanisms are merely depressed, not destroyed, donor–host interaction finally leads to difficulty for the host. The major reaction seems to be of the host to the transplanted tissue, but the reverse is also possible. In any event, even though the animal has survived the lethal consequences of irradiation it may not survive the delayed results of the treatment when incompatible tissues attempt to destroy one another (Congdon, 1971).

The first symptoms of what is termed "secondary disease" appear after the period of radiation mortality. Extreme constitutional disturbances develop as a metabolic consequence of the immune reaction. Even animals which respond with an increased food intake lose weight until they are emaciated, suffering from diarrhea and dermatitis at the same time. Death may occur from a sort of metabolic starvation for which the biochemical alterations need to be determined.

We need to learn much more about the immunological basis of tissue compatibility. At present, clinical use may be justified only as experimental, and upon the basis that any improvement in survival is desirable following known lethal exposure, regardless of later consequences. Permanent marrow grafts were not achieved in the Yugoslavian patients and we do not know whether the treatment helped them. Dog, pig, and monkey experiments have not shown the clear-cut benefits which appeared with rodents. Persistence of marrow cells has occurred in a human survivor of an industrial accident in which the body re-

ceived 600 R, but his donor was an identical twin with complete his-
tocompatibility. In the absence of an identical twin to serve as donor,
the problem of obtaining a matching source of differentiated marrow is
serious. Further work on the transplantation of fetal bone marrow may
prove helpful. If difficulties can be overcome, clinical applications of
marrow transplantation will include not merely cases of exceptional
accidental radiation exposure, but also routine usage following chemo-
or radiotherapy of malignancies.

Late Effects

Cancer Induction. One of the most disturbing features of radiation
exposure is that damage of a malignant nature may become apparent
long afterward. Many of the early investigators inadvertently overex-
posed their hands before this danger was recognized, and skin cancer
claimed the lives of an appreciable number of pioneer radiologists. We
now accept this form of cancer to be related to previous radiation, and
especially because of the published fate of watch-dial painters we do
not question its part in causing bone cancer. For other types of human
cancer, the evidence is largely statistical. Surveys demonstrated a
higher incidence of leukemia among early radiologists than among
other professional groups. Also, leukemia is more prevalent in Japanese
survivors of the atomic bombing than in the general population. Except
for chronic lymphocytic leukemia, dose-related increases occurred in all
forms of leukemia although the frequency depended upon the type of
radiation exposure, age at the time of exposure, and type of leukemia.
Overall, the risk is about 20 cases per million people per year per rad.
However the actual numbers of individuals is small for doses under 100
rads. The incidence in Hiroshima was higher, presumably a result of
the neutron component. An RBE of 5 has been suggested but even
higher estimates may be made for lower doses.

The incidences of other forms of radiation-induced cancers have been
estimated in terms of cases per million people per year per rad: 1.2 for
thyroid, 2.1 for breast, and 2.0 for lung. Since these types have appeared only after 25 years, the latent period is longer than that for
leukemia. The years 1950 to 1954 were peak ones for leukemia. Subsequently there has been a decline, but leukemia incidence has not yet
returned to preexposure levels.

Experimentally, radiation has proved more universal in action than
other agents by producing cancers in practically all tissues of all species

of investigated mammals. In 1936, Furth and Furth reported that in x-rayed mice ovarian tumors were increased 15 times. Bone marrow and lymphoid tissue cancers were also much more frequent in x-rayed mice than in control mice. Several years later, Lorenz (1950) demonstrated an increased percentage and earlier onset of neoplasms at all doses while evaluating the maximum permissible dose of chronic gamma irradiation. Subsequently, a multitude of investigators have played a part in expanding this area of research. Lymphoid leukemia turned out to be one of the most widely recognized and investigated carcinogenic actions of ionizing radiation. Characteristically the period intervening between irradiation and the earliest detectable evidence of cancer is an appreciable part of the life span, up to 30 months for mice and as long as 30 years for man.

Localized irradiation may produce local lesions as an obvious indication of tissue damage which precedes cancer formation, but whole-body irradiation produces no obvious precursory signs. When the entire organism is exposed, incidence and cancer site depend upon genetic makeup and physiological variables plus character and dose (Alexander and Connell, 1960) of radiation. Figure 14.3 contrasts the

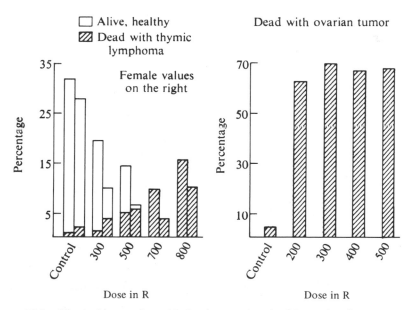

Figure 14.3. The incidence of two kinds of cancer in mice 30 months after exposure to ionizing radiation from a nuclear explosion. (Based on Furth *et al.*, 1954; with permission of the Radiological Society of North America, Inc.)

incidence of thymic leukemia in different strains of mice after x irradiation.

In a comparison with x rays based on absorbed dose, neutrons proved effective for inducing neoplasms in rats but, more important, indicated a situation too complicated to warrant extrapolation to low doses. Furthermore, it seems that more than one cell may be involved in the inductive process (Rossi and Kelleher, 1972).

Genetically uniform mice were used for the first experimental investigation of the late effects of radiation from a nuclear detonation (Furth *et al.*, 1954). Large groups of equivalent age were placed at various distances from the hypocenter along with devices for monitoring the intensity of exposure. After early mortality had been scored, the animals were transported to Oak Ridge where they were individually caged until death. An increase in thymic lymphomas in proportion to the dose became apparent and, to a lesser extent, other types of leukemia became more frequent. The incidence of ovarian and mammary gland tumors increased and tumors of lung, liver, kidney, and other organs were present occasionally. Unanticipated were tumors of the pituitary and harderian gland, the latter previously unreported in mice.

Most of the research on carcinogenesis has been performed using radiations delivered from outside the organism. Except on the induction of bone and thyroid tumors there is little information on internal isotopes as carcinogens. Here too, as in Chapter 10, tissue affinity as well as the character of radiation are important considerations. Thus bone-seeking alpha emitters are potent skeletal carcinogens. One comparison of plutonium and polonium demonstrated that the former tripled the incidence of bone tumors, while the latter doubled the incidence of soft tissue tumors (Finkel, 1958).

Despite extensive investigation, the mechanism of carcinogenesis remains unknown. Our attitude toward permissible occupational exposures will depend upon whether there is a threshold dose of radiation needed to initiate a cancer or whether minute increases to the accumulated dose contribute to the possibility of cancer. The abnormality occurs in the mechanism that determines the territorial limits of a cell type, and involves a loss of controlled cell multiplication. Classified on a tissue basis, there are three main groups of cancers: carcinoma, sarcoma, and leukemia–lymphoma. Further classification by organs gives about 100 varieties. However, the cause of uncontrolled cellular growth remains obscure. One theme features mutation in which ionizing radiations (a) cause gene mutations in somatic tissues, or (b) cause mutation or gene inactivation in a virus, or (c) cause chromosome aberrations which are a prevalent feature in cancer cells. Other concepts involve tissue damage which might promote infection by an extraneous virus or upset some delicate balance within the organism. The latter theme includes such ideas as that the ionizing radiation may (a) cause a precancerous lesion in which regeneration leads to cancer, or (b) damage an endocrine gland (e.g., pituitary) so that a hormonal effect leads to cancer at another site (e.g., ovary), or (c) depress the immune response which normally performs a surveillance function.

No matter which proves to be the critical step in induction, the result is a self-perpetuating cell abnormality, because autonomous growth occurs upon transplantation into a normal host. Also, the existence of a latent period suggests that the "acquisition of the malignant state" involves more than one step. Irradiation may exert influence to a greater or lesser extent upon each stage. Furthermore, radiation is only one of a number of environmental causative factors now identified. To what extent chemical and physical agents are additive is unknown.

Life Span. The aging and death of mammals have always received attention because low chronic doses produced less life span shortening than acute irradiation (Mole, 1957). A change of the slope of the line plotted for the Gompertz function (the rate at which animals of a population are dying) is the prime observation to be explained. Over the years, at least six mathematical treatments advanced theoretical interpretations. Strehler's (1962) book discusses the various theories which incorporated concepts such as decay in vitality, accumulation of damage, and expenditure of energy to restore altered systems. Life shortening is still not completely understood, but cell dysfunction and attrition are involved to a considerable extent (Lamb, 1977).

The evidence for radiation-induced life shortening in humans is derived from studies of the exposure of radiologists and the Japanese survivors. The mean age of death of U.S. radiologists was 5 years less than that of other physicians in a study of those dying between 1940 and 1960. However, those radiologists dying more recently did not have a shortened life span. Similarly, a study of British radiologists failed to show a decrease in life expectancy. The discrepancy is apparently related to the exposure dose: the early U.S. radiologists absorbed extremely high doses compared to present day exposures. Thus far, the Japanese study of A-bomb survivors does not show any evidence of radiation-induced aging. The reduction in life span results from certain diseases, especially neoplasia. Numerous tests of neurologic, neuromuscular, and physical functions have failed to show any radiation effect. The only pathological change is a suggestion of tubular sclerosis. However it is quite possible that effects may be seen in individuals exposed at an early age.

The plotted results from significant experiments will help us appreciate the pattern in life-shortening after whole body exposure to radiation. Figure 14.4 shows selected curves which present mortality in large numbers of mice exposed to an experimental nuclear detonation. Figure 14.5 shows curves obtained from chronic gamma irradiation. From these examples we percieve that a family of curves results. At higher doses of radiation, the pertinent curves are displaced forward in time and the slopes become steeper. The same S-shaped curves are obtained with x rays and other types of rays. However the magnitude of effect depends on how a dose is delivered. A chronic exposure over a prolonged period is much less effective than an acute dose for shortening lives. The reduction for acute exposure is 5 to 10% per 100 rads and less than 1% for a chronic exposure. In the study by Furth and associates (1954), all mice receiving more than 700 R were dead within thirty months, while twice as much radiation was required when spread out through time in the Lorenz experiment. Recovery processes are operating. Other evidence along the same line is provided by fractionation experiments with x rays. The acute lethal dose is unchanged if several weeks intervene between it and the last sublethal dose.

There is difficulty in dissociating the process of aging from that of

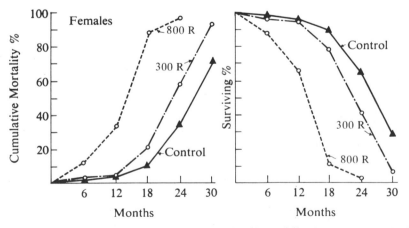

Figure 14.4. Two ways of representing live and dead mice following exposure to ionizing radiation from nuclear detonation. This type of exposure is very brief, practically instantaneous. (Based on Furth *et al.*, 1954; with permission of the Radiological Society of North America, Inc.)

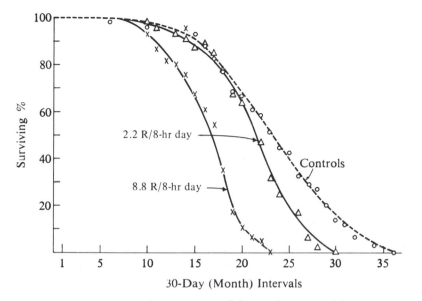

Figure 14.5. Mortality curves for mice exposed during their entire life span to gamma rays from radium sources. (From Lorenz, 1950; courtesy of Thomas, Springfield, Illinois.)

injury when one attempts interpretation of mortality or survival curves. The carcinogenic aspects of radiation contribute significantly to the reduction of life span in mice. Degenerative diseases in which radiosensitive cells are killed and blood vessels are damaged account for a smaller proportion of deaths. Kidney failure is one such defect which typifies reaction to irradiation by certain strains of mice. However, when death due to all obvious causes has been excluded, the average lifespan of irradiated animals is decreased. Even if no deaths occur within several months after irradiation, exposure of a mammal to an acute whole-body dose of more than 100 R shortens the average life span. Age-specific mortality rates and major pathological lesions are discussed in the book edited by Fry *et al.* (1970).

Irradiation and Aging. Does radiation induce a new factor or does it merely accelerate normal aging processes? We should not be willing to accept either alternative without experimental evidence. Even experimental evidence must be viewed with suspicion when irradiation causes "aging" processes not evident in the absence of radiation. For example, it seems inappropriate to interpret radiation-induced graying of hair as accelerated aging in a strain of mice which does not exhibit senile graying (Walburg, 1975).

Life span studies of adult holometabolous insects provide information on the response of organisms characterized by nondividing somatic tissue cells. Whether this can assist us to arrive at an explanation of reduced life span in mammals remains to be seen. The persistent weight loss of irradiated mammals is consistent with cell destruction involving mitotic difficulties. This feature is missing for insects.

In wasps where haploid and diploid types can be compared, the pattern of death due to normal aging and that which is radiation-induced do not seem comparable. Ordinarily, differences in life span are related to sex and nutritional pattern but not to genome number. In radiation experiments, life span is markedly influenced by genome number. In other words, there is evidence for damage of a genetic nature (Clark et al., 1963).

Tissue changes in aging and irradiated insects are now being studied. Most obvious is the increased deposition of urates, an end product of purine metabolism, in specialized cells of the wasps' fat-bodies. This process is known as a storage type of "excretion." Ionizing radiations increase the rate of urate accumulation. In Drosophila, the degenerative changes found in most tissues of senescent flies (100 to 120 days) do not appear in groups dying 30 to 40 days after ^{60}Co γ rays. Miquel et al., (1972) consider this an indication that radiation-induced death is due to a syndrome unrelated to aging, which may involve increased sponginess of the CNS neuropil, focal cytoplasmic edema in other tissues, and virus accumulations.

A decade ago, the somatic mutation theory stimulated many experiments by offering a common basic cause of aging in all species. This postulated aging to be due to the accumulation of mutations in nondividing, nonreplaceable somatic cells. Radiation was a prime candidate for the inducing agent, but the identification and quantification of mutations is difficult in this type of cell. In cells where chromosome aberrations can be observed, x-ray doses with little influence on life span produce more aberrations than are necessary to explain life shortening. A vestige of the idea persists in the suggestion that cumulative mutations in the genome could prevent the proliferation of needed stem cells.

In mammals, several interrelated tissue changes appear at an earlier age in irradiated individuals. Along with an alteration in the ratio of parenchymal cells to connective tissues, the fine vasculature decreases (Casarett, 1968). This histopathological combination is believed to impede the transfer of gases and metabolites between the blood and an organ's functional cells. Also, wastes may accumulate, or large molecular products of both normal and abnormal reactions may be synthesized at a rate more rapid than that at which they can be removed in an aging tissue. Thus lipofuscin has come to be regarded as more than merely an embellishment of old age.

However lipofuscin accumulation is another classical senescent event which is refractory to irradiation. Collagen changes and declining neuromuscular function are additional physiological aspects of normal aging not significantly changed in mammals given realistic doses of radiation.

Molecular biology has contributed a number of aging theories, but not yet has it been possible to demonstrate a causal relationship between a metabolic change at the cellular level and the shortening of the metazoan life span. A progressive cross-linkage of molecules, possibly caused by free radicals, could lead to correlated deterioration of biochemical performance. Among the favored candidates for experimental investigation of cellular aging are the regulatory mechanisms of protein synthesis. However, integrated theories must not be ignored in attempts to explain the progressive decline in functional reserves and adaptive powers which involve immunological reactions, stress responses and cybernetic interrelations (Hart and Carpenter, 1971). In an organism there are feedback systems at the organ level that provide self-aggravation to the aging process.

Lethal Dose. A radiation exposure which shortens life span is no less a lethal dose than one which renders an animal irreversibly unconscious. Furthermore, sigmoid mortality curves reflect the fact that irradiated individuals in an apparently uniform population do not show an identical survivorship response. In mammals, the standard approach of 50% dead in 30 days provides a stable centering point for a high degree of variability. To accomplish LD_{50} in 30 days for adult mammals, the dosage of total-body x radiation ranges from 200 to 800 R. Within this range are included, in order of sensitivity, guinea pigs, swine, dogs, goats, monkeys, mice, hamsters, and rabbits. Cited references contain the results of experiments on this matter, but no absolute values can be listed here because the specific dose depends upon strain, conditions of exposure, and maintenance. In addition, species differ in normal life span so that 30 days is not necessarily an equivalent period of living. A value which is optimum as an index for a small fast-breeding species may be a poor representation of conditions for a large slow-breeding type.

There are other considerations which complicate determination and interpretation of the lethal dose. While they remain at a cold temperature, hibernating mammals show little indication that a serious dose has been exceeded. The damage becomes apparent upon return to a warm temperature. Figure 14.6 (Kunkel *et al.*, 1957) compares survival curves for the dormouse *Glis glis*, but observations have also been made on hibernating ground squirrels, bats, marmots, and frogs (Schmidt, 1967). The serious consequences of a dose evidently lethal at ordinary temperatures may be undetectable in biological terms while hibernation persists. Cell hypoxia and an accumulation of cells in radiotolerant stages of their cycle are factors that partially explain the situation. The delay in the appearance of damage is closely associated with the resumption of cell division.

Some of the cold blooded vertebrates are as radiosensitive as mammals. The LD_{50} for several species of snakes is between 300 and 400 R, but other reptiles are more tolerant (Cosgrove, 1971). Turtles have an LD_{50} near 1000 R, and the acute lethal dose for lizard species ranges from 1000 to 2000 R. At the same level or above are lethal doses reported for frogs and newts. Marine teleost fish have LD_{50}s as high as 5500 R. The few birds studied to date are as sensitive as mammals, but an adequate picture of responses in types with high body temperatures and metabolic rates is not available.

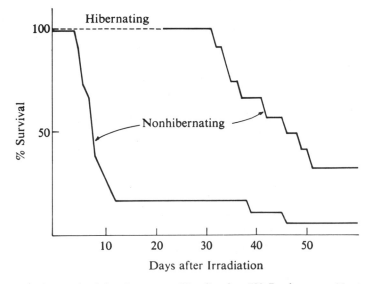

Figure 14.6. Survival of the dormouse *Glis glis* after 700 R of x rays. No irradiated animals died during a 3-week period of hibernation at 3°C. On day 22 they were moved to 20°C. Radiation damage apparently remained latent until after wakening. (Kunkel *et al.*, 1957; by permission of Oliver & Boyd, Edinburgh, and J. D. Abbatt, ed.)

Instead of a 30-day base, the more gradual and prolonged tissue changes necessitated the use of a 90-day period for snakes and 120 days for turtles. Even more instructive–than LD_{50}s are mean lethal-dose–time curves for describing radiation tolerance.

For lethal dose studies with invertebrates, no single fixed period has been adopted as the significant length of time for survival. This is fortunate because the normal life span ranges from hours for microorganisms to decades for many coelenterates, molluscs, and crustacea. The life span for some forms may even exceed that of man. However, very few invertebrates have been studied from the standpoint of adult reactions to irradiation. Among widely scattered representatives from a variety of phyla and classes, there are examples requiring doses comparable to those which kill insects. Even among Insecta only a few insect types have been studied adequately. The results show a wide range of radiation tolerance among different species. Doses which produce 100% lethality for more susceptible species have no demonstrable effect on the most resistant types. As yet no generalization can be made relating the differences to taxonomy, type of metamorphosis, nutrition, or habitat. Most probably the importance of some aspect of nuclear cytology will soon be revealed as it has been for plants (see Chapter 8).

For comparison with the dose range mentioned for mammals, one insect example may be instructive. In the wasp *Habrobracon*, decreases in life span become obvious only when adults have received between 2500 and 10,000 R. Above this, up to 50,000 R, there is little additional decrease, but then effects become pronounced under the proper conditions. Finally, at doses of more than 100,000R, a conflicting influence, induced lethargy, appears. This feature may be the forerunner of the obvious knockdown doses of twice or three times the magnitude. Wasps and other insects which normally live only a few weeks may appear more resistant than other organisms because natural death may ensue before a radiation syndrome has a chance to develop fully. This is a particularly significant consideration for holometabolous insects in which the adult somatic tissues are typified by nondividing cells.

Extension of Life Span. Acute dose *Habrobracon* experiments (Figure 14.7) (Sullivan and Grosch, 1953) refocused attention on the neglected discovery by Davey (1919) that irradiated flour beetles may survive their controls. Cork (1957) has since sought and found a favorable chronic dosage for beetle investigations, and other investigators have demonstrated the phenomenon for additional types of insects. However, this provides no evidence for assuming that ionizing radiation can be bene-

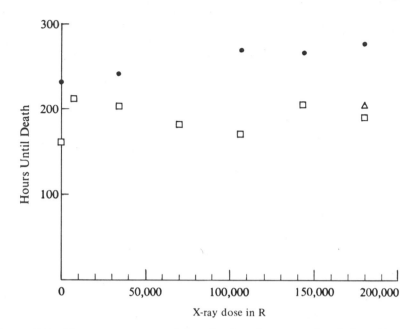

Figure 14.7. The average amount of time elapsing after acute x-irradiation of braconid wasps before death occurs. Circles, females; squares, males; and triangle gives the average for 47 diploid males. (Data of Sullivan and Grosch, 1953).

ficial. Although they were not dead, the irradiated insects were not alert specimens at the peak of their physical ability. Their behavior, as well as that of uncoordinated *Drosophila* observed in other experiments, suggests radiation vulnerability of the insect nervous system.

The acute-dose wasp experiments were run under starvation conditions where radiation-induced lethargy becomes an important factor decreasing the expenditure of energy and the utilization of stored reserves (Grosch, 1956). In the beetle experiments, starvation was not the sole cause of death. Since experimental methods are inadequate for measuring the rate of aging and tissue changes, postulated explanations have been tinged with optimism. The possibility of adaptive organ system response has been suggested along with the hyperstimulation of repair mechanisms which might more than offset the destructive effects of radiation.

A stimulation of renovation processes after mild injury has also been advanced to explain the results of a rat experiment (Carlson *et al.*, 1957). Rats living at 25° and at 5°C received ^{60}Co gamma rays at 0.1 R/hr for 8 hr daily throughout adult life. Irradiated animals at both temperatures had an increased life expectancy, as shown by significant displacement of mortality figures. In the warmer temperature, the lst rat of the irradiated group died at 600 days, in comparison with the last of the controls which died at 460 days.

On the other hand, it has been possible to demonstrate a concrete basis for the better life expectancy of female mice recieving 300 R or less of x rays. Here, the hazards of giving birth to young were reduced due to the poor reproductive performance of irradiated females (Gowen, 1960). Elimination of these hazards outweighted the generally damaging effects of irradiation at lower doses, and life span was extended. In female insects, the doses employed for lifespan extension are adequate for ovarian destruction, and the relation of ovipositional activity to life span is well established. No equivalent change in irradiated males is known, although a modified intensity of the mating urge might have important consequences.

Concluding Remarks

This chapter demonstrates that sickness and death of the organism involve many complex systems. Shielding certain areas or organs may modify the outcome of radiation exposure, and there are tantalizing therapeutic aspects to the almost successful implantation of tissue from unexposed sources. The genetically important nucleic acids and the chromosomes containing them are involved to varying degrees in both early and late effects. Therapeutic approaches by way of DNA systems are only speculative. Enough unknown factors exist to justify continued anxiety about the consequences of adding undue radiation to our environment. This will be the next topic considered.

References

Alexander, P., and Connell, D. I., (1960). Shortening of the life span of mice by irradiation with x rays and treatment with radiomimetic chemicals. *Radiat. Res.* **12**, 38–48.

Andrews, G. A. (1962). Criticality accidents in Vinca, Yugoslavia and Oak Ridge, Tennessee. *J. Am. Med. Assoc.* **179**, 191–197.

Bender, M. A., and Gooch, P. C. (1962). Persistent chromosome aberrations in irradiated human subjects. II. $3\frac{1}{2}$ year investigation. *Radiat. Res.* **16**, 44–53.

Bender, M. A., and Gooch, P. C. (1966). Somatic chromosome aberrations induced by human whole body irradiation: The Recuplex criticality accident. *Radiat. Res.* **29**, 568–582.

Butler, J. A. V. (1956). The action of ionizing radiations on biological materials. *Radiat. Res.* **4**, 20–32.

Carlson, L. D., Scheyer, W. J., and Jackson, B. H. (1957). The combined effects of ionizing radiation and low temperature on the metabolism, longevity and soft tissues of the white rat. *Radiat. Res.* **7,** 190–197.

Casarett, A. P. (1968). Late effects of radiation. In "Radiation Biology," Chapter 12. Prentice-Hall, Englewood Cliffs, New Jersey.

Clark, A. M., Bertrand, H. A., and Smith, R. E. (1963). Life span differences between haploid and diploid males of *Habrobracon serinopae* after exposure as adults to x rays. *Am. Nat.* **97,** 203–208.

Cole, L. J., Haire, H. H., and Alpen, E. L. (1967). Partial shielding of dogs: Effectiveness of small external epicondylar lead cuffs against lethal x-radiation. *Radiat. Res.* **32,** 54–63.

Congdon, C. C. (1971). Bone marrow transplantation. *Science* **171,** 1116–1124.

Cork, J. M. (1957). Gamma radiation and longevity of the flour beetle. *Radiat. Res.* **7,** 551–557.

Cosgrove, G. E. (1971). Reptilian radiobiology. *J. Am. Vet. Med. Assoc.* **159,** 1678–84.

Cronkite, E. P., and Bond, V. P. (1960). Diagnosis of radiation injury and analysis of human lethal dose of radiation. *U.S. Armed Forces Med. J.* **11,** 249–260.

Davey, W. P. (1919). Prolongation of life of *Tribolium* apparently due to small doses of x rays. *J. Exp. Zool.* **28,** 447–458.

Ellinger, F. P. (1955). Newer concepts of radiation sickness and its treatment. *Proc. Rudolf Virchow Med. Soc. City N.Y.* **14,** 9–24.

Finkel, M. P. (1958). Induction of tumors with internally administered isotopes. *Ann. Symp. Fundam. Cancer Res.* **12,** 322–335.

Ford, C. E., Hamerton, J. L., Barnes, D. W. H. and Loutit, J. F. (1956). Cytological identification of radiation chimaeras. *Nature (London)* **177,** 452–454.

Fry, R. J. M., Grahn, D., Griem, M. L., and Rust, J. H., eds. (1970). "Late Effects of Radiation." Taylor & Francis, London.

Furth, J., and Furth, O. B. (1936). Neoplastic diseases produced in mice by general irradiation with x rays. *Am. J. Cancer* **28,** 54–65.

Furth, J., Upton, A. C., Christenberry, K. W., Benedict, W. H., and Moshman, J. (1954). Some late effects in mice of ionizing radiation from an experimental nuclear detonation. *Radiology* **63,** 562–570.

Glasstone, S., ed. (1962). "The Effects of Nuclear Weapons." U.S. Govt. Printing Office, Washington, D.C.

Gowen, J. W. (1960). Lengthening of life span in mice in relation to two deleterious agents. *Am. Inst. Biol. Sci. Publ.* **6,** 188–191.

Grosch, D. S. (1956). Induced lethargy and the radiation control of insects. *J. Econ. Entomol.* **49,** 629–631.

Haley, T. J., and Snider, R. S., eds. (1962). "Response of the Nervous System to Ionizing Radiation." Academic Press, New York.

Hart, J. W., and Carpenter, D. (1971). Toward an integrated theory of aging. *Am. Lab.* **D,** 31–40.

International Atomic Energy Agency (1962). "Effects of Ionizing Radiation on the Nervous System." IAEA, Vienna.

Jacobson, L. O., Marks, E. K., Gaston, E. O., Robson, M., and Zirkle, R. E. (1949a). The role of the spleen in radiation injury. *Proc. Soc. Exp. Biol. Med.* **70,** 740–742.

Jacobson, L. O., Marks, E. K., Gaston, E. O., Robson, M., and Zirkle, R. E. (1949b). The effect of spleen protection on mortality following x irradiation. *J. Lab. Clin. Med.* **34,** 1538–1543.

James, W. T., Peacock, L. J., and Rollins, J. B. (1966). The effect of satiation on the value of the conditioned salivary response. *Acta Biol. Exp. (Warsaw)* **26,** 245–250.

Korner, B. (1959). Antibiotic therapy of endogenous and experimental infections in x irradiated mice. *Prog. Nucl. Energy, Ser. 6* **2**, 265–277.

Künkel, H., Höhne, G., and Maas, H. (1957). Radiobiological investigation on the hibernating Loir *(Glis glis)*. *Adv. Radiobiol.*, pp. 176–179.

Lamb, M. J. (1977). "Biology of Aging." Wiley (Halsted), New York.

Lorenz, E. (1950). Some biologic effects of long continued irradiation. *Am. J. Roentgenol., Radium. Therapy Nucl. Med.* [N.S.] **63**, 176–185.

Maisin, J., Dunjic, A., Maldaque, P., and Maisin, H. (1958). Delayed effects in rats subjected to a single dose of x rays. *Int. Conf. Peaceful Uses Atom. Energy 2nd,* **22**, 57–64.

Miller, D. S. (1962). Audiogenic convulsive seizures in mice. *In* "Response of the Nervous System to Ionizing Radiation" (T. J. Haley and R. S. Snider, eds.), pp. 513–531. Academic Press, New York.

Miquel, J., Bensch, K. G., Philpott, D. E., and Atlan, H. (1972). Natural aging and radiation-induced life shortening in *Drosophila melanogaster*. *Mech. Ageing Dev.* **1**, 71–97.

Mole, R. H. (1957). Shortening of life by chronic irradiation: The experimental facts. *Nature (London)* **180**, 456–460.

Riley, A. L., and Baril, L. L. (1976). Conditional taste aversions, a bibliography. *Anim. Learn. Behav.* **4**, Suppl., 1S-13S.

Rosen, D., and Dawson, K. D. (1960). Search for immediate effects of x radiation on frog nerve–muscle preparations. *Radiat. Res.* **12**, 357–370.

Rossi, H. H., and Kelleher, A. M. (1972). Radiation carcinogenesis at low doses. *Science* **175**, 200–202.

Saenger, E. L., ed. (1973). Medical Aspects of Radiation Accidents," Handbook. U.S. At. Energy Comm., Washington, D.C.

Schmidt, J. P. (1967). Response of hibernating mammals to physical, parasitic, and infectious agents. *Mamm. Hibernation 3, Proc. Int. Symp., 1965* pp. 421–438.

Selye, H. (1973). The evolution of the stress concept. *Am. Sci.* **61**, 692–699.

Strehler, B. L. (1962). "Time, Cells and Aging." Academic Press, New York.

Sullivan, R. L., and Grosch, D. S. (1953). The radiation tolerance of an adult wasp. *Nucleonics* **11**(3), 21–23.

Upton, A. C. (1957). Ionizing radiation and the aging process. *J. Gerontol.* **12**, 306–313.

Van Cleave, C. D. (1963). "Irradiation and the Nervous System." Rowman and Littlefield, New York.

Walburg, H. E., Jr. (1975). Radiation-induced life-shortening and premature aging. *Adv. Radiat. Biol.* **5**, 145–179.

Wilson, B. R. (1963). Survival studies of whole body x irradiated germ free (axenic) mice. *Radiat. Res.* **20**, 477–483.

Zeman, W. (1961). Radiosensitivities of nervous tissues. *Brookhaven Symp. Biol.* **14**, 176–199.

PART V

ECOLOGY: PURE AND APPLIED

The earlier sections of this book contain accounts of investigations that stretch back to the discovery of ionizing radiations. Early research appraised induced pathologies in individual organisms and their offspring. Only in recent decades has attention shifted from individuals to populations, and finally to the interrelated populations of different species in the natural environment.

Each living organism has become adapted to survive in some particular kind of environment and has developed relationships with other living organisms in its immediate vicinity. We shall now consider how radiations may disrupt such ecological systems. Disruption may be undesirable if it interferes with our health and welfare. On the other hand, selective damage may be desirable if food supplies are improved or if pests and parasites are destroyed. In the following chapters, each of these main interests is discussed.

The emphasis here will be on alterations from damaging exposures. Detailed quantitative treatment of the passage of isotope-labeled compounds through food chains and webs is beyond the scope of this book.

CHAPTER 15   Radiation Effects on Life in Contaminated Areas

We, as well as all other living organisms, are constantly exposed to small amounts of radiation. This is inescapable. From their prehistoric beginnings, through geological periods of time, living organisms have been irradiated. Much of the radiation from the sun is necessary so life can continue. Some natural radiation is unnecessary and may be potentially harmful. Included in this category are cosmic rays, body burdens of ^{14}C and ^{40}K, and the gamma radiation from earth, rock, and the structural materials of our buildings (Eisenbud, 1973). From time immemorial these have been part of the natural environment, and presumably adaptation to their influences has occurred. Figure 15.1 (Folsom and Harley, 1957) demonstrates that the variation in natural dosage is large, depending upon the habitat. Any radiation dose which is small in comparison with the background may be of trivial biological importance and may be accepted as part of the normal hazard of living. On the other hand, we wish to avoid environmental contamination which might alter the natural balance of plant and animal life (Table 15.1).

In this matter our attention must be directed to naturally aggregated groups of populations. Such investigations have had their beginnings in studies of a selected few plant communities: mixed oak–pine forest, granite outcrops and hardwood stands, old fields, shortgrass plains, and a tropical rain forest. A plant community is an assembly of plant species occupying a given area of landscape, the members of which share many features of the microenvironment. The presence of the plant assemblage has resulted through natural plant succession. In association are the animal types adapted to the plant community. A convenience for organizing diverse information is the concept of trophic level, which indicates how far a species is removed from feeding upon the primary producers. In order, the trophic levels are (1) the producers, the green plants; (2) plant eaters; (3) carnivores which eat herbivores; and (4) secondary carnivores. In addition to these four niches which make up food webs or chains, an ecosystem also may include scaven-

279

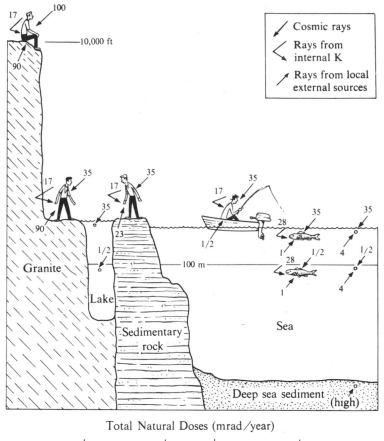

Total Natural Doses (mrad/year)

Man over Granite		Man over sedimentary rock	Man over sea	Large fish in sea		Microorganism in sea	
10,000 ft	m.s.l.			at surf	100 m	at surf	100 m
207	142	75	52	64	30	39	5

Figure 15.1. Variation in natural doses of radiation. (After Folsom and Harley, 1957; courtesy of the authors.)

gers which feed on dead organic matter, decomposers, transformers, and parasites. Let us consider them in order.

First Trophic Level: Lower Plants

Studies on the suspended microbiota of bodies of water in areas near atomic energy installations should reveal the effects both of radiation from external sources and from incorporated radioisotopes. Lackey's

1957 report on the Clinch River and adjacent Tennessee waters contained the interesting observation that seepage pits were continuously green with algae in spite of radiation as high as 400 mR/hr. Along the same lines are occasional reports of profuse bacterial growth in the water of a reactor (Anellis, 1961). In other words, aquatic microscopic biota persist and even thrive in a highly radioactive environment.

In radiation-denuded areas of shortgrass plains, the soil microflora, actinomycetes and fungi, persisted through three years of continuous irradiation, although they were not as numerous as in control plots. Some bacteria flourished, reaching densities in excess of the populations present in control areas (Fraley and Wicker, 1973a,b).

Regardless of high or low background radiation, microorganisms accumulate radioactive substances in a nonvolatile state, suggesting the use of algae and other forms as decontaminating agents. Modern texts on sewage disposal recommend the removal of radioisotopes by "slimes." In the Clinch River, algae with a concentration factor as high as 10,000 times greater than water were found. Experiments to determine the most effective means of removing ^{32}P from Columbia River water at Hanford, Washington, employed algae which concentrated the isotope to 300,000 times that of the water concentration.

The accumulation of radioactivity by an organism depends upon the biochemical processes by which an organism selects or discriminates against the various elements available for assimilation and incorporation. Each organism requires a particular combination of elements for growth and development; however, in nature the elements usually occur in proportions different from those found within the organism. Uptake may be direct or through a food chain, and elements may be either concentrated or diluted during the course of events. The experimental culture of algae in the presence of a variety of radioisotopes demonstrates clearly that the efficiency in concentration of a particular element depends upon the species of algae. Such diverse chemical behavior has been found among plankton, that the safest generalization seems to be that for any given chemical element there will eventually be found at least one plankton species capable of concentrating it spectacularly (Boroughs et al., 1957).

The fate of nuclides taken up by plankton depends upon whether they pass into the food chain or, upon decay, form sediment. Water of the Clinch River showed no detectable radioactivity within a short distance below Oak Ridge. In contrast, the Columbia River has been reported to retain radioisotopes even until its mouth 362 miles below Hanford (Perkins and Nielson, 1960). The difference appears to be in the efficiency of trapping by organisms and silt.

No malformations or abnormal types have been detected. If muta-

TABLE 15.1

Radiation Released to Our Natural Environment[a]

Source	Kinds of radiation	Duration of exposure	Dose to environment	Secondary activity induced	Heat and blast effects	Total area involved	Significant direct effects	Incorporated in natural cycles
Natural (background) radiation	Alpha Beta Gamma	Several billion years	0.1–0.5 R per year	No	No	The earth	No	Yes
Medical and occupational		Not normally delivered to man's environment						
Gamma Fields up to 4,000 Ci ^{60}Co	Gamma	Chronic, several years	Up to several thousand R per hour	No	No	Thousands of acres	Yes	No
Shielded reactor	Mixed gamma-neutron	Intermittent	Up to several times background	Negligible	No	Acres	No	Negligible
Unshielded reactor	Mixed gamma-neutron	Intermittent	Up to 100,000 rads per hour	Yes	No	Hundreds of acres	Yes	Negligible
Reactor effluents	Alpha Beta Gamma	Continuous	Above background	No	No	Hundreds of square miles	No	Yes
Waste disposal	Alpha Beta Gamma	Continuous	Slightly above background	No	No	Hundreds of acres	No	Potentially
Accidental explosions	Alpha Beta Gamma	Acute	Up to several thousand rads/hour	No	Yes	Acres	Yes	No
Nuclear detonations (220 announced to date)	Alpha Beta Gamma	Acute	Up to several billion rads/hour	Yes	Yes	Hundreds of square miles	Yes	No

282

Fallout from above two sources	Alpha Beta Gamma	Chronic, thousands of years	Up to several times background	No	The earth	No	Yes
Thermonuclear war (projected)	Alpha Beta Gamma	Acute	Up to hundreds of millions of rads/hour	Yes	Thousands of square miles	Yes	No
Fallout from thermonuclear war (projected)	Alpha Beta Gamma	Chronic, thousands of years	Up to several rads/hour	No	The earth	Yes	Yes

[a] From Platt, 1963, by permission of Van Nostrand-Reinhold, Princeton, New Jersey.

tions have been induced they were either missed in the sampling, or the growth of biota was sufficient to make up for individuals lost through the expression of lethals. A study of marine algae a year after the Bikini tests resulted in similar conclusions. Blinks (1952) could detect no injurious genetic effects. Furthermore, although various physiological activities were studied, no significant alterations were detectable except an *increase* in catalase activity ascribable to enzymatic adaptation to an increase of H_2O_2 in the environment. Some algae were radioactive, others were not. Nevertheless there was appreciable external radiation absorbed by all algae as shown by the significant increase in counts per unit time when an algal mass was stripped from a rock surface. Subsequent comprehensive studies of the algae of the Pacific proving ground have not revealed anomalous individuals.

Less attention has been given to mosses and lichens, although their radiotolerance has been established. Diffuse "meristems" and small chromosomes in both fungal and algal components confer on lichens the ability to survive in irradiated zones where all vascular plants have been killed. In the Enterprise, Wisconsin, forest (Zavitkovski, 1977), *Parmelia sulcata* withstood up to 100 krad, and above this level damage was not manifested until the spring of the year following irradiation. Furthermore, no evidence of damage appeared in tests with several other species until environmental conditions made demands upon them for growth.

Forest moss and liverworts have a range of tolerance between the lichens and vascular plants. The radiotolerance of mat or cushionlike growths is fortunate because their greater surface area per unit of dry weight results in more radioactivity accumulated from fallout than that of most higher plants (Gorham, 1959). Both the alpine and the arctic tundra lichens collect and retain radioisotopes in impressive amounts.

First Trophic Level: Higher Plants

Although algae and bacteria include some of the most radioresistant plants, higher plants are more sensitive. Coniferous gymnosperms have proved to be at least as sensitive as mammals to radiation damage. Dicot angiosperms are more resistant and monocots most resistant. On this basis we expect moderate exposure to eliminate coniferous forests, or at least to make them more sensitive to disease. Deciduous forests would show less damage. In complex systems, by reducing the diversity of species, radiation would simplify the ecosystem and alter the time course of succession, but homogeneous stands of herbs, grasses, and important food grains might give only subtle evidence of radiation exposure.

Near the Nevada test sites, bunch grass survived in areas where trees and shrubs were destroyed (Rickard and Shields, 1963). However, these observations were difficult to interpret because of the heat and shock accompanying atomic detonations (Shields and Wells, 1962). More instructive were Cowan and Platt's (1963) studies of an isolated natural environment containing an intentionally unshielded reactor, and Woodwell's (1962) observations on the area around a Brookhaven-type gamma source installed in a forest ecosystem. In these situations, the radiation is entirely free of heat and blast. The growth of pine trees was inhibited by as little as 2 R/day, in contrast to such grasslike herbs as the sedges, which withstood up to 350 R/day from the ^{60}Co source. Within 1000 feet of the unshielded reactor, all pine trees were killed during the first year, the cumulative dose reaching 4000 R. At greater distances their growth was aberrant. The leaves of herbs and hardwoods fell one to three weeks earlier than in control stands, and this zone extended for several hundred feet beyond the dead pine trees. In the spring, the same trees comprised a leafless island 3000 feet across in a forest which had already achieved full leaf, although beyond 700 feet most leafing-out lagged by only about one month. In general, the period of dormancy proved proportionate to radiation dose. Thus with an earlier fall and prolonged dormancy, the net result was a shortened growing period.

Within 700–800 feet, the terminal buds of woody vegetation were killed. Therefore trees and shrubs had to depend upon the adventitious buds on wood several years old. In time, these growing tips are killed and ultimately plant starvation and death results for oaks, hickory, and similar trees.

In several studies, the herbacious vegetation of old fields proved to be 5 to 10 times as resistant as temperate forests which are comprised predominantly of vascular species. Differential sensitivity to radiation was also apparent in the shifts in predominant plant types of abandoned fields near the reactor. Furthermore, shortened growing periods were seen for annuals which accumulated 10,000 R or more. They completed their life cycles up to a month earlier than usual.

Barring scatter or deflection effects, woody vegetation and irregular terrain have shielding ability. Vegetation below the brow of a hill or behind a substantial man-made structure will not experience the same dosage nor show the damage of plants directly in a line-of-sight to the reactor (Figure 15.2). Vines and adventitious buds of stems on the far side of tree trunks more than a foot in diameter have not shown the same damage as more exposed structures. These considerations, of course, apply to radiations from an external source.

Line of sight

Shielding effects from terrain

Unshielded reactor → 1000 ft — 1300 ft → 2000 ft → 3000 ft

Effects of Distance ⟩ Differences in resistance of types of trees   Terrain permitting mixed gamma-neutron field extends 3000 feet

Generalized Scheme for Field Studies

Air Dose in Rads 15-90 Days	Developmental Stages								
	Herb			Shrub			Tree		
	Year of Development								
	Year abandoned	1st	2nd	3rd	4th	5th	7th-12th	12th-50th	Oak Hickory Pine
							Pine domination		Climax
0-1,000	Minor effects			Some damage to pine					
1,000-3,000									
3,000-6,000				Pine seedlings killed			Pine killed; hardwoods released; succession accelerated		Pine killed
6,000-10,000									
10,000-20,000	Shift in dominance			Hardwood seedlings killed			Hardwoods killed; reversion by sprouts to hardwood seedling stage		
20,000-50,000									
50,000-100,000				Reversion to earlier herb stage			All trees killed; reversion to herb stage		
100,000-300,000									
300,000 and over	Mixture from well shielded seeds, corms, etc.								

Figure 15.2. Ecological effects. Top: Effects on vegetation of an unshielded reactor placed in a wooded natural area. Bottom: A summary of Emory University studies of short-term radiation exposure of temperate ecosystems in north Georgia and the Upper Piedmont Plateau. Doses are plotted against developmental stages from abandoned agricultural fields to climax forests. (Data by courtesy of R. B. Platt.)

More recently, results were published for cesium source exposures of a shortgrass plain community in Colorado (Fraley and Wicker, 1973a,b), and the El Verde rain forest in Eastern Puerto Rico (Odum, 1970). In the former, a 3-year continuous irradiation from 8750 Ci ^{137}Cs lowered the density of several shrubs and demonstrated that the most resistant species were among the herbaceous plants. After 2 years of intensive preirradiation studies, the El Verde site was irradiated for only 92 days by a 10,000 Ci ^{137}Cs source, and rocks, ravines, and trees provided protected habitats. Nevertheless, in the first year after exposure an area of bare ground appeared, along with a fall of green and yellow leaves out to 25 m from the source. The leaf fall continued for 2 years, by which time a carpet of regenerative growth had covered the denuded area. Still, palms were dying at 30 m, the 5 kR perimeter. In general however, the tropical rain forest was not more sensitive than temperate forests, and it recovered faster. Most striking was a simplification of the community following radiation damage. In addition, there was an increase in crownless plants and alterations in crown shape.

For the quantitative evaluation of differences in communities, ecologists have devised composition indices, calculated vegetation density, evaluated species diversity, and measured productivity (Wicker and Fraley, 1974). The same approaches can reveal changes induced in an area if it is studied periodically after irradiation. Although the threshold dose to reduce the coefficient of community composition to 50% of the original differs according to the community irradiated, above this the decline is linear when plotted against the log of exposure rate. Species composition progressively becomes dissimilar to that of the original community with increases in time and radiation intensity. This results from the differential mortality of species and shifts in their numerical importance. The trend may be toward ecosystem instability if diversity is required for needed potential to adjust to stress and change.

Productivity is the rate at which organic material is created per unit area. Net primary productivity is defined as the amount available for consumption by herbivores after that utilized for plant respiration has been subtracted. Ionizing radiation can alter productivity, but not necessarily as a simple overall decrease. Poor performance by radiosensitive species may be offset by growth of more resistant types. Furthermore, the actual harvest by man or herbivore is selective. Despite luxuriant foliage, a garden or pasture taken over by pest species or impalatable weeds is a deleterious change.

Indices which depict trends but do not serve as absolute measures of productivity include biomass, percent of ground covered, leaf size and number, and plant height. Changes in some of these have been presented in Chapter 9. Woodwell (1962) and staff obtained the patterns of decreased biomass along the chronic gamma radiation gradient in fields as well as in pine–oak forests. At one isodose contour (1 kR/day), vegetative biomass increased due to the growth of *Digitaria*, a radioresistant annual characteristic of recently disturbed areas. Above this level, biomass dropped sharply. At a similar dose level, biomass production increased for the logging roads of the Enterprise, Wisconsin, forest (Zavitkovski, 1977). Fraley and Wicker (1973a,b) obtained a straightforward pattern from the chronic irradiation of Colorado grasslands, but considerable fluctuations resulted from short seasonal exposures. The invasion by broad leafed weeds was a problem, but revegetation of desirable grass also contributed to a variable pattern. In the El Verde tropical forest, the opening created by irradiation promoted the growth of plants benefiting from increased light intensity and temperature, but the situation was of short duration. Recovery began with an explosive growth of seeds, fast shoot regeneration from shielded root systems, and lateral growth from individuals on the periphery. Results in the control experiment were consistent with the response of vegetation on Bikini. In less than 10 years, vegetation became so dense that investigators had to hack their way inland from the beach. Despite die-back, defoliation, and tree death, on Rongelap and Rongerik atolls extensive clearing was necessary before resettlement.

A general pattern emerging from exposures to radiation in experimental forests indicates that biomass studies (Table 15.2) reveal a similar order of radiosensitivity for plant types as that obtained from studies scored by direct observations of the plants in the stand. The slightly higher doses tabulated for biomass depression result from analyzing the Enterprise data by 10-m zones. Indeed, when crown growth of individual trees was taken as the end point, dose ranges for recognizable damage were identical to those obtained in other studies.

Incorporated Radioisotopes. In a contaminated area, the vegetation becomes radioactive and internal sources contribute to the dosage. In the Marshall Islands, within 6 weeks, the sap of coconut trees reached a level of 1 μCi/liter due to the uptake of fission products. After longer periods of time, appreciable levels of radioactivity were attained by edible portions of plants. In Oak Ridge, Tennessee, plants of the X-9 area such as cattail, wild lettuce, and curly dock are many times more radioactive than the water in which they grow. Also in Oak Ridge, plants have taken up radioisotopes in their invasion of the drained basin of White Oak Lake, a unique, heavily contaminated study area

TABLE 15.2

Radiosensitivity of Plant Components of Terrestrial Ecosystems after 3 Months[a]

Northern forest of Enterprise, Wisconsin	Exposure (in kR) to produce depression of biomass production (%)			Other studies	Exposure (in kR) to produce growth inhibition and lethality		
	10–25	25–50	35–60		Minor	Intermediate	Severe
Deciduous trees	5–10	10–35	35–60	Coniferous trees	0.1–1	1–2	2–10
				Deciduous trees	1–5	5–10	10–15
				Tropical rain forest	4–8	8–10	10–15
Shrubs	3–5	5–20	20–60	Shrubs	1–5	5–20	20–60
Herbacious							
Under forest	20–40	40–60	60–160	Herbaceous rock outcrop	8–10	10–40	40
Logging road	40–60	60–160	160–200	Old field annuals	3–10	10–100	100
				Grassland	8–10	10–100	100–200
Lichen	60–100	100–200	200 +	Moss and lichen	10–50	50–500	500–?

[a] Based on Zavitkovski, 1977.

289

(Auerbach, 1957). Nevertheless, within five years succession gave rise to a profuse growth of complex woody vegetation. Subsequently the distribution of some of the major elements in plants and soil has not changed in over 30 years.

Agricultural experiments in the White Oak Lake bed using three species of forage crops—millet, sudan grass, and fodder cane (sorghum)—revealed an influence of accumulated nuclides and yield. Millet, the crop with the highest concentration, had the lowest yield. This is a deleterious effect expected by radiobiologists but contrary to certain traditions. Since the discovery of radioactivity, claims have been made that plant growth is stimulated by radioactive substances. Although the idea is persistent, it gains no support from careful field plot experiments carried out by the U.S. Department of Agriculture with a representative variety of crops in a number of states (Alexander, 1950). Radium, uranium, and a commercial product were used with a dolomite carrier as three separate treatments providing the same number of alpha particles per unit area as 300 μg of radium.

In the state of Washington, a comprehensive study has been perpetuated on the trace amounts of radioisotopes present in farm produce irrigated by the Columbia River. From our standpoint, perhaps the most significant result is the demonstration that direct foliar absorption from sprinkler-irrigated crops plays an important role in the uptake of many isotopes. In established forests, the root mass and its shared mycorrhyzal fungi contribute to the movement of nuclides. Radioisotopes introduced into the stumps of red maples were found in the leaves of 19 other woody species up to 24 ft from the donors.

Second Trophic Level: The Primary Consumers

Field studies using a fixed gamma source are not as feasible for animals as they are for plant communities. The decline in exposure with distance is too sharp, and mobile animals do not remain in concentric patterns around the irradiator. Much of the research above the first trophic level has been concerned with radioisotope accumulations and transfers through the food web. Because trace amounts of isotopes are usually involved, there are few instances of obvious damage.

Second Trophic Level: Water Animals

Before White Oak Lake was drained, the region of highest contamination had only half as many genera as related uncontaminated regions

(Krumholz, 1956). Unfortunately, heavy sedimentation as well as radiation contributed to this unproductive situation. Among the littoral and sublittoral bottom fauna, which were mostly worms and aquatic insect larvae, concentration factors above 100,000 were noted, but no obvious morphological consequences were detected. A unique opportunity for studying chromosomal damage was provided by the *Chironomus* larvae which live in the radioactive sediments of the creek which drains the waste disposal area and most of the experimental locations in the Oak Ridge reservation. By the time Blaylock (1965) made a definitive survey, the chironomid populations had been exposed for over 20 years of radioactive wastes. The average dose of radiation at 230 rad/year was about 1000 times background. Nevertheless, no quantitative difference in chromosomal polymorphism was demonstrable. The chromosome aberrations from irradiated populations amounted to 53.1%, as compared to 55.0% in controls. Against a background of endemic inversions, qualitative differences appeared as nine unique inversions observed once, and one new inversion noted five times in the irradiated populations. One was a rare pericentric example. Periodic collections demonstrated that chromosomal types disappear from both control and irradiated populations. Conceivably, most of the new aberrations which arose through the years were eliminated rapidly by selection or genetic drift.

A difference between marine and terrestrial food chains is the small range in size of the herbivores. The planktonic euphasids and salps filter large volumes of water while feeding. Because of their size, they reach equilibrium quickly and can serve as biological monitors of the environmental radiation. Among larger animals, crustacea such as brine shrimp, true shrimp, and crabs, and molluscs such as oysters, clams, and scallops can accumulate radiostrontium from sea water, but when radioactive algae were supplied, accumulation was much more rapid and impressive. This emphasizes the sequential interrelationships of trophic levels.

Although shellfish can accumulate alkaline earths in their shells, the long-lived isotopes of greatest public concern are found only in low amounts in marine organisms studied under field conditions. The radioactive forms of Mn, Fe, Co, and Zn account for almost all the radioactivity found in marine organisms. This pattern, first noted at Bikini, was confirmed at Eniwetok, and extended by repeated ocean surveys. However, any release of radioactive products sets up a biological reaction peculiar to the place, season, and condition of the release itself (Templeton *et al.*, 1970). The variables are manifold and the situation can be assessed only by a comprehensive on-site ecological study.

The *Tilapia* is among the few fish which can be considered in the second trophic level; it is predominantly an herbivore. When fed ^{89}Sr, the order in which radioactivity developed in the organ systems was skeleton, integument, gills, muscle, and visceral organs; this order is also demonstrable for pelagic fish of higher trophic levels (Boroughs *et al.*, 1956, 1957). From the human viewpoint, this is encouraging because the structures of highest radioactivity are not used for food. Incidentally, small sluggish fish excrete isotopes much more slowly than do pelagic fish. Also, water is involved to some extent in radioisotope uptake by marine fish since they swallow water continually.

Here we cannot detail the overwhelming volume of research on radioisotope distribution in aquatic organisms. This was impressively demonstrated by Polikarpov (1966), who reviewed both the Slavic and English publications. His book on radioecology contains 190 pages on the migration and accumulation of the various elements, but only 17 pages on radiation injury. Even this chapter on damaging exposures relied heavily on acute lethal dose determinations delivered from outside the organism. Another dozen pages surveyed the evidence for the radiosensitivity of embryos.

Ten years later, the 1976 summary of International Atomic Energy Agency (IAEA) panel meetings of Effects of Ionizing Radiation on Aquatic Organisms and Ecosystems reported a similar predicament. That is a tremendous gap between the sizable acute doses used in experiments, and the small chronic doses that aquatic organisms can receive in nature. The natural background of the marine environment contributes less than 40 μrad/hr. Even in the vicinity of radioactive waste discharges, the maximum dose is only 25 mrad/hr. No deleterious effects on populations are expected at these levels. The 1976 report from the IAEA panel cites nearly 400 papers which contain recent studies on a variety of aquatic organisms. Those which deal with teratogenesis or lethality usually concern the effect of hundreds or thousands of rads delivered at high dose rates. With this qualification, the most sensitive aquatic organisms proved to be salmonid teleost fish, especially the embryos and young fry.

At Bikini, more than 1000 species of organisms were exposed, but 1 year later a careful search by competent specialists from all of the biological disciplines turned up no evidence of aberrant forms. Tens of thousands of specimens were examined. Even the sea urchins from the most heavily irradiated portion of the reef were reproducing normally (Hines, 1962). Numerous worms and sea cucumbers were burrowing into and ingesting the highly radioactive bottom mud. Presumably, high reproductive potentials enabled the organisms to pay the price of selection against disadvantaged genotypes in the population. The destruction in a large atoll like Bikini amounts to only a small proportion of the total animal life. An increased utilization of reproductive capacity can maintain a population at preirradiation density (Templeton *et al.*, 1970).

Second Trophic Level: Land Animals

In the Oak Ridge National Laboratory (ORNL) reserve, muskrats and woodchucks became more radioactive than raccoons and squirrels, presumably because of living and dietary habits (Bustad, 1960). A muskrat's diet features the stems and roots of aquatic vegetation. One specimen, reported by Oak Ridge plant guards of the X-10 area, had a useless rear leg and carried more than 1 μCi of ^{90}Sr per gram of bone. The difficulty proved to be an advanced osteogenic sarcoma which had developed at the proximal end of the tibiofibula with metastasis to both kidneys and lungs. Although captured at the height of the breeding season, the female was not gravid (Krumholz and Rust, 1954).

Subsequently, the radioisotope burdens in muskrats from the ORNL have been followed carefully. The high concentration of ^{137}Cs in muscle may be the aspect of most concern to humans, since this is the tissue used for food. Indeed, calculations have indicated that if a person had based one meal per week upon muskrat dispersed from the setting basin, he would have exceeded the permissible dose rate before the end of the second meal. Obviously we need to determine the extent of movements of radioactive animals from controlled areas to uncontrolled areas.

In general, small mammal succession on the drained White Oak Lake bed was similar to plant succession in that more species and greater total populations were present in later years than in the first year. Over a period of years the cotton rat established itself as the dominant species. Except for one individual with a white nose, no freaks were noticed. The incidence of external injuries did not differ significantly from that in a nonradioactive old-field study area. The only differences demonstrable between populations were associated with reproduction. Notable was the fact that in the late fall there was a lack of pregnant females and of males with descended testes. Also, the average litter size in the lake bed was 5.4 as compared with 7.7 in the old field (Dunaway and Kaye, 1963). However, follow-up surveys disclosed fluctuations in weather conditions severe enough to decimate populations every few years and obscure distinctions based on reproductive performance. Subsequently, a search for pathological conditions in cotton rats and two other rodent species was unsuccessful. No significant differences attributable to radiation were seen in organ weights, microscopic necropsy, erythrocyte volumes, differential leukocyte counts or incidence of parasitic infection. Early deaths from natural causes seem to nullify opportunity to observe the late effects of chronic irradiation demonstrated in laboratory colonies.

As an approach to larger fauna, biologists at the Hanford laboratories selected jack rabbits for study because their food habits are similar to those of the large range animals (Hanson, 1960). In their tissues, concentrations of mixed fission products were relatively stable, presumably because equilibrium with the daily intake had been attained. Feces and bone showed similar concentrations while liver was consistently lower. When increases to higher plateaus occur, they are due to rainout of bomb test debris. An immediate change becomes apparent in feces. However, no visible changes occur in the liver for 30 days or in the bone for 60 days. An especially sensitive index of radioactive debris is supplied by ^{131}I in the thyroid, provided that the seasonal and developmental pattern of iodine concentration has been established. A tenfold increase in ^{131}I concentration with little station-to-station variation occurred in rabbit thyroids after one series of distant tests of nuclear devices. Sheep, cattle, and other herbivores appear to react similarly.

Perhaps the only long-term study of a community exposed to significant local fallout has been that made on Rongelap Island. Pigs and chickens sacrificed at various times following the incident confirmed ingestion to be the more important route of entry. The body burden of tissue products was roughly proportional to the gamma dose rate on each island of the Marshall group. Ninety-nine percent of the internal activity was associated with the skeleton, especially with the growing ends of the bones. However, no pathological changes ascribable to radiation were detected in the 66 domestic animals collected up to two months after the start of fallout. Rats that lived two years on the island also yielded negative pathological results. Late effects on humans are discussed below.

Although terrestrial invertebrates play an important role in biological cycles, they have not received commensurate attention in radiation ecology. Fortunately, their habitat often contributes to invertebrate radiotolerance. The cotton rats of the White Oak Lake bed received only about 2.9 rad/week. Jar populations of Collembola became infecund only after 5 rad/hr in sand coated with $^{90}Sr-^{90}Y$. ^{60}Co gamma doses in excess of 10 krads were required to alter the populations of mixed woodland soils containing earthworms, myriapods, mites, and insects.

Decreases were observed by following the populations for several months. Sometimes when predators were more radiosensitive than their prey, the latter responded by increasing their numbers. In the absence of bone for the deposit of alkaline earths, the persistence of radioisotopes depends on the makeup of other tissues, especially on the binding of metallic cations by tissue proteins.

In radiation areas, damage to the insects themselves may not be the only influence on their frequency. Induced changes in food quality or abundance, or destruction of the vegetation needed for cover or habitat, contribute to fluctuations in insect populations. After the trees of the Brookhaven forest died, there was a significant increase of invading insects subsisting on dead wood and associated fungi.

Omnivores: Birds, Lizards, and Crabs

Some organisms ingest such a variety of foods that they participate in the food chain at several trophic levels. Birds are in this category. Furthermore, their seed–fruit–insect diet is so analogous to the grain–fruit–meat diet of man that investigations of the uptake of radionuclides of passerine birds provide information at a trophic level of direct interest to man.

Birds frequenting the White Oak Lake basin reached ^{90}Sr levels higher than we would want to risk in man (Willard, 1960). A variety of opinions exist on the maximum permissible concentration in man, but the average value of 172 pCi/gm of bird bone is well up in the range of 25–250 pCi/gm expressed for humans. The maximum found in these birds, 1487 pCi/gm of bone, is greatly in excess of any concentration deemed permissible for humans, although at present we do not know whether these levels are harmful for birds. Nesting birds were found in Nevada test sites after nuclear detonations (Rickard, 1961).

The appreciable difference between average and maximum values for strontium also occurs with ^{137}Cs and other isotopes. Differences in diet and habit are involved. Birds which keep to the tops of shrubs, feeding on berries, or remain high in the trees, feeding on insects, exhibit only a tenth or less of the tissue radioactivity of birds feeding near or on the ground. The greatest intake results when birds probe into the mud for seeds and ingest contaminated soil as well as radioactive seeds. The seasonal availability of food plays an important role in this regard.

As indicated in earlier chapters, reproductive effectiveness is more critical for the survival of irradiated populations than somatic attributes or longevity. Further evidence is afforded in fenced rodent and lizard

populations in southern Nevada, where the largest ^{137}Cs source without
a cooling requirement (33,000 Ci) provided continuous exposure
(Turner, 1975). Within the enclosure, the tissue dose ranged from 1 to 5
rad/day. Five years after the experiment started, mature female
Crotophytus lizards ceased display of the coloration typical of the breeding season. In the next population census, no yearling lizards appeared.
Autopsies of a few females revealed the absence of ovaries accompanied
by hypertrophied fat body.

Female sterility appeared in three other lizard species in the irradiated area, but no comparable condition has occurred in control
areas. The species which take longer to mature and produce fewer eggs
in the single clutch per season drifted to extinction in the test plots. *Uta*
lizards have survived, presumably because they begin reproducing
when only 8 to 9 months old, which is before they accumulate a sterilizing dose. Second, third, and fourth year classes do not play an important role in *Uta* population maintenance. The majority of the *Uta* population is replaced annually.

On Eniwetok Atoll, the 50 land crabs populating Belle Island survived
despite tests which repeatedly destroyed vegetation and left a litter of
dead birds and fish. Quick withdrawal into the shell and a tendency to
hide under debris decreased their exposure to radiation. As omnivo-
rous scavengers, they subsisted on washed up detritus. Reproductive
performance was not studied. Tissue samples showed a rate of decline
in radioactivity approximating the decay of mixed fission products
during the first 150 days. Later, ^{137}Cs and ^{90}Sr accounted for more than
80% of the total radioactivity of crabs, although these two isotopes
comprised only 35% of the island's activity. On Rongelap, concentrations of ^{90}Sr remained high in the coconut crabs even after 15 years.
In fact, the 700 pCi/gm Ca in the flesh of these crabs is identical with the
average value for ^{90}Sr in Oak Ridge birds of the disposal area.

Omnivores: Humans

Only in the Marshall islands has there been an adequate opportunity
to study the consequences of fallout on humans. Many inhabitants ate
surface-contaminated food and drank water from open containers in the
two day period before evacuation. The conglomerate of ingested
isotopes delivered 3 mCi to the average digestive tract; this dose proved
too low for acute effects. At first ^{131}I and ^{140}Ba made major contributions
to the dose but they have short half-lives. The body burden of radioac-

tive material decreased rapidly in a few months. After two years, radiochemical analysis of urine showed only slight activity due to ^{144}Ce–^{144}Pr and ^{90}Sr. The estimation that body burdens were well below permissible levels was borne out by determinations on ashed tissue from a man who had died of heart disease (not due to radiation damage). Even his bones proved to be within the range of ^{90}Sr content typical of American bone. By the time 3 years had elapsed, other sources of fallout were contributing more to the body burden of Marshallese than the original exposure.

After 3½ years of optimum nutrition and medical care on Kwajalein, the Rongelap natives were returned to their island. A summary published 15 years after the incident recounts their temporary early responses and the appearance of late effects (Conard et al., 1970b). The skin burns of the first weeks left some residual scarring and pigmentation but no evidence of malignancy. Changes detected by precursor and peripheral blood studies disappeared within a decade. Most remarkable was a delayed high incidence of thyroid pathomorphism including benign nodules, cancers, and atrophy. An associated problem was the growth retardation in exposed children (Conard et al., 1970a). Lenticular imperfections, biochemical suggestions of accelerated aging, have emerged in later years. One case of acute myelogenous leukemia was identified 18 years after exposure.

In contrast, during their return to Japan the 23 fishermen of the contaminated Fukuryu Maru lived for 13 days under crude conditions in intimate contact with the most radioactive environment man has yet survived. The one early fatality appeared to be due to hepatitis of undetermined origin. Normally in developed countries, food, water, and medical attention are carefully supervised, but in times of catastrophic emergency, primitive conditions are likely to occur. In addition, blast, heat, and fire damage complicate interpretations of the sequellae from nuclear explosions to persons near the site.

Third Trophic Level

With the exception of fish, carnivores of the higher trophic levels are not used for food by civilized man. Nearly a dozen species of marine fish have been used for studying the uptake, concentration, and loss of common radionuclides. Fast swimmers excrete ingested ^{89}Sr relatively rapidly, retaining injected ^{89}Sr somewhat longer. In either case, soft visceral tissues lose alkaline earth elements soon, whereas bony structures, gills, and integument retain it for long periods. Muscle is inter-mediate. In contrast, cesium accumulation is typical of muscle, brain, and the gonads, but not of bone (Boroughs et al., 1956).

In the tissues of fresh water fish from the Hanford area, similar patterns of radioisotope distribution occur. Bone shows the highest concentration of $^{89-90}Sr$, related elements, and other minerals. Muscle and generalized soft tissues take on ^{137}Cs and other alkali metals. Glands and specialized tissues may be characterized by specific isotopes, for example the spleen's ^{60}Co, the blood's ^{51}Cr, and the retina's ^{65}Zn. A species of duck that feeds almost exclusively on invertebrates from the Columbia River bottom exhibits body burdens of radionu-clides much like those of fish living on similar food.

Neither the most nor the least radioactive fish are found at the third and fourth trophic levels. Whitefish, which prey upon herbivorous aquatic insects, exemplify the third level, and squawfish, which eat other fish and crustacea, belong to the fourth level. They are less radioactive than suckers of the second level which feed directly upon sessile algae. Scavengers like sturgeon were the least radioactive of Columbia River fish.

Studies of terrestrial carnivores are of ecological interest. In the southeastern United States, radionuclide burdens (especially ^{137}Cs) of predators and prey have been determined with a whole-body counter (Jenkins et al., 1969). Animals from the coastal plains showed consider-ably more radioactivity than those from the Piedmont, which reflects the difference in soils. Wildcats, entirely carnivorous, accumulated more ^{137}Cs than foxes with a more varied diet. Consistently, wildcats exceeded the standard body burden set for man, while foxes averaged about a third of that value. Predator/prey ratios reached a high 15.9 for bobcat/rabbit and 5.6 for gray fox/cotton rat. These exceed the ratios of 3 for cougar/deer and wolf/caribou determined in the far north.

Earlier chapters have discussed the radiopathology of mammals. Fisheries research reveals patterns of radiation-induced damage similar to those found in mammalian tissues, with gonads and hemopoietic tissues again the most sensitive. Surveys in the waters around Pacific test sites yielded equivocal data except for thyroid tissue. Clear evi-dence of ^{131}I damage was obtained in 79 species of fish from the Eniwetok lagoon. The degree of thyropathy was well correlated with proximity to the explosion site. In tropic waters, weakened individuals quickly fall prey to carnivores, or if they die decompose rapidly (Hines, 1962). Therefore the fate of more seriously injured fish is difficult to determine.

Food Chains

Living organisms are tied together in the ecosystem through steps in the food chain (or web) built on the capture of solar energy by green plants. A radioisotope introduced into such a scheme ultimately appears throughout the ecosystem, at some levels building up with surprising rapidity to an impressive degree, depending in part upon the rates of cycling and of decay in radioactivity (Davis and Foster, 1958). However, studies of radioisotope movement through food chains have provided few instances of radiation damage, because trace amounts are intentionally low.

The degree to which organisms concentrate elements from the environment is expressed as a concentration factor for each element. Concentration factors tend to be higher and more variable for freshwater than for marine forms, because the marine environment is relatively rich in minerals and more uniform. Marine ecosystems form a continuum in a sense not approached in fresh water or on land (Templeton et al., 1970). Movement of materials is freer and exometabolites of any particular form become available to all others. Contributing to this are passive planktonic drift with the water currents and long migrations of the large forms of the higher trophic levels. The general oceanic pattern of phytoplankton–zooplankton–higher forms is well established, but the intimate details for specific organisms are not all known.

In the Columbia River, one biological chain which concentrates radionuclides consists of algae → insect larvae → young carp → trout. Other chains involve other animals such as snails, crustacea, and salmon. Seasonal differences in water temperature control metabolic rate and influence radioisotope uptake (Fig. 15.3). With short-lived isotopes such as ^{24}Na, or even ^{32}P, radioactivity may not persist through a long chain even though the element has been passed along. This may occur especially in cold weather when movement through the chain may be slowed. On the other hand, ^{65}Zn with its half-life of months, and ^{90}Sr with its half-life of years, do not show seasonal fluctuations in the higher trophic levels.

Fortunately, more than five times the radioactivity found anywhere in the Columbia River would be required to produce demonstrable effects on fish. Furthermore, a conservative attitude is taken toward release of radioisotopes into any habitat. However, in our desire to emphasize the possible consequences of concentration factors, let us consider water which contains a radionuclide at the maximum permissible concentration as given by the National Bureau of Standards hand-

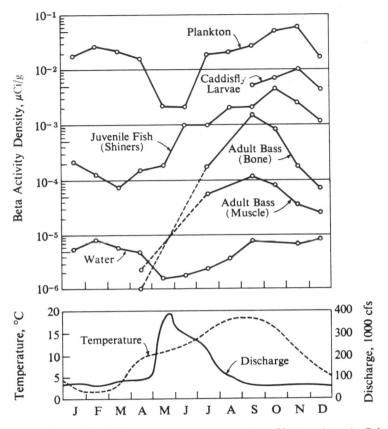

Figure 15.3. Seasonal variation on average concentration of beta emitters in Columbia River organisms and water. River discharge and temperature are shown for comparison. (Henderson and Foster, 1957; by courtesy of the authors and the American Fisheries Society.)

book. A human might drink several pints of such water per day without exceeding the allowable body burden, yet if the water contains fish that have concentrated an isotope by a factor of 1000, few pounds can be eaten without exceeding the allowable body burden. In the light of 10^4 and 10^5 concentration values for many isotopes at certain trophic levels, this concentration factor of 10^3 is a moderate one.

Interested readers may consult ecology texts for depictions and discussions of the variety of food webs. Also, ecology journals are beginning to publish papers on radioecology. For our example, we shall consider one of the earliest radioisotope experiments of this type.

On July 1, 1948, staff from Dalhousie University distributed the 100 mCi contents of a single vial of $KH_2{}^{32}PO_4$ to the surface of an 0.8-acre lake, thereby increasing the natural store of phosphorus by only 2%. Subsequently, the water content, mud content, and uptake by plants and animals were followed by Geiger-Müller counting techniques (Coffin et al., 1949). In spite of discharge by an outlet stream, 80% of the ^{32}P found its way into lake organisms. Within hours it had been taken up strongly by floating plankton, by sponges, and by the sphagnum which made up most of the lake margin. Within a few days it had reached the bodies of fish, and within 2 weeks it had built up in their bones. The importance of food-incorporated radioisotope is indicated by the failure to demonstrate ^{32}P in fish until 2 days had elapsed. In spite of a continuous stream of water through the mouth to the gills, ^{32}P had to become associated with plankton, and the plankton ingested, before the fish showed demonstrable changes.

When the various organisms were considered from the standpoint of absolute uptake, lower plants took up more than higher plants; higher animals more than lower animals; and animals more than plants. However, the movement up the food chain does not necessarily mean continued concentration of an isotope. In lake organisms on a basis of unit wet weight, copepods attained the "hottest" rating. They became 40,000 times as radioactive as the water. In comparison, although belonging to a higher trophic level, fish had tissue merely 13,000 times as radioactive as water. In part this reflects the short generation time of microscopic forms which leads to rapid turnover of materials. Fish not only have relatively long generations but they also have a slow turnover of skeletal phosphate. In terms of relative uptake per grams of total P in the organism, copepods prove to be 10 times as high.

Naturally, the chemical characteristics of an isotope are important in these matters as is also the physical half-life. Not all isotopes will follow a pattern determined for ^{32}P. With half-lives of months (^{65}Zn) or years (^{90}Sr), longer-lived isotopes persist at a high level through food chains which require considerable periods for consummation. A study of ^{137}Cs in the components of an aquatic community showed herbivores ranging from one-third to several times as radioactive as the algae on which they fed. The vertebrate predators of the third, fourth, and fifth trophic levels concentrated ^{137}Cs to higher levels than found in their prey.

Biological Surveys and Environmental Programs

In an Atomic Age, food chains are a matter for national and international concern. Also, the protection of workers in nuclear industries and the safeguarding of surrounding areas are matters for legislation authorizing surveillance and enforcement. Measures taken at Hanford, Los Alamos, Oak Ridge, Argonne, Knolls, and other installations have been detailed in U.S. Atomic Energy Commission (AEC) reports. Let us consider Hanford's waste management practices, since with its complex of production reactors, Hanford discharged more than 90% of all low and intermediate-level radioactivity so disposed in the United States. This was accomplished in commendable fashion with no permissible limit exceeded at any point of exposure, however near to or remote from the point of discharge.

A staff of site surveyors was continuously in the field measuring radioactivity and collecting samples of air, water, earth, vegetation, and animal life from the northwestern states. This resulted in literally thousands of measurements each month. In addition to area monitoring designed to demonstrate as precisely as possible where discharged radioactive materials went, research was performed to determine the effects of radioactive wastes on plant and animal life (Hanson and Kornberg, 1956). Studies included determination of (a) routes, rates, and quantities of specific radioisotopes transferred through different aquatic and terrestrial ecosystems; (b) influences of environmental factors upon transfer and accumulation in ecological systems; and (c) ways of retarding or accelerating the movement of radiocontaminants by manipulation of ecological factors.

The concern over water-borne wastes results in a study of weekly samples from 11 points on the Columbia River and five on the Yakima River. Less frequently, water samples were taken from other points, including the ocean at the river mouth. Equally important was the program of aquatic biology to detect alterations in the river system's natural balance of plant and animal life. In addition, a continuous sample of the effluent destined for the river was pumped into an aquatic biology laboratory for toxicity texts on living organisms. High-level liquid wastes are in a class by themselves since they are stored in tanks, for years if necessary.

In addition to weapons-test fallout, the monitoring of land areas checks upon the content of gaseous wastes. In 1947, radioactive particles were discovered near the separations plant stacks, and workers were required to wear masks when in the area. Subsequently, redesign eliminated the problem and the principal constituent of concern became ^{131}I. Even here drastic reduction was achieved, partly by modifying operating procedures, but especially by scheduling in accordance with meteorological conditions. This points up the importance of a knowledge of atmospheric patterns and phenomena where gaseous fission products may be released or where nuclear reactors are air cooled.

Solid wastes, including contaminated construction and production items, are easily controlled. In Hanford they were isolated from the environment by burial well above the water table in an area with practically no rainfall and hence no percolation. Until 1963 the AEC took care of low-level solid wastes by shallow burial on government sites. Subsequently, private companies were licensed to operate waste burial grounds. The optimum geological sites for storing high-level solidified wastes are still a matter for debate. Originally these came from the production of plutoneum for military purposes, but after 20 years the Hanford works was gradually shut down. The high-level wastes of the future are expected to derive from the reprocessing of spent fuel from nuclear power stations.

Ironically, relaxed vigilance of outdated equipment blemished the Hanford image of successful waste control long after eight of the nine production reactors were "mothballed." Leaking waste-storage tanks were undetected or not reported immediately. An especially big leak in 1973 forced reassessment of the supervisory program.

Strontium 90 in United States Milk

A type of food-chain research and an aspect of environmental programs which concerns the whole nation, and not merely areas influenced by Atomic Energy establishments, is the determination of ^{90}Sr and other radionuclides in milk. The responsibility for radiation surveillance of this sort is assigned to the U.S. Environmental Protection Agency. Milk was chosen, not only because of predominance in the diet of infants, but especially because it is one of the most important components of the diet available in all regions at all seasons. It can provide a useful index of trends in a changing environment, not only in itself but also in other foods and for soils.

An original network of five raw-milk sampling stations was expanded for a while to 12 strategically located stations. In 1960, the Public Health Service established a second sampling program for processed milk consisting of 60 stations (Knapp, 1961). This provided at least one sampling point within each state, to measure the levels of radioactivity in milk of the type consumed by the public. The ^{90}Sr concentration in milk declined from the 1963 peak until all of the strontium blasted into the upper atmosphere prior to the test ban returned to earth by 1970.

The concern about fallout was abating by 1971, when 156 stations were operating. Pesticide contamination had entered the scene as a more serious environmental threat reflected in milk samples. The development of new instrumentation enables simple measurements of a number of substances. Among the nucleotides, ^{131}I peaks appear in the United States soon after bomb tests in China. A correlation between the ^{131}I in milk and thyroid content is well established.

In 1976, there were 65 nationwide sampling sites in the EPA's monitoring system supplying monthly samples of pasteurized milk to a national analytical laboratory (which also analyzes air and water samples provided by the network). Milk is analyzed for ^{131}I, ^{140}Ba, ^{137}Cs, total K, ^{89}Sr, and ^{90}Sr. In addition, as a collaborative program, the Pan American Health Organization developed a sampling network for the South American countries.

Most discussions of ^{90}Sr in food chains use the strontium unit (SU), defined as the ratio of 1 pCi ^{90}Sr/g Ca. At the 1965–1966 peak, the bones reached a maximum of 7 SU in children under 4 years old. A decade earlier, the value was 1–2 SU, while in adults maturing before 1945 it was only 0.19 SU. For comparison, 80 SU was generally accepted as an amount which probably could be tolerated for a lifetime without medically detectable damage.

Fortunately, in animals and man there is metabolic differentiation between Sr and Ca so that of 1 SU in the soil only 0.13 SU appears in milk and 0.032 in human bones. Figure 15.4 emphasizes this pattern by showing discrimination barriers. A vegetable diet may result in as much as 0.25 SU passed along to human bone from each SU of the soil when Sr and Ca are present in uniform mixture. In fact, when all dietary sources of ^{90}Sr were considered for 1968, vegetables and grain products each contributed more to the yearly human intake than milk. Furthermore, the dietary intake of ^{90}Sr in the Soviet Union was significantly higher than in New York due to the unrefined flour used for Russian dark bread.

Resumption of atmospheric testing by the French and Chinese has maintained the dietary intakes of ^{90}Sr for almost a decade since 1968. The pattern of dietary sources was also continued. For 1973, in New York City 67% and in San Francisco 75% of the yearly intake of ^{90}Sr was from vegetables, fruit, and grain products. Dairy products accounted for only 31% and 21% in the same cities, respectively.

In addition to Sr levels, ^{131}I, ^{140}Ba, and ^{137}Cs have been routinely determined in milk and their levels have consistently been a mere fraction of the permissible levels. A similar statement might also be made for a variety of foods purchased from a few local markets for study

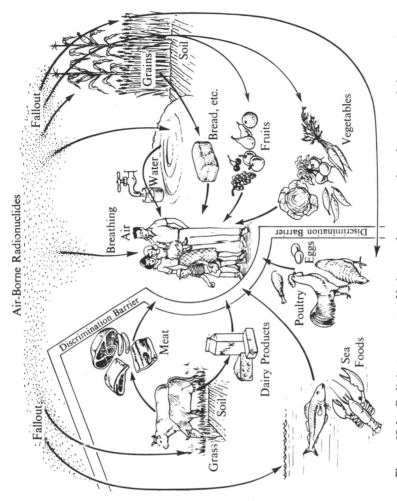

Figure 15.4. Radioisotope routes. Various pathways may be taken to reach human tissue. However, the processes of animal physiology discriminate against chemically related elements in favor of the normal dietary constituent. For example, there is a discrimination factor for ^{90}Sr of 2 to 4 in respect to Ca.

by the Public Health Service, especially the Cincinnati station. However the actual responsibility for commodities lies with the Food and Drug administration. As yet they have not had to take legal action against any foods. For purpose of reference, radioactivity data are available for all basic foods produced before 1945. The current status of the problem is reflected in monthly reports of radiological health data prepared by the U.S. Public Health Service.

An additional step toward human protection was taken in 1974, when Congress passed legislation to require federal regulation of drinking water. The supplier is legally responsible for the quality of the water fed into public water systems. The act required the Environmental Protection Agency (EPA) to establish contaminant levels to ensure the health of the U.S. population.

Concluding Remarks

In this chapter, ecological damage has been discussed and the "healing powers of the natural environment" have been revealed. These two aspects were observed consistently in the vicinity of experimental radiation sources, areas of waste disposal, and the sites of nuclear explosions. Biologists who witnessed the severe destruction of the Pacific proving ground "failed to find evidence of gross population or morphological change . . . ascribable to the effects of residual radioactivity alone" (Hines, 1962). Presumably, organisms with high reproductive potential could afford the loss of defective gametes and zygotes without showing phenotypic change or decrease in population size. The chapter closes with comments on food chains and environmental safeguards aimed especially at minimizing the human intake of radionuclides.

References

Alexander, L. T. (1950). Radioactive materials as plant stimulants, field results. *Agron. J.* **42,** 252–255.

Anellis, A. (1961). Radioresistance of a *Pseudomonas* species isolated from the Omega West Reactor. *Radiat. Res.* **15,** 720–723.

Auerbach, S. I. (1957). Waste pit area studies. *Health Physics Div. Ann. Prog. Report,* ORNL-2384. Oak Ridge National Laboratory (see reports for 1950–1970).

Blaylock, B. G. (1965). Chromosomal aberrations in a natural population of *Chironomus tentans* exposed to chronic low-level radiation. *Evolution* **19,** 421–429.

Blinks, L. R. (1952). Effect of radiation on marine algae. *J. Cell. Comp. Physiol.* **39,** Suppl. 2, 11–18.

Boroughs, H., Chipman, W. A., and Rice, T. R. (1957). Laboratory experiments on the uptake, accumulation and loss of radionuclides by marine organisms. (Chapter 8 of a committee report on Effects of Atomic Radiation on Oceanography and Fisheries). *N.A.S.–N.R.C., Publ.* **551,** 80–87.

Boroughs, H., Townsley, S. J., and Hiatt, R. W. (1956). The metabolism of radionuclides by marine organisms. *Biol. Bull. (Woods Hole, Mass.)* **111,** 336–351 Sr-89 (I) and 352–357 Y-91 (II).

Boroughs, H., Townsley, S. J., and Hiatt, R. W. (1957). The metabolism of radionuclides by marine organisms. III. The uptake of calcium in solution by marine fish. *Limnol. Oceanogr.* **2,** 28–32.

Bustad, L. (1960). Significance of nuclear industry effluents in animal populations. "Radioisotopes in the Biosphere," pp. 243–254. University of Minnesota Press, Minneapolis.

Coffin, C. C., Hayes, F. R., Jodrey, L. H., and Whiteway, S. G. (1949). Exchange of materials in a lake as studied by the addition of radioactive phosphorous. *Can. J. Res., Sect. D* **27,** 207–222.

Conard, R. A., Dobyns, B. M., and Sutow, W. W. (1970a). Thyroid neoplasia as late effect of exposure to radioactive iodine in fallout. *J. Am. Med. Assoc.* **214,** 316–324.

Conard, R. A., Meyer, L. M., and Sutow, W. W. (1970b). "Medical Survey of the People of Rongelap and Utirik Islands 13, 14, and 15 Years After Exposure to Fallout Radiation," BNL 50220 (T-562). U.S. Brookhaven Natl. Lab., Upton, New York.

Cowan, J. J. and Platt, R. B. (1963). Radiation doses in the vicinity of an unshielded nuclear reactor. "Radioecology" (V. Schultz and A. W. Klement, Jr., eds.), pp. 318–355. Van Nostrand-Reinhold, Princeton, New Jersey.

Davis, J. J., and Foster, R. F. (1958). Bioaccumulation of radioisotopes through aquatic food chains. *Ecology* **39,** 530–535.

Dunaway, P. B., and Kaye, S. V. (1963). Effects of ionizing radiation on mammal populations on the White Oak Lake bed. *In* "Radioecology" (V. Schultz and A. W. Klement, Jr., eds.), pp. 333–338. Van Nostrand-Reinhold, Princeton, New Jersey.

Eisenbud, M. (1973). "Environmental Radioactivity," 2nd ed. Academic Press, New York.

Folsom, T. R., and Harley, J. H. (1957). Comparison of some natural radiations received by selected organisms. *N.A.S.–N.R.C., Publ.* **551,** 28–33.

Fraley, L., Jr., and Wicker, F. W. (1973a). Response of shortgrass plains vegetation to gamma radiation. I. Chronic irradiation. *Radiat. Bot.* **13,** 331–342.

Fraley, L., Jr., and Wicker, F. W. (1973b). Response of shortgrass plains vegetation to gamma radiation. II. Short term seasonal irradiation. *Radiat. Bot.* **13,** 343–353.

Gorham, E. (1959). A comparison of lower and higher plants as accumulators of radioactive fallout. *Can. J. Bot.* **37,** 327–329.

Hanson, W. C. (1960). Accumulation of radioisotopes from fallout by terrestrial animals at Hanford, Washington. *Northwest Sci.* **34,** 89–98.

Hanson, W. C., and Kornberg, H. A. (1956). Radioactivity in terrestrial animals near an atomic energy site. *Proc. Int. Conf. Peaceful Uses At. Energy, 1st, 1955* Vol. 13, pp. 385–388.

Henderson, C., and Foster, R. F. (1957). Studies of smallmouth black bass (*Micropterus dolomieu*) in the Columbia River near Richland, Washington. *Trans. Am. Fish. Soc.* **86,** 112–127.

Hines, N. O. (1962). "Proving Ground." Univ. Washington Press, Seattle.

Jenkins, J. H., Monroe, J. R., and Golley, F. B. (1969). Comparison of fallout ^{137}Cs accumulation and excretion in certain southeastern mammals. *Symp. Radioecol., Proc. Natl. Symp., 2nd, 1967* Conf. 670503.

Knapp, H. A. (1961). The effect of deposition rate and cumulative soil level on the concentration of Strontium-90 in U.S. milk and food supplies. *U.S.A.E.C. Div. Tech. Info.* **TID-13945.**

Krumholz, L. A. (1956). Observations on the fish population of a lake contaminated by radioactive wastes. *Bull. Am. Mus. Nat. Hist.* **110,** 281–368.

Krumholz, L. A., and Rust, J. H. (1954). Osteogenic sarcoma in a muskrat from an area of high environmental radiostrontium. *AMA Arch. Path.* **57,** 270–278.

Lackey, J. B. (1957). The suspended microbiota of the Clinch river and adjacent waters, in relation to radioactivity in the summer of 1956. *Oak Ridge Natl. Lab. (U.S.)* **ORNL-2410.**

Odum, H. T. ed. (1970). "A Tropical Rain Forest: A Study of Irradiation and Ecology at El Verde, P.R.," TID-24270. U.S.A.E.C., Div. Tech. Inf., Washington, D.C.

Perkins, R. W., and Nielson, J. M. (1960). "Radioactivity in Foods Resulting from Columbia River Water Radioisotopes." Radiol. Chem. Operation, Semiannu. Rep. HW63824, pp. 25–38. Hanford Lab.

Platt, R. B. (1963). Ecological effects of ionizing radiation on organisms, communities, and ecosystems. *In* "Radioecology" (V. Schultz and A. W. Klement, Jr., eds.), pp. 243–255. Van Nostrand-Reinhold, Princeton, New Jersey.

Polikarpov, G. G. (1966). "Radioecology of Aquatic Organisms." Van Nostrand-Reinhold, Princeton, New Jersey.

Rickard, W. H. (1961). Notes on bird nests found in a desert shrub community following nuclear detonation. *Condor* **63,** 265–266.

Rickard, W. H., and Shields, L. M. (1963). An early stage in the plant recolonization of a nuclear target area. *Radiat. Bot.* **3,** 41–44.

Shields, L. M., and Wells, P. V. (1962). Effects of nuclear testing on desert vegetation. *Science* **135,** 38–40.

Templeton, W. L., Nakatani, R. E., and Held, E. E. (1970). Radiation effects. *In* "Radioactivity in the Marine Environment," Chapter 9. Comm. Oceanog., NAS–NRC, Washington, D.C.

Turner, F. B. (1975). Effects of continuous irradiation on animal populations. *Adv. Radiat. Biol.* **5,** 83–144.

Wicker, F. W., and Fraley, L., Jr. (1974). Effects of ionizing radiations on terrestrial plant communities. *Adv. Radiat. Biol.* **4,** 317–366.

Willard, W. K. (1960). Avian uptake of fission products from an area contaminated by low level atomic wastes. *Science* **132,** 148–150.

Woodwell, G. M. (1962). Effects of ionizing radiation on terrestrial ecosystems. *Science* **138,** 572–577.

Zavitkovski, J., ed. (1977). "The Enterprise, Wisconsin, Radiation Forest Radioecological Studies," TID-26113-P2. Tech. Inf. Cent., Oak Ridge, Tennessee.

CHAPTER 16   Pest Control, Food Treatment, and Other Applications

Our discussion now turns to applications which may be commercially profitable as well as practical. Here we will limit ourselves to biological matters. Chemical, civil, electrical, and metallurgical engineering are beyond the scope of our discussions, although certain general considerations apply here as well as there. From a safety standpoint, in addition to the necessity of reliable controls and the desirability of economic shielding, the radiation should not induce radioactivity in the material exposed. However, radiation sources must supply an output adequate for the operation at a reasonable cost for equipment and installation. At present, executives consider the capital expenditure prohibitive for the equipment needed for safe supply of doses adequate for fast-flowing materials like grain, water, or sewage.

Food processing, an area in which new technology often finds application, is one of the oldest of human endeavors. From prehistoric times man has sought ways of escaping malnutrition in lean years or nongrowing seasons, but dry foods are subject to insect infestation and moist foods to decay microorganisms. Preservation by the selective destruction possible with radiation has suggested itself as an alternative to the heat processing which dates from Napoleonic times, and the quick-freeze, low-temperature techniques of the last decade.

The desired goal is decay-free storage without refrigeration. An ability to store and ship fresh food without refrigeration would be a great advantage in catastrophic emergencies—or even normally in parts of the world which lack power supplies for adequate temperature control. However, many problems must be solved. Figure 16.1 indicates dose ranges which have been found effective, along with an indication of the doses which destroy vitamins and induce discoloration, odors, and off-flavor.

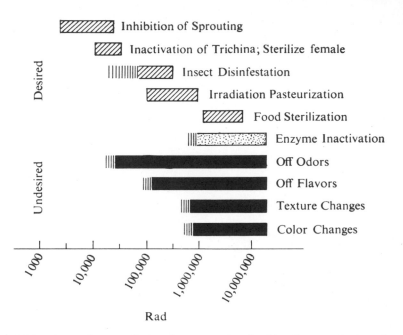

Figure 16.1.   Approximate radiation dose ranges involved in effects on foods and products.

Historical Notes

As early as 1943, food-radiation research was under way at the Massachusetts Institute of Technology (M.I.T.), but in the next five years only two other laboratories became interested. Between 1959 and 1960 when government support made itself felt, 31 university and college laboratories, 8 foundations and institutes, 4 government agencies, and 52 industrial firms were involved in research. In all fairness, we must recognize that two-thirds of the industrial and foundation funds were of private origin, although federal funds had conditioned the environment. Beginning with 1954, when over a million dollars were expended, nearly the entire government program of food treatment with ionizing radiation was under Army auspices (U.S. Army, 1961). In 1951, the Quartermaster Corps had started their research program, which at one time promised to culminate in a giant center at Stockton, California. However, support of the program was withdrawn in 1959. During the succeeding decade, the Army moved nearly all of its research efforts to its Natick, Massachusetts, laboratory, conveniently close to M.I.T. In

1969 there were nearly 300 papers published on irradiated foods, but within 5 years the international output dropped to less than 100 research reports. Many of these were final summaries. Two factors contributed to this situation: the U.S. Atomic Energy Commission's mission and name changed, and industry recognized discouraging aspects (to be explained below). The AEC's successor agency, the Energy Research and Development Administration (ERDA), has an urgent, less diversified mission. Fortunately, the international effort has been sustained by the joint efforts of the United Nations Food and Agriculture Organization (FAO) and the International Atomic Energy Agency (IAEA). In 1970 a five-year agreement was signed by 19 supporting countries, which later was extended through 1978 by 23 countries. The Federal German authorities made a particularly important contribution by providing host center facilities at their Research Institute for Nutrition at Karlsruhe.

The entire scientific world paid tribute to the pioneering research of United States investigators at the FAO-organized meeting on the Use of Ionizing Radiations for Food Preservation. Held in November 1958 at Harwell, England, participants included 176 representative of 17 European governments and 14 international organizations (European Meeting, 1959). They surveyed the status of food irradiation and critically evaluated its potentialities. Appreciation of the exploratory United States investigations was unanimous.

Key publications summarizing similar subsequent meetings include U.S. Atomic Energy Commission (1965), Hickman (1966), and International Atomic Energy Agency (1973a). Also see IAEA Vienna panel proceedings on the irradiation of particular types of foods (IAEA, 1968, 1970a, 1973b).

Basic Principle

Regardless of whether it is food treatment or some other application, fundamentally the problem resolves itself to one of breaking the life cycle of an infesting organism. If there is a weak link in the biology of a particular pest, it must be exploited. Merely from a dosage standpoint this makes sense. An attack aimed at a radiosensitive stage requires much less radiation. Furthermore, if nature has been enlisted in the undertaking, the desired outcome is assured. The outstanding example of successful radiation control of an unwanted organism has been in the protection of food and by-products during production rather than in storage. We shall discuss this next.

Screw-Worm Control

From 1933 until 1959 in the southeastern United States, normal birth and routine castration of livestock were hazardous due to the presence of a calliphorid called the screw-worm fly. The adult female is attracted to any open wound, shingling the area with about 200 eggs. In less than a day, larvae emerge to form a feeding mass which literally eats the host alive. A small scratch, even a tick bite, can serve as a fatal attraction.

The pest, introduced into the southeast through shipment of infested cattle from Texas, found the Florida climate suitable for overwintering. Annually, from here the flies spread over the southeastern states during the summer months. It became evident that if the flies could be eliminated from the winter range, at least five states would be freed of their summer depredations. As we shall see, extinction was accomplished by breaking the life cycle in the embryonic stage through the introduction of dominant sperm-borne genetic situations which were lethal. Irradiated males conveyed these sperm. Inspection stations along the Mississippi guard the southeast against reinfection (Knipling, 1960).

The job was an impressive one. Fifty thousand square miles of Florida required the release of more than fifty million sterile flies per week. To produce enough insects, a plant was constructed at Sebring, Florida, which used 40 tons of ground whale and horse meat for the rearing slurry. Twenty airplanes were required to distribute the product of this factory.

E. F. Knipling, R. C. Bushland, A. W. Lindquist, and other staff members of the U.S. Department of Agriculture's Entomological Research Branch are the heroes of the 1959 Florida screw-worm conquest. Earlier in 1954 they had demonstrated that the method would work on the island of Curacao of the Netherlands Antilles.

The approach was to promote species self-destruction by the sustained release of sterile males which compete for mates with the existing fertile males. Table 16.1 demonstrates the population trend expected in an area if sterile males are distributed in numbers adequate to dominate the natural population. As shown, an initial 2:1 ratio is considered desirable. In subsequent releases, the original number of sterile males is employed.

Factors Considered in "Sterile" Male Release

There are a number of factors to consider in appraising the feasibility of the method. The released stage should be nondestructive yet the

TABLE 16.1

Population Trend of an Insect in an Area if Sterile Males Are Distributed in Sufficient Numbers to Dominate the Natural Fertile Male Population Initially by a Ratio of 2:1

Assumed population of virgin females	Ratio of sterile to fertile males competing for each virgin female	Percentage of females mated to sterile males
1,000,000	2:1	66.7
333,333	6:1	85.7
47,619	42:1	97.7
1,107	1,807:1	99.95
Less than 1		

[a] 2,000,000 sterile males would be released in each generation over the four generations shown. (After Knipling, 1955, with permission.)

males and their sperm should be fully capable in competition with the normal. An economic procedure for rearing enormous numbers of insects may need to be developed along with sure techniques of dispersal. A finite area adequately isolated from reinfection is preferred. In the southeast, effective natural barriers are provided by the Gulf of Mexico and the winter temperatures of the Gulf states.

In Texas, eradication has not been considered a practical goal since screwworm flies can migrate from Mexico. Nevertheless, in view of a 25-million-dollar annual loss, control measures were desirable. In the fall of 1962, 63,000 square miles were being supplied with sterile males at the rate of 400 males per square mile per week. The second phase of control, instituted early in 1963, included the establishment of a buffer zone 100 miles wide along the Mexican border. This was achieved by releasing 100 sterile males per square mile per week.

The program was so successful that ranchers relaxed surveillance and the treatment of wounds, but in 1972 a breakdown in buffer-zone control occurred, due mainly to evolutionary divergence between the mass-reared factory strain and the wild-type invaders. Bushland obtained assistance from professors at the University of Texas, who identified several genetic differences. Most important was a change in an enzyme involved in flight activity [α-glycerol phosphate dehydrogenase (α-GDH)]. The α-GDH variant is less active at the temperature range experienced in nature. To be competitive, released males must fly well from early morning to late afternoon. Until the plant was shut down for complete destruction of its flies, every new strain brought in deteriorated genotypically within six months. The constant high temperature of the accelerated rearing scheme favored the altered behavior of the α-GDH variant. Additional complications included a shift to a more artificial diet due to the high price of fresh meat and whole blood. Also, in nature an outbreak of wound-causing pests (such as ticks) favored screw-worm infestation.

A new barrier belt at the narrow Tehuantepec Isthmus would be much easier to maintain, and the United States–Mexico problem eliminated if all territories north of the belt could be cleared of screw-worm. To this end, an international agreement was signed enabling the construction of a new mass rearing plant in Mexico which began production of sterile flies in 1978. However, Richardson (1978) emphasized that it would be most prudent to make a detailed taxonomic and genetic study of the wild flies before implementing a sweeping control program. He also warned that the role of the weather in population increases has not been adequately investigated.

Meanwhile, there have been several successes on a moderate scale. Sterile males were chiefly responsible for the 1971–1974 eradication of screw-worms from Puerto Rico and the Virgin Islands. However, progress was expedited by a vigorous supportive program of inspection and pesticide treatment of affected animals (Williams *et al.*, 1977). In 1977 a 6-year-old reinfestation of Curacao yielded to sterile male release after the population was suppressed by 3 months of bait-toxicant trapping (J. W. Snow, Screwworm Research Lab., Mission, Texas, personal communication).

The screwworm successes have inspired entomologists in various parts of the world to consider similar methods for controlling other pests (International Atomic Energy Agency, 1970b, 1975). Exploratory experiments have been performed with virtually every destructive insect, and many of them were found to possess biological features causing them to be less amenable to radiation sterilization than Dipteran insects. Lepidoptera and Hemiptera have holokinetic chromosomes. Therefore fragments are not lost at the division following induced breakage. The boll weevil, a Coleopteran, has a radiosensitive gut which is severely damaged at sterilizing doses.

Even when amenable species have been attacked, successful eradication has been accomplished primarily in situations of geographical or habitat isolation such as islands, mountain valleys, and focal outbreaks in a new country. A more practical goal may be pest management of well-established populations. With this intent, the pendulum has swung toward integrated control in which radiation may be used adjunctively.

Other Germ Line Approaches to Control

In addition to the induction of dominant lethals in sperm, there are a number of alternate approaches which can employ radiation (Davidson, 1974). These include the destruction of gametogenic cells, which is more easily accomplished in female insects. Also, there is the production of laboratory strains with chromosomal translocations which result in sterile heterozygotes from interbreeding with the wild strain. A third possibility is the incorporation of conditional lethal mutations into pest populations to render them incapable of surviving temperature extremes.

Direct Killing of Insects

Instead of contriving ways to influence fertility, undesirable organisms may be eliminated directly if lethal doses of radiation are provided. Except for strictly genetic studies, more has been written on killing insects than on any other aspect of radiation experiments. Results with representative pests have been consistent with the results from other species studied. We will not take the space to detail these findings (see Cornwell, 1965). The relatively high lethal dose for adult insects and the vulnerability of immature stages have been discussed in earlier chapters. Fortunately for radiation control, at any given time, a large proportion of an insect population may be made up of immature stages.

The annual insect damage to stored products in the United States alone has been estimated at over a billion dollars. Many of these cannot be subjected to heat; and insecticide treatment, particularly of foodstuffs, is undesirable. Even if applicable, chemical fumigation is ineffective on insect eggs, yet this stage of the life cycle is the most sensitive to radiation.

Bulk fission waste or spent reactor fuel elements have been suggested as a source of gamma rays to reach deep into timbers, boxes, packages, and bags where they destroy insects. However, a matter of practical concern is supplying an adequate dose at the handling rate typical of the product or commodity. At present, the capital expenditure for obtaining and installing an adequate source may be prohibitive.

Foods such as grain, dried fruits, beans, nuts, spices, and confections are subject to insect attack. Especially liable to infestation are packaged military rations or similar food reserves which are often stored for considerable periods in suboptimum environments. Prevention is costly, and sometimes impossible when infestation is carried over from the raw materials to the finished product. Irradiation extermination of units protected by insect-proof packaging offers a solution to the problem.

When wood borers are considered, the treatment of infested timbers in buildings of historical and architectural value might pose problems in shielding an adequate source and supporting the heavy result. On the other hand, portable antiques such as furniture can be transported to permanent installations for irradiation. New timbers intended for furniture or structural use can be pretreated with radiation (Bletchly and Fisher, 1957).

Control of Trichinosis

In addition to insects there are other unwanted invertebrates such as the worms which contaminate food and give rise to disease. Nearly a dozen helminthic diseases of man are food-borne, and although thorough cooking can destroy the infective form, preferences in flavor and texture make the approach ineffective. Control of trichinosis, a prevalent helminthic disease, has received considerable research by way of meat irradiation. The principle is to break the life cycle of the parasite by delivering radiation to larvae encysted in the meat. A dose of 1,000,000 rep will kill encysted *Trichinella*, but this dose produces objectional flavor changes in meat. Lower doses to inhibit larval development (15,000 rep) or to sterilize females (5000 rep) are more in order since they do not alter palatability (Alicata *et al.*, 1951). A few experiments performed with tapeworms suggest that the same range of doses will be effective as those used for the trichina worm.

We shall take space to give detailed consideration to only one set of experiments, performed to verify the efficacy of ^{60}Co gamma ray doses. Rats were fed irradiated *Trichinella* larvae in quantities greater than the number of unirradiated larvae known to cause fatal infections. Some of the results are shown in Table 16.2. The average length of survival for rats receiving such massive doses of worm larvae was 11 days. In contrast, rats receiving irradiated larvae typically survived the test period of 31 days and appeared active and healthy. In addition to the tabulated observations, rat muscle was digested after necropsy, and counts were made of the number of larvae recovered. Whereas thousands of larvae were obtained from unirradiated controls, the count averaged only 226 in the 10,000 R experiment. After 18,000 R, encysted larvae were exceptional. Furthermore, related experiments demon-

TABLE 16.2

Sequellae of Feeding Massive Number of *Trichella* Larvae to Rats[a]

Radiation delivered to *trichinella* larvae (R)	No. rats fed	No. larvae fed each rat	Rats with diarrhea	Weight loss	30-Day check for adult worms in intestine
10,000	12	12,000	6/12	Temporary	1/12
18,000	10	12,000	0	0	0
18,000	10	24,000	1/10	1/10	0

[a] Based on Gould *et al.*, 1955, by permission of American Association of Pathologists and Bacteriologists.

strated that irradiated larvae disappear from the host's intestine quite rapidly. From this we may infer that a person would suffer little or no ill effect from eating undercooked pork if it had received at least 18,000R.

During processing, the hog carcass is split and spread for a cooling period before cutting. This period has been regarded as a most suitable time for irradiation, and University of Michigan investigators have demonstrated that ^{60}Co, ^{137}Cs, and reactor fuel slugs may be used effectively. One detailed cost study revealed that a plant could process 2000 hog carcasses per day with 30,000 roentgen equivalent physical (rep) for less than one-quarter cent per pound. Processing in more compact pieces would reduce the cost.

Inhibition of Sprouting in Root Crops

A step beyond damaging living parasites in dead meat is the destruction of embryonic tissue in live roots in order to extend their storage life. Figure 16.2 shows examples from a potato experiment which demonstrated that sprouting and concomitant shrinking can be greatly reduced by 5000 R and completely inhibited at 20,000 R of ^{60}Co gamma rays (Sparrow and Christensen, 1954). Higher doses resulted in excessive weight loss and wrinkling; also, a majority of the members of a taste panel reported a sweet flavor. Subsequent investigation has revealed differences in responses between varieties, but there is no question about the efficiency of the method. Storage tests sponsored by the Army Quartermaster Corps provided impressive records of bulk storage over several years.

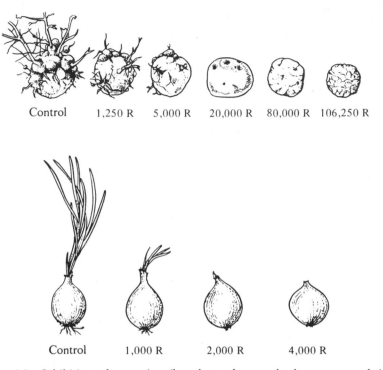

Control   1,250 R   5,000 R   20,000 R   80,000 R   106,250 R

Control   1,000 R   2,000 R   4,000 R

Figure 16.2. Inhibition of sprouting (based on photographs by courtesy of A. H. Sparrow). Top: Potatoes 15 months after receiving gamma radiation from ^{60}Co (Sparrow and Christensen, 1954). Bottom: Onions 5 months after receiving gamma radiation from ^{60}Co (Dallyn *et al.*, 1955).

Figure 16.2 also depicts sprout inhibition for onion bulbs (Dallyn *et al.*, 1955). Unlike the potato where the sprout starts from tissue close to the surface, an onion shoot arises from meristematic tissue deep within the center of the bulb. Although there is more tissue around this focus of growth, inhibition was quite successful even in larger onions. Indeed smaller bulbs usually have a greater tendency toward sprouting.

Irradiation also successfully prevents sprouting of carrots (Madsen *et al.*, 1959), red beets, turnips, and the so-called Jerusalem artichoke. However, there was a high incidence of rotting. With carrots, this could be decreased by washing, cleaning, and storage in plastic bags. Possibly damage and death of outer cell layers reduces the resistance to rot. Consistent with this hypothesis is the finding that radiation interferes with periderm-formation and wound-healing in potatoes. The rapidity of decay depends in part upon the temperature of storage.

Microorganism Control

Two dose levels are employed in the radiation preservation of food. In the previous paragraphs, we have been considering doses of less than 1,000,000 rads; that is, doses less than a megarad. High doses—higher than a megarad—are necessary to kill all microorganisms. However, such doses alter the flavor and odor. Accordingly, even though fungal and bacterial control serve as goals, lower doses may be employed. This procedure has been termed "pasteurization" because it destroys some bacteria and inhibits others. The term "radurization" has been coined to distinguish the process from conventional dairy methods (Goresline et al., 1964). "Radicidation" is synonymous with bactericidal effect. "Radappertization" implies a total destruction of microflora, which requires a dose adequate to cause a 12-log destruction of *Clostridium botulinum* spores.

Milk is perhaps the most sensitive of all foods to radiation-induced changes in flavor and odor. An M.I.T. group worked on the problem for years and developed a procedure to provide sterile milk indistinguishable from fresh milk. The procedure requires vacuum irradiation plus simultaneous distillation to remove off-flavor compounds. Although this success is of great theoretical interest, the procedure is not competitive with well-established commercial pasteurization processes.

The wholesomeness of food has its microbial, nutritional, and toxicological aspects (Reber et al., 1966). The evaluation of toxicity has stimulated considerable investigation of irradiated food components in the last decade. Although the data from simplified model systems of single carbohydrates, fats, or proteins cannot fully explain the reactions in complex foods, they revealed that the substances formed are similar to those obtained by other treatments. Free-radical reactions occur during the heating, autoxidation, and freeze-drying of foods as well as during irradiation. No new or novel products caused by radiation have been identified. The concentrations of the most abundant of the radiolytic substances are in parts per million (ppm) with radiation doses typical of food processing, and they fall off considerably if the dose can be reduced (Diehl and Scherz, 1975; Elias and Cohen, 1977).

Poultry, Meats, and Seafoods

Considerable research has been directed toward inhibiting microbial spoilage of poultry products and meats from domestic animals. Although *Salmonella* are destroyed, irradiation has little application for the preservation of fresh eggs because of flavor and form changes. Fortunately, naturally clean eggs seldom go bad under ordinary storage conditions. Our main concern is with another matter. Spray-drying after irradiation eliminates the undesirable aspects and could be a feasible method to control cross-transfer of pathogens in the bulk egg products used by bakers, confectioners, and food caterers.

The bacterial species ordinarily associated with the spoilage of chicken meat appear to be well controlled by 100,000 rad. In addition, uncooked chicken shows improved flavor at high temperature storage, more than observed for any other meats. However, there is a limitation in that yeasts persist at pasteurization doses and higher doses affect acceptability.

Until it was established that pork can stand a higher dose without losing acceptability, beef research took precedence. Shelf life at temperatures as high as 38°C was extended for weeks over unirradiated control samples. Early reports (1945–1947) suggested that irradiation enabled the storage of raw beef for almost a year at room temperature. However, it soon became evident that all types of radiation, delivered in appreciable quantity, induced changes objectionable to the senses. Steak, for example, is unacceptable after doses above 40,000 rad. Prepared and cooked meats offer more promise. Ham was acceptable even after 500,000 rads. Furthermore, higher doses can be delivered to spiced and flavored products (like sausage, bologna, and salami) without detectable consequences because spices mask odor and flavor changes.

The perishability of seafoods which complicates delivery in prime condition has dictated a relatively low consumption inland. Thus, they were among the earliest foods to be experimentally irradiated. Unfortunately, they have provided some of the more spectacular disappointments. Against a background of mild and subtle flavor, alterations are readily detected. About 2 megarads are required to produce commercially sterile fish. This is more than enough radiation to alter flavor and modify pigmentation. Oily lipids and delicately tinted flesh are vulnerable characteristics of prized seafoods.

Encouragement comes from demonstration that radurization has proved selective against the pseudomonads which are the most active in fish spoilage. Their elimination may confer remarkable extension in shelf life at chill temperatures (0°–5°C). One example was cod fillets which were acceptable up to 100 days later. Radurization also greatly improves the keeping qualities of blanched oysters, cooked crab, and shrimp. Unirradiated control samples spoiled in about two weeks of ordinary refrigeration, whereas less than half a megarad enabled storage from two to four months. On the strength of these findings, the Bureau of Commercial Fisheries dedicated an irradiator in Gloucester, Massachusetts. In 1964, the optimistic view was that radurized marine products would soon join pasteurized milk in the family refrigerator (Kaylor and Slavin, 1965). Despite supporting studies in most of the developing countries, which established that dozens of species of fin fish and shellfish profit by an extended shelf life if irradiated and refrigerated, commercial distribution is only a hope. Production and sale of irradiated food was forbidden by law in the six countries of the European Economic Community. In the United States, approval of the Food and Drug Administration was deferred until completion of a multilaboratory investigation of botulism hazards (Anon., 1965). Also, efficacy of the process under commercial shipping conditions was questioned. Before these aspects could be settled, a national concern about carcinogens developed.

Fruits and Vegetables

The aim of irradiating fresh fruit and vegetables is to inhibit postharvest disease by reducing the microbial surface flora, thus minimizing storage problems at any temperature. Fruits more than any other food are preferred in their natural state. Because of the low pH, bacteria give little difficulty. Molds and yeasts are the problem. In general, doses less than a megarad have increased shelf-life up to 10 times. Odor and flavor changes are slight, tending toward sharp, astringent qualities. Loss of quality due to texture and color changes determine the dosage limitations. Textural changes result from radiation breakage of macromolecules such as pectin and cellulose. Oxidative changes of the flavonoid pigments are as much a problem in classical methods of fruit preservation as in radurization. Above 250 krad, the concentration of total and reducing sugars may fall; above 1500 krad, glucose is degraded into glycolic and other acids.

Experiments on the preservation of mangoes, guavas, sapotas, bananas, and other tropical fruits have been performed. Also, considerable research has been done with citrus fruits, irradiating them not only after ordinary harvest procedures but also after inoculation with dense mold suspensions. Spoilage can be controlled, but a technical problem stems from the susceptibility of characteristic oils. Storage time may also be increased for berries, grapes, peaches, cherries, peppers, and tomatoes. In some cases, delayed ripening may contribute to success. Apples, peaches, and pears belong to the climateric class of fruits which are prone to physiological decay. Once the ripening process is initiated, 250 to 400 krad did not inhibit it.

Tough-textured leafy vegetables and podded seeds stand up well under doses adequate to decimate a microbial population. Cabbage, spinach, asparagus, and broccoli are examples of types which respond well to radiation. Exposure of beans, peas, and corn before storage can be advantageous. In all these experiments, the nature of subsequent handling and the type of packaging is very important if storage is to be prolonged without seriously modifying acceptability.

Acceptability of Irradiated Products

We have already mentioned the difficulty with milk, and implied that there have been problems with other substances. It seems impossible to discuss the radiation preservation of food without considering organoleptic qualities, that is, the impressions made on the senses. In all cases, sensory acceptability places a limit on the dose of radiation which can be used.

Except for changes in fatty meats to which the word rancid usually applies, descriptions of odor and flavor changes vary. However, people invariably find them unattractive. For example, there is the term "goaty" which is applied to the odor of irradiated meat; the tastes "bitter" and "burnt" are also frequently mentioned. At sterilizing doses all common species of fish develop "metallic" or "rubbery" odors.

Discolorization and moisture loss are problems in sprout inhibition. An additional problem with white potatoes is one of accelerated sweetness. Irradiated potatoes reach top sugar content in about half the time required by controls, but this is an exception. In general, the effect of ionizing radiations on the flavor of uncooked plant material is to reduce natural flavor rather than to induce new flavors. Nevertheless, this plus effects on texture are as limiting as off-flavor and off-odor in the processing of animal products. We shall not take the space to catalog all the different kinds of vegetables, berries, and fruit in which flat taste has been induced, nor will we identify special cases of unexplained tastes. The latter cases may trace to the nature of the packaging used for storage convenience and to guard against reinfection. Polyethylene is near the top of a list of materials which give off-odors.

When irradiated foods are packaged in impermeable sealed containers, gaseous radiolytic products are trapped in the "head space." The amount depends upon the type of food. Canned green beans yield twice the amount of head-space gas as the same volume of ground beef, while canned cherries give much less gas. Irradiated clam meat provides the greatest variety of head-gas components including H_2S, methyl mercaptan, several organic sulfides, acetone, toluene, butene, pentene, and a group of aldehydes (Elias and Cohen, 1977).

Improper packaging can result in undesirable changes more severe than those induced by radiation. The normal respiration of fruits and vegetables cannot take place in sealed plastic bags. In contrast, cooked foods require airtight packaging. However, bland products do absorb flavors from some materials. For instance, bread receiving only 50,000 rad acquired an acid flavor from polymer-coated cellophane, whereas bread in ordinary cellophane was unaffected. We should mention here that bakery products are not a homogeneous class. Although bread reacts well to radiation, pastry reacts poorly because of its fat content.

The things that people eat are as varied as man's imagination and ingenuity. Most foods have been or will be irradiated. We will mention only a few of the more common items not yet discussed. Spices withstand irradiation without detectably unpalatable results. Even after 1,500,000 rep, little change except toward mildness has been reported. Pepper, for example, lost some of its bite.

Results with complicated colloidal systems like mayonnaise are poor because irradiation tends to break down the emulsion. A related area is the decreased berry juice viscosity which is presumably due to the degradation of peptic substances. Radiation has been reported to cause bleaching, off-flavor, and denatured protein in ale and stout. In spite of this, the artificial aging of beer and other alcoholic beverages has been proposed.

Wholesomeness

A matter not necessarily related to color, odor, or taste is whether irradiated food is good for human consumption. So far as induced radioactivity is concerned, the phenomenon is energy-dependent rather than dose-dependent. Early in the course of research on radiation preservation, energy threshold values were verified as safe for all elements known or suspected to be present in food.

Let us go on then to biochemical aspects. Even at sterilization doses, only about 0.003% of the compounds of radiated food are affected. Thus nutritive value cannot be greatly influenced except (a) by destroying micronutrients or (b) by creating toxic substances (Hannan, 1956). The former change has been demonstrated to comprise vitamin deficiencies in rat experiments at several different institutions, but can easily be alleviated by supplements. The second possibility is more difficult to determine, but both short- and long-term feeding studies have been in progress. Growth rate, food consumption, lactation, litter size, viability, and life span were scored along with carcinogenic tests, hematology, and other clinical studies.

Short-term, 8-week tests demonstrated that food given sterilizing doses furnishes a macronutritionally adequate diet for laboratory rodents. In addition, studies lasting four generations were performed with rats. Mice, dogs, and monkeys have also been employed by several institutions in testing 18 sterilized foods and four types which have been irradiated at pasteurization doses. Typically these animals maintained excellent health. In a few cases, improved growth on irradiated food has been reported. To account for this, speculation has recognized both the possibility of better protein utilization as well as the possible depolymerization of cellulose to increase food value.

Considerable time and money was expended on these experiments. Figure 16.3 summarizes the results of a four-generation test of irradiated wheat fed to rats, performed at the University of Michigan. The data on which the figure is based was presented in detail in a clearance petition submitted to the U.S. Food and Drug Administration.

Forty irradiated foods making up 35, 65, 80, and 100% of their dietary calories have been fed to human volunteers, without effects demonstrable in periodic complete physical examinations (Levy, 1957). Subsequent to their separation from the project, these individuals have also had annual follow-up examinations which have verified their general good health. Furthermore, no toxic reactions have been experienced by the thousands of people who have sampled irradiated foods, including guests at the historical dinner of June 26, 1956, when members of the Joint Congressional Committee on Atomic Energy were served a complete dinner of irradiated foods. The menu included both low- and high-dose items.

A more extreme type of experiment can be performed by using as food, organisms which have been killed by radiation. At Oak Ridge, Tennessee, growing dogs were fed for four months on the flesh of lethally irradiated cows and sheep. No differences from controls were demonstrable in weight gain (Table 16.3), nor did the dogs differ in hematological or other tissue characteristics.

Carcinogenesis

Despite decades of research, the wholesomeness of irradiated foods remains questionable, mainly because of a lingering apprehension

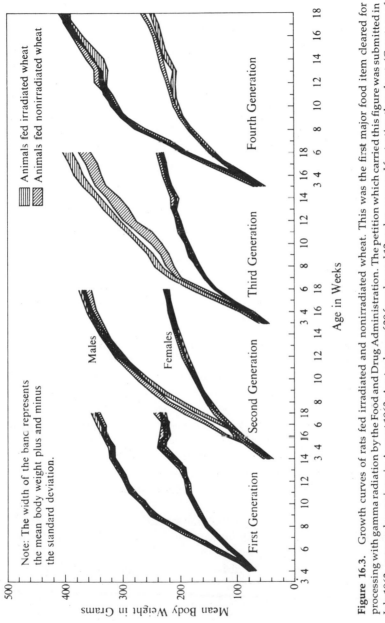
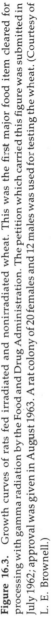

Figure 16.3. Growth curves of rats fed irradiated and nonirradiated wheat. This was the first major food item cleared for processing with gamma radiation by the Food and Drug Administration. The petition which carried this figure was submitted in July 1962; approval was given in August 1963. A rat colony of 20 females and 12 males was used for testing the wheat. (Courtesy of L. E. Brownell.)

325

TABLE 16.3

Summary of Experiments in Which Puppies Were Fed the Flesh of Lethally Irradiated Animals[a]

Trial	Breed	Source of meat	Number of animals	Average initial weight (kg)	Average final weight (kg)	Average daily gain (g)	Standard error of mean
I	Greyhound	Irradiated sheep	4	2.7	20.0	135	±3
I	Greyhound	Control sheep	3	3.0	20.1	134	±2
I	Beagle	Irradiated cattle	4	1.4	7.4	47	±7
I	Beagle	Control cattle	3	1.4	6.8	42	±3
II	Beagle	Irradiated cattle	4	2.1	8.6	50	±3
II	Beagle	Control cattle	4	2.3	8.3	46	±5

[a] Dog growth was followed for 128–129 days (Wasserman and Trum, 1955, by permission of the AAAS and the authors.)

about carcinogens and mutagens. In 1965 an unchallenged opinion endorsed by the U.S. Army's Surgeon General culminated in a favorable review by the Food and Drug Administration of a petition for irradiated bacon. Although cleared for unlimited human consumption, within 3 years the FDA revoked its approval of radappertized bacon when the original bacon data was cited in a petition for clearing ham.

Demonstrations that radiation-induced toxic compounds are below 0.01 mg/100 g were no longer satisfactory in a period when the Delaney Amendment to the Food and Drug Act was interpreted to ban foodstuffs which contain any substance shown to produce cancer at any dose in any experimental animal.

Laboratories in several countries have studied the biological effects of irradiated fats. There is general agreement that the initially formed peroxides of lipids are cytotoxic, but they are so short-lived that they are not likely to be a problem in irradiated foods. On the other hand, radiation produces an appreciable yield of dimeric products in soybean and corn oils. In both vegetable and animal fats, members of the hydrocarbon series containing one or two carbon atoms less than the major component fatty acids are formed in relatively large amounts. In addition small amounts of aromatic hydrocarbons and short-chain aldehydes, ketones, alcohols, and esters have been identified after irradiation. However, the natures of the compounds produced by radiation and heat treatment are mostly similar, but far more decomposition products have been obtained from heated or thermally oxidized fats.

The irony of the situation is that fats may have been falsely accused. The source of the causative agent is in doubt because most of the tumors appeared in rats fed both fruit compote and bacon. Other investigators have raised questions about the kinds of molecules formed by irradiating carbohydrates. The radiolytic products of sugars are capable of inducing chromosomal abnormalities in *Vicia* and *Tradescantia*. Also similar effects occur in plant cells grown in irradiated media. Furthermore, radiation-sterilized dextrose or fructose contained products cytotoxic to bacteria and cultured mammalian cells. The situation is further complicated by unconfirmed reports of mutations in *Drosophila* reared on irradiated media. Other laboratories have failed to duplicate the fly results. Nevertheless, biochemical studies indicate that cytotoxic sucrose solutions can inhibit coupled phosphorylation, which in turn can inhibit lipid, protein, and nucleic acid synthesis.

Under the circumstances, commercial development of irradiated foods seems unlikely. The FDA has adopted a wait-and-see attitude. Irradiated foods are now in a class requiring more expensive testing than any other commodity in the history of the food industry. After early abortive subsidization, industry decided to let the government agencies carry development to the point of commercialization. This mission has a very low priority in a time of austere federal research budgets.

Surgical Supplies and Pharmaceuticals

In addition to food preservation, there are related areas of microorganism control in which taste, flavor, and nutritional value are not problems. Antibiotics can be sterilized by irradiation without altering their potency. Although it was somewhat altered in color, procaine was unchanged in anaesthetic assay after radiation sterilization. Other applications, including the sterilization of drugs, blood, and tissues intended for transplantation may come into common usage in the near future. In advertising, one commercial company, the High Voltage Engineering Corporation of Burlington, Massachusetts, has featured a photograph of electron-beam sterilization of polyethylene surgical tubing within the final container. This was a pioneering application in the surgical-supply industry, extended also to sutures and intravenous feeding sets. Unfortunately, not all pharmaceutical preparations are unchanged. The potency of vitamin preparations is decreased, the drug content of alkaloid preparations is decreased, and the potency of organometallic compounds is altered.

Water and Sewage Treatment

A procedure in use for over two decades for specialized industrial purposes, such as manufacturing pharmaceuticals, is the sterilization of water by exposure to ultraviolet lamps. Low penetrability is a limitation. Water must be clear and exposed with large surface and small volume. More penetrating ionizing radiations could sterilize large volumes of drinking water (Lowe et al., 1956). However, this expectation of the optimistic 1950s has not materialized. Instead of γ-ray sources becoming standard water works equipment, the procedure has restricted usage in the 1970s (Tebbutt, 1973).

The sterilization of sewage by irradiation could also become economically feasible (Narver, 1957). However, because of the suspended matter, sewage presents additional problems. Doses above 65,000 R have been shown to increase the settling, and doses above 350,000 R increased the amount of suspended solidified material. On the credit side is the advantage of bactericidal action independent of pH, which is unlike chlorination. A study made for the city of Los Angeles demonstrated the radioresistance and persistence of coliform bacteria. Cost comparisons were discouraging because a short ocean outfall associated with an adequate irradiation facility was not competitive in price with a long outfall combined with diffusers.

Concluding Remarks

The early optimism for a wide variety of peaceful uses of atomic energy has been tempered by economic necessity. This chapter recounts the exploratory investigations and indicates that research in the applied areas has fallen off. Insect control has been perhaps the most rewarding application, yet even there temporary setbacks occur. Rethinking the possibility of cancer induction and the necessary safeguards against it has dampened the enthusiasm of private industry for developing food treatment facilities. In general, the unsettled energy situation makes prediction of the future impossible.

References

Alicata, J. E. (1951). Effects of roentgen radiation on *Trichinella spiralis*. *J. Parasitol.* **37**, 491–501.

Anonymous (1965). Future looks cloudy for irradiated food. *Chem. & Eng. News* **43**, No. 25, 32.

Bletchly, J. D., and Fisher, R. C. (1957). Use of γ-radiation for the destruction of wood boring insects. *Nature (London)* **179**, 670.

Cornwell, P. B., ed. (1965). "The Entomology of Radiation Disinfection of Grain." Pergamon, Oxford.

Dallyn, S. L., Sawyer, R. L., and Sparrow, A. H. (1955). Extending onion storage by gamma irradiation. *Nucleonics* **13**(4), 48–49.

Davidson, G. (1974). "Genetic Control of Insect Pests." Academic Press, New York.

Diehl, J. F., and Scherz, H. (1975). Estimation of radiolytic products as a basis for evaluating the wholesomeness of irradiated foods. *Int. J. Appl. Radiat. Isot.* **26**, 499–507.

Elias, P. S., and Cohen, A. J., eds. (1977). "Radiation Chemistry of Major Food Components." Elsevier, Amsterdam.

European Meeting (1959). On the use of ionizing radiation for food preservation. Summary report and proceedings. *Int. J. Appl. Radiat. Isot.* **6**, 1–317.

Goresline, H. E., Ingram, M., Macúch, P., Mocquot, G., Mossel, D. A. A., Niven, C. F., Jr., and Thatcher, F. S. (1964). Tentative classification of food irradiation processes with microbiological objectives. *Nature (London)* **204**, 237–238.

Gould, S. E., Gomberg, H. J., Bethell, F. H., Villella, J. B., and Hertz, C. S. (1955). Studies on *Trichinella spiralis*. *Am. J. Pathol.* **31**, 933–963.

Hannan, R. S. (1956). "Research on the Science and Technology of Food Preservation by Ionizing Radiations." Chem. Publ. Co., New York.

Hickman, J. R. (1966). United Kingdom irradiation programme—wholesomeness aspects. *Food Irradiat., Proc. Int. Symp.*, IAEA STI/PUB/127, pp. 101–117.

International Atomic Energy Agency (1968). "Preservation of Fruit and Vegetables by Radiation," STI/PUB/149. IAEA, Vienna.

International Atomic Energy Agency (1970a). "Preservation of Fish by Irradiation," STI/PUB/196. IAEA, Vienna.

International Atomic Energy Agency (1970b). "Sterile Male Techniques for Control of Fruit Flies," STI/PUB/276. IAEA, Vienna.

International Atomic Energy Agency (1973a). "Radiation Preservation of Food," STI/PUB/317. IAEA, Vienna.

International Atomic Energy Agency (1973b). "Improvement of Food Quality by Irradiation," STI/PUB/370. IAEA, Vienna.

International Atomic Energy Agency (1975). "Sterility Principle for Insect Control," STI/PUB/377. IAEA, Vienna.

Kaylor, J. R., and Slavin, J. N. Irradiation big advance in preserving seafood. *Fish. News Int.* **4**, 147–151.

Knipling, E. F. (1955). Possibilities of insect control or eradication through the use of sexually sterile males. *J. Econ. Entomol.* **48**, 459–462.

Knipling, E. F. (1960). The eradication of the screw-worm fly. *Sci. Am.* **203**(4), 54–61.

Levy, L. M. (and Army unit). (1957). "An Assessment of the Possible Toxic Effects to Human Beings of Short-term Consumption of Food Sterilized with Gamma Rays," A.M.N.L. 203. Army Med. Nutr. Lab., Denver, Colorado.

Lowe, H. N., Jr., Lacy, W. J., Surkiewicz, B. F., and Jaeger, R. F. (1956). Destruction of microorganisms in water, sewage and sewage sludge by ionizing radiations. *J. Am. Water Works Assoc.* **48,** 1363–1372.

Madsen, K. A., Salunkhe, D. K., and Simon, M. (1959). Certain morphological and biochemical changes in gamma irradiated carrots and potatoes. *Radiat. Res.* **10,** 48–62.

Narver, D. L. (1957). Is sterilization of sewage by irradiation economical? *Civ. Eng. (N.Y.)* **27,** 618–619.

Reber, E. F., Raheja, K., and Davis, D. (1966). Wholesomeness of Irradiated Foods/An annotated bibliography. *Fed. Proc., Fed. Am. Soc. Exp. Biol.* **25,** Pt. I, 1529–1579.

Richardson, R. H., ed. (1978). "The Screwworm Problem." Univ. of Texas Press, Austin.

Sparrow, A. H., and Christensen, E. (1954). Improving storage quality of potato tubers after exposure to ^{60}Co gammas. *Nucleonics* **12**(8), 16–17.

Tebbutt, T. H. Y. (1973). "Water Science and Technology." Barnes & Noble, New York.

U.S. Army (1961). "Preservation of Food by Low-dose Ionizing Energy," Off. Tech. Serv., U.S. Dept. of Commerce, Quartermaster Res. Eng. Cent., Natick, Massachusetts.

U. S. Atomic Energy Commission (1965). "Radiation Preservation of Foods." Proc. Int. Conf., Boston, Massachusetts, 1964. N.A.S.–N.R.C., Publ. 1273.

Wasserman, R. H., and Trum, B. F. (1955). Effect of feeding dogs the flesh of lethally irradiated cows and sheep. *Science* **121,** 894–896.

Williams, D. L., Gartman, S. C., and Hourrigan, J. L. (1977). Screwworm eradication in Puerto Rico and the Virgin Islands. *World Anim. Rev.* FAO No. 21-1, 31–35.

Subject Index

A

Abscopal effect, 216, 233
Accidental exposure, 197, 253, 261, 296
Acne, 195
Actinomycetes, 62
Action
  direct, 19, 244
  indirect, 19, 238
Activated water, 18
Active transport, 32, 172
Adaptive value, 148, 150
Adrenal, 256–257
Aging, 265, 267–269
Air/nitrogen ratio, 83
Algae, 281, 284
Alpha rays, 7, 34, 40, *see* specific emitters
Aminothiols, 233, 237–242
Amoeba, 36, 40
Anemia, 183, 196–197, 253, 259
Angiosperms, 169, 284
Antibiotics, 257–258
Antibodies, 257–258, 260–262
Aquatic plants, 288
Arbacia, 38, 41–42
Artemia, 21–22, 152
Arteries, 198
Ascorbic acid, 233, 234
Aspermy, 197, 213–215
Asterias, 37
Atom bomb, 4, 146, 172, 186, 251, 282, 284–285, 291, 296, 306
Atomic structure, 8
Atomic waste, 302–303
ATP synthesis, 232
Audiogenic seizure, 255
Autoradiography, 58
Auxin, 166

B

^{140}Ba, 296, 304
Background radiation, 279, 280, 282
Bacteria
  control in food, 309, 319–322
  infection by, 257–258
  mutation studies, 117, 133, 240
  sewage and water, 328
Bacteriophage, 26, 116
Barley, 133, 134, 169, 234–235
Bats, 270
Beta rays, 6, *see* specific emitters
Bikini, 146–147, 172, 284, 288, 291, 292
Biological survey, 301–303
Bird
  embryology, 180
  gonads, 219
  isotope burdens, 295
Birth weight, 183
Blister, 194
Blood
  cells, 32–34, 195–197
  counts, 196–197, 253, 294
  forming tissue, 196, 199, 203–204
  plasma, 32–34
  vessels, 198
Bone
  growth, 202–203
  marrow, 98, 203–204
  marrow injection, 260–261
Bone-seeking isotopes, 204–206, 295
Bracon, see Habrobracon
Brine shrimp, *see Artemia*
Burn, 4, 194, 258
Burro, 201